Disease Progression and Disease Prevention in Hepatology and Gastroenterology

FALK SYMPOSIUM 150

Disease Progression and Disease Prevention in Hepatology and Gastroenterology

Edited by

P.R. Galle
University Clinic
Mainz
Germany

G. Gerken
University Clinic
Essen
Germany

W.E. Schmidt
St Joseph Hospital
Bochum
Germany

B. Wiedenmann
Charité Medical University
Berlin
Germany

*Proceedings of the Falk Symposium 150 held in Berlin, Germany,
October 3–4, 2005*

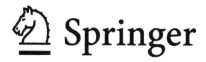

Library of Congress Cataloging-in-Publication Data is available.

ISBN-10 1-4020-5109-3
ISBN-13 978-1-4020-5109-8

Published by Springer,
PO Box 17, 3300 AA Dordrecht, The Netherlands

Sold and distributed in North, Central and South America
by Springer,
101 Philip Drive, Norwell, MA 02061 USA

In all other countries, sold and distributed
by Springer,
PO Box 322, 3300 AH Dordrecht, The Netherlands

Printed on acid-free paper

Printed and bound in Great Britain by MPG Books Limited, Bodmin, Cornwall.

Contents

PANCREATIC CARCINOMA
Chair: WE Schmidt, B Wiedenmann

SECTION LIVER I: DIAGNOSIS AND SURVEILLANCE IN LIVER DISEASE
Chair: A Lohse, G Ramadori

SECTION LIVER II: METABOLIC LIVER DISEASE
Chair: HE Blum, A Pietrangelo

List of principal contributors

F Berr
Department of Medicine I
University Hospital Salzburg
Müllner Hauptstr. 48
A-5020 Salzburg
Austria

K Bosslet
Schering AG Berlin
Müllerstr. 171–178
D-13353 Berlin
Germany

CE Broelsch
Department of General Surgery and
    Transplantation
University Hospital Essen
Hufelandstr. 55
D-45147 Essen
Germany

MC Carey
Department of Medicine, Thorn 1430
Brigham and Women's Hospital
75 Francis Street
Boston, MA 02115
USA

DW Cox
Department of Medical Genetics
8–39 Medical Sciences Building
University of Alberta
Edmonton, Alberta, T6G 2H7
Canada

CP Day
School of Clinical Medical Sciences
The Medical School
Framlington Place
Newcastle upon Tyne
NE2 4HH
UK

AM Diehl
Duke University Medical Center
Gastroenterology Division
Box 3256, Snyderman/GSRB-1
595 LaSalle Street
Durham, NC 27710
USA

H Friess
Department of General Surgery
Heidelberg University Hospital
Im Neuenheimer Feld 110
D-69120 Heidelberg
Germany

GJ Gores
Mayo Clinic College of Medicine
200 First Street SW
Rochester, MN 55905
USA

S Kubicka
Gastroenterologie/Hepatologie
Medizinische Hochschule Hannover
Carl-Neuberg-Str. 1
D-30625 Hannover
Germany

F Lammert
Department of Internal Medicine I
University Hospital Bonn
University of Bonn
Sigmund Freud Str. 25
D-53127 Bonn
Germany

KN Lazaridis
Center for Basic Research in
Digestive Diseases
Mayo Clinic College of Medicine
200 First Street SW
Rochester, MN 55905
USA

R Lencioni
Division of Diagnostic and
Interventional Radiology
Department of Oncology,
Transplants and Advanced
Technologies in Medicine
University of Pisa, Via Roma 67
I-56126 Pisa
Italy

MM Lerch
Innere Medizin A
Universitätsklinikum Greifswald
Friedrich-Loeffler-Str. 23A
D-17485 Greifswald
Germany

J-M Löhr
Molekulare Gastroenterologie
Universitätsklinikum Mannheim
Theodor-Kutzer-Ufer 1–3
D-68167 Mannheim
Germany

M Lu
Institüt für Virologie
Universitätsklinikum Essen
Hufelandstrasse 55
D-45122 Essen
Germany

J Mössner
Universität Leipzig
Medizinische Klinik und Poliklinik II
Philipp-Rosenthal-Str. 27
D-04103 Leipzig
Germany

P Neuhaus
Allgemein- und Viszeralchirurgie
Charité Universitätsmedizin
Campus Virchow Klinkum (CVK)
Augustenburger Platz 1
D-13353 Berlin
Germany

JA Odin
1 Gustave L Levy Place
Box 1123
New York, NY 10029
USA

A Pietrangelo
Center for Hemochromatosis and
Hereditary Liver Diseases
Department of Internal Medicine
University of Modena and Reggio
Emilia Policlinico
Via del Pozzo 71
I-41100 Modena
Italy

P Schirmacher
Institute of Pathology
University of Heidelberg
Im Neuenheimer Feld 220
D-69120 Heidelberg
Germany

M Schuchmann
Medizinische Klinik I
Universität Mainz
Langenbeckstr. 1
D-55101 Mainz
Germany

A Stiehl
Innere Medizin IV
Klinikum der Universität
Im Neuenheimer Feld 410
D-69120 Heidelberg
Germany

R Thimme
Innere Medizin II
Universitätsklinikum Freiburg
Hugstetter Str. 55
D-79106 Freiburg
Germany

SS Thorgeirsson
Laboratory of Experimental
Carcinogenesis
Center for Cancer Research, NCI
37 Convent Drive, Building 37,
Rm 4146
Bethesda, MD 20892-4262
USA

List of chairpersons

HE Blum
Innere Medizin II
Universitätsklinikum Freiburg
Hugstetter Str. 55
D-79106 Freiburg
Germany

WO Böcher
Innere Medizin I
Klinikum der Universität
Langenbeckstr. 1
D-55131 Mainz
Germany

PR Galle
I. Department of Internal Medicine
University of Mainz
Langenbeckstr. 1
D-55131 Mainz
Germany

M Geissler
Allgemeine Innere Medizin
Städtische Kliniken
Hirschlandstr. 97
D-73730 Esslingen
Germany

G Gerken
Gastroenterologie/Hepatologie
Universitätsklinikum Essen
Hufelandstr. 55
D-45147 Essen
Germany

GJ Gores
Mayo Clinic College of Medicine
200 First Street SW
Rochester, MN 55905
USA

JM Llovet
Division of Liver Disease
RM Transplantation Institute
Mount Sinai School of Medicine
1425 Madison Avenue, 11F-70
Box 1104
New York, NY 10029
USA

AW Lohse
Innere Medizin I
Universitätsklinikum Eppendorf
Martinistr. 52
D-20251 Hamburg
Germany

G Otto
Klinikum der Universität
Transplantationschirurgie
Langenbeckstr. 1
D-55131 Mainz
Germany

A Pietrangelo
Policlinico di Modena
Clinica Medica III
Divisione di Medicina Interna
Via del Pozzo 71
I-41100 Modena
Italy

G Ramadori
Gastroenterologie
Universitätskliniken
Robert-Koch-Str. 40
D-37075 Göttingen
Germany

T Sauerbruch
Innere Medizin I
Universitätsklinikum Bonn
Sigmund-Freud-Str. 25
D-53127 Bonn
Germany

WE Schmidt
Innere Medizin I
St.-Josef-Hospital
Ruhr-Universität Bochum
Gudrunstr. 56
D-44791 Bochum
Germany

B Wiedenmann
Hepatologie/Gastroenterologie
Charité Universitätsmedizin
Campus Virchow-Klinikum (CVK)
Augustenburger Platz 1
D-13353 Berlin
Germany

Preface

Chronic inflammatory, malignant and metabolic diseases of the liver, pancreas and bile system account for substantial morbidity and mortality. Thus, new strategies to prevent, diagnose and treat such diseases are urgently needed.

These issues were addressed during the Falk Symposium 150, entitled 'Disease Progression and Disease Prevention in the Gastrointestinal Tract', held on October 3–4, 2005, in Berlin.

The meeting focused on the biliary system, pancreas and liver. Pathogenic processes were described as well as primary and secondary prevention and treatment of disease. Scientific and clinical experts offered a broad understanding and paved the ground for extensive interdisciplinary discussions. In this sense, this symposium generated new aspects contributing to 'translation research' developing also – at least in some aspects – new perspectives on the various different pathogenic mechanisms in gastrointestinal organs. The present monograph summarizes the state of the art in these different disease entities, as presented at the meeting.

On this occasion, the members of the organizing committee thank all speakers and chairpersons for their valuable contribution to the success of this symposium. In addition, we are grateful to the Falk Foundation e. V., Freiburg, Germany, in particular to Dr. Martin Falk, making this meeting and its publication possible.

P.R. Galle
G. Gerken
W. Schmidt
B. Wiedenmann

Cholelithiasis and biliary cancer

Chair: G. OTTO and T. SAUERBRUCH

1
Molecular mechanisms controlling bile metabolism in health and disease

M. C. CAREY

INTRODUCTION

Apart from its role in distributing immunoglobulins and antioxidants throughout the small intestine, bile's lipid secretory functions are also particularly important in health and disease[1,2]. Bile promotes 'exocrine' lipid secretion, especially quantitative cholesterol elimination from the body as itself and its major catabolic products, the bile salts. Bile facilitates dietary lipid absorption from the upper small intestine by micellar solubilization of otherwise insoluble fat digestion products, thereby promoting their absorption as monomers. Through its phospholipid components, mostly phosphatidylcholine in humans, bile promotes intraluminal solubilization of cholesterol and fat-soluble vitamins as well as enterocytic synthesis of the monomolecular emulsifier coats of chylomicrons. Through bile salt detergency, bile is essential for the micellar solubilization and monomeric absorption of all lipo-(fat soluble) vitamins, A, D, E, and K. Bile is the principal conduit for excretion of endobiotics, principally bilirubin conjugates as well as xenobiotics (e.g. lipophilic drugs) and exhibits a particular affinity for drugs with molecular weights in the 300–400 range[3]. This chapter will deal mainly, but not exclusively, with the molecular mechanisms controlling bile metabolism in health and in one common disease, namely, cholesterol gallstones[4].

COMPOSITION OF BILE

Four dissimilar lipids are dissolved in an aqueous colloidal solution in animal biles[1]. In humans in decreasing quantitative order they are bile salts, a group of structurally similar detergent-like molecules with solubilizing, antibacterial, and signalling functions; a phospholipid mixture mostly phosphatidylcholines, principally the *sn*-1 palmitoyl species, unesterified cholesterol with traces of phytosterols, chonchosterols and cholesterol precursors and bilirubin conjugates principally di- and monoglucuronates and small amounts ($\approx 5\%$)

of hetero-glucuronate, xylose and glucose conjugates. Despite theoretical objections[5], bilirubin conjugates can be considered soluble lipid amphiphiles as inferred from Small's 1968 classification of lipids based of their surface and bulk interactions with water[6] because all bilirubins and their conjugates exhibit self-aggregating properties[7]. Apart from a low monomeric concentration of bile salt (circa 1 mM), all lipid components of bile are heteroaggregated via hydrophobic interactions into simple micelles which contain no phospholipids plus mixed micelles containing all biliary lipids including phospholipids. In the 'supersaturated' state, unilamellar vesicles composed principally of phosphatidylcholine and cholesterol are also present, hence supramicellar concentrations of cholesterol constitute a two-phase system[1]. The detergency of bile salts is responsible for solubilizing phospholipids and sterols in bile and solubilizing the products of dietary fat (principally triglyceride) hydrolysis, namely fatty acids and monoacylglycerols plus lipovitamins and unesterified sterols in the upper small intestine[8]. Bile salts also act as high-affinity binders for bilirubin conjugates: these lipopigment molecules bind with high affinity to the exterior surfaces of biliary lipid aggregates in bile, thereby abolishing their otherwise high osmotic activity[7]. Some bile salt species possess strong bactericidal properties[9] responsible, in part, for the conventional 'sterility' of hepatic and gallbladder bile.

PHYSIOLOGY AND BIOCHEMISTRY OF BILIARY LIPID SECRETION

Most (>98%) bile salts secreted into bile are in the process of completing an enterohepatic circulation, that is, movement of molecules from liver to bile to intestine, from whence the molecules traverse ileocytes of the distal small intestine to return to the liver[1]. All bile salts return to the liver in portal blood and no traces are found in lymph[1]. Bile salts can be modified by microbial organisms in the distal ileum by hydrolysis of their taurine or glycine side-chains; the bacterial enzymes are known collectively as cholyl-glycylamidases[1,2]. These deconjugated bile salts also return to the liver by the active transport system of ileocytes. However, nuclear modification of deconjugated bile salts by selective anaerobic metabolism occurs only in the colon, principally by *Eubacteria* and *Clostridia* species[11], including sp. nov. *Clostridium hylemonae* isolated from human faeces[12]. These organisms ingest deconjugated bile acids by a specific energy-requiring transport system and then through a series of oxidoreductive steps controlled by a bile salt inducible operon, selectively remove the 7 OH group of cholate and chenodeoxycholate, forming deoxycholate and lithocholate respectively. These are, in turn, effluxed by a second bacterial membrane transport system[10,11]. The secondary bile acids constitute the principal bile acids in faeces, which amounts to 250–450 mg/day in humans[1]. Bile acid molecules are absorbed from the colon in part, are carried in portal blood to the liver where they are extracted efficiently and reconjugated with taurine or glycine in a 1:3 ratio prior to resecretion into bile. In addition, lithocholate is mostly sulphated at the 3-OH position by the human liver[13], forming a sulphate ester. The taurine and glycine conjugated lithocholate sulphates utilize the canalicular MRP3(ABCC2) transport

system[14,15] to exit the hepatocyte; moreover, because they are trivalent anions, the molecules resist recapture by ileocytes and hence break their enterohepatic circulation after one cycle[13]. Consequently, human bile is a mixed conjugated bile salt system containing the primary bile salts synthesized directly from cholesterol and the secondary bile salts that were bacterially modified. A fifth bile salt, ursodeoxycholate, is also a secondary (sometimes called a tertiary) bile salt and is formed from 7-ketolithocholic acid, a product of colonic anaerobic metabolism of chenodeoxycholic acid[11]. This keto intermediate is reduced and epimerized to a 7β-hydroxyl function either by colonic bacteria or following return to the liver by hepatic enzymes, and secreted into bile after amidation with taurine or glycine[11]. In a number of animals, particularly the Ursidae[16], Hystricidae[17] and possibly their New World counterparts, the Erethizontidae[17], ursodeoxycholate is a primary bile acid. In contrast to humans the rodent liver is capable of further modifying the nucleus of secondary as well as many primary bile acids with the addition of one or more OH groups in α or β orientations on the steroid nucleus[13].

The principal phospholipids of human and many laboratory animal biles are a phosphatidylcholine mixture[5,18]. They are not derived to any major extent from the phospholipid surface monolayers (the 'emulsifier') of plasma lipoproteins despite receptor-mediated endocytosis of the intact particles by the liver[19,20]. Most biliary phospholipids are synthesized *de novo* in the liver from diacylglycerol via the CDP-choline or Kennedy pathway[21]. A lesser amount of biliary PC is made on the inner leaflet of the canalicular membrane by the trimethylation of phosphatidylethanolamine[22] – a process that may be increased in the lithogenic state (unpublished observations). Most (80%) biliary phosphatidylcholines are the *sn-1* palmitoyl and 20% of the *sn-1* steroyl species[18]. In descending rank order of frequency the *sn-2* fatty acid of biliary PC is linolenic (C18:2), linoleic (C18:1), oleic (C18:1) and arachidonic (C20:4)[23,24]. The hepatic selection mechanism is not well worked out, but the phosphatidylcholine transfer protein of liver which is highly selective for phosphatidylcholines may play a crucial role in their transport from the endoplasmic reticulum, their site of synthesis, to the canalicular membrane[25,26]. Canalicular transport is selective for phosphatidylcholines and only small amounts (< 5%) of other phospholipids, mostly phosphatidylethanolamines, appear in human bile[23]. Their fatty acids are usually similar to those of biliary phosphatidylcholines[23,27], and since they are fully miscible with each other they probably are removed 'accidentally' in the exovesiculation of phosphatidylcholines from the outer leaflet of the canalicular membrane[28].

Cholesterol molecules enter bile from all lipoprotein sources[29,30]; biliary and dietary cholesterol return to the liver in chylomicrons remnants – both hepatic synthesized and peripherally synthesized cholesterol reach the liver in VLDL, IDL, LDL, and HDL, which are taken up[19,20] by endocytosis (VLDL, IDL, LDL) or, in the case of HDL, selective lipid extraction[19]. Although cholesterol synthesis occurs in the liver, apparently very little enters bile directly in health[31]. There is experimental evidence that the cholesterol of HDL selectively enters bile very rapidly[32–35], apparently by diffusion within the plasma membranes of the liver[32,33], whereas the cholesterol ester of HDL enters bile as cholesterol following ester hydrolysis and vectorial movement within the cell to the canalicular membrane[19,36,37]. There is also evidence from modelling studies that the cholesterol ester of LDL mostly traverses the liver in part to enter bile salt synthetic pathways[38,39] but when apolipoprotein B/E receptors are overexpressed pharmacologically by oestrogen therapy cholesterol derived from LDL can also enter bile directly as the unesterified sterol[40,41]. Biliary cholesterol may or may not be a reflection of the dietary intake in humans depending, among other factors, on the genetic make-up of an individual, but certainly is a reflection of total body pools of cholesterol in obesity[31]. In the mouse biliary cholesterol secretion is under the control of multiple *Lith* genes[42–44] and in humans most likely by their *LITH* gene counterparts[45–47]. Biliary cholesterol homeostasis is also controlled, either directly or indirectly, by several other mechanisms including hormones, principally thyroid hormone, oestrogen, leptin, and insulin[48–56].

Although technically a soluble emphiphilic lipid, the hepatic routing of bilirubin conjugates, the most important endobiotic lipigment, will not be detailed here. Bilirubin uptake, conjugation, synthesis and secretion are well defined[57] and little new information is available apart from the fact that a cytoplasmic transcription factor CAR (NR1I3) has been characterized as well as the pregnane X receptor (PXR, NR1I2), which is normally located in the nucleus of hepatocytes, as crucial in the control of hepatic bilirubin clearance including the conjugation steps[58,59]; moreover, the primary active canalicular transport pump ABCC2 (MRP2) is essential for the biliary secretion of bilirubin conjugates[60].

MECHANISMS OF UPTAKE

Based principally on rodent studies, molecular mechanisms for the major pathways of bile salt, phosphatidylcholine, cholesterol uptake, metabolism and secretion by the liver are well worked out[1,2,13–15,61–63]. On the basolateral membrane, chylomicron remnants (primarily ApoB/E receptor) and HDL (SRBI receptor) are the primary sources of cholesterol for bile[64,65], whereas LDL (ApoB/E receptor) provides cholesterol for *de-novo* bile salt synthesis[35,36]. The biliary phospholipids are *de-novo* synthesized by the diacylglycerol pathway with smaller quantities from trimethylation of phosphatidyl-ethanolamine on the canalicular membrane[21,22]. Bile salts returning to the liver are recaptured principally by an Na^+ coupled SLC (solute carrier) 10A1 (NTCP)[14,61–63]; and at least four other SLC exchangers (OATP) have been identified; perhaps two of which transport bile salts[14]. SLC22A1 is an organic cation transporter[66] contributing choline to the hepatocyte, aiding but not essential for phosphatidylcholine synthesis via the diacylglyceride Kennedy pathway[67].

SECRETION AND RECAPTURE

The multiplicity of exit transporters on the canalicular membrane for lipids are rate limiting in bile formation[15,61–63]. All transporters are of the ABC (ATP-binding cassette) family with two molecules of ATP being hydrolysed during their functioning in primary active transport[15]. Individual transporters exist for monovalent bile salts (ABCB11, BSEP), phosphatidylcholine (ABCB4, MDR2/3), divalent bile salts plus bilirubin conjugates (ABCC2, MRP2), and sterols (ABCG5/G8). At least one other transporter is responsible for cholesterol secretion in the mouse, but is not yet characterized (unpublished observations). In the distal small intestine, bile salts are recovered actively from the intestinal lumen by apical, transcellular and basolateral membrane transport systems of distal ileocytes, thereby maintaining the enterohepatic circulation of bile salts[68,69]. The three components include an electrogenic Na^+ coupled apical transporter, SLC10A2 (ASBT), an FABP6 (IBABP) shuttle for bile salts within the cytoplasm[68,69], and an OSTα/β antiporter on the basolateral membrane[69,70] which exchanges bile salt molecules with bicarbonate ions. Bile salts are delivered to the liver in portal blood bound to albumen (hydrophobic bile salts) and HDL (hydrophilic bile salts)[1].

HEPATIC REGULATORY FACTORS

In the liver, bile salts activate FXRα, a nuclear transcription factor which associates with its obligate heterodimer partner RXR, and having entered the nucleus exhibits a variety of pleiotropic effects of the lipidologic regulation of biliary lipid events[14,15,62,63]. FXRα activation is responsible for increased conjugation and secretion of bile salts from hepatocytes and decreased basolateral uptake via SLC10A1 and especially biosynthesis of bile salts, via an intermediary nuclear transcription factor SHP1, through down-regulation of CYP7A1 (rate-controlling enzyme in the 'neutral' pathway for bile salt synthesis) and CYP8B1 (the 12α-hydroxylase that leads to cholic acid). In the small intestine, FXRα activation results in increased FABPB-IBABP expression and decreased ASBT (SLC10A2) expression, facilitating loss of bile salts from the enterohepatic circulation. Similarly, activation of CAR and PXR (by bilirubin), LXRα (by oxysterols) and PXR (by xenobiotics) all up-regulate phase II metabolism of their ligands as well as their canalicular secretion into bile[58].

CHOLESTEROL GALLSTONES

In the Western world the disease most frequently attributed to bile dysfunction is cholesterol gallstones[71,72]. Most afflicted individuals exhibit hypersecretion of hepatic cholesterol, and less commonly, hyposecretion of bile salts plus phosphatidylcholines[1,4]. Irrespective of the secretory cause, the end-result is supersaturation of gallbladder bile with cholesterol. Pathogenesis of cholelithiasis has genetic, environmental, dietary, and microbial components[73]. Studies in the inbred mouse have revealed 23 *Lith* loci[42–44,71] (also unpublished observations), but to date none of the *Lith* genes has been unequivocally identified. Candidate genes include all of the canalicular lipid transporters as well as FXRα, ABCG5/ABCG8[74] and Megalin[75] (a member of the LDL receptor family – LDL related protein 2 – LDLRP2) expressed in gallbladder epithelium[76].

Lith and *LITH* genes

Rarely do human *LITH* genes cause monogenic, i.e. Mendelian, cholesterol gallstone disease[73]. Syndromes defined to date include defects in ABCB4 which cause 'low phospholipid-associated cholelithiasis' or LPAC, and defective CYP7A1, which causes cholesterol gallstones and hypercholesterolaemia resistant to HMG-CoA reductase inhibitors[73]. Two other monogenic causes of cholesterol gallstones involve genes that are highly expressed in the gallbladder[73]. Megalin, a candidate gene for the murine *Lith1*[75], in conjunction with cubilin, mediates endocytic uptake of a variety of substrates including ApoAI bound to phospholipid and cholesterol. It is expressed in the gallbladder epithelium[76] and could possibly be also expressed on large cholangiocytes and may be responsible for decreasing the levels of cholesterol supersaturation in hepatic as well as gallbladder bile. The second defect involves the CCK1 receptor responsible for motility of the gallbladder and also small intestine[73]. A number of case reports have shown that CCK1 receptor dysfunction is associated with cholesterol cholelithiasis as a consequence of gallbladder paralysis and hypomotility of the small intestine. The former facilitates mucin accumulation and cholesterol crystal nucleation, whereas the latter engenders increased cholesterol absorption and augmented deoxycholate formation with its subsequent hyperabsorption from the intestine[77,78]. Nonetheless, in the vast majority of cholesterol gallstone subjects the disease is polygenic, but to date none of the responsible *LITH* genes has been definitively identified[73].

Enterohepatic helicobacters

An exciting recent discovery is that cholesterol gallstones occur with high prevalence rates in a well-defined mouse model, only when the distal small intestine, caecum and colon are infected with one or more cholelithogenic enterohepatic *Helicobacter* spp.[79]. These non-*H. pylori* helicobacters are apparently crucial for nucleating supersaturated bile in mice, and have been shown to be extremely potent inducers of cholesterol crystal phase separation from liquid crystals in supersaturated bile[79]. Since humans are known to be infected with a wide variety of enterohepatic helicobacter strains[80], it remains to be determined what their cholelithogenic potentials are employing a suitable infected murine model.

The adaptive immune response

One possible explanation for the cholelithogenic potential of certain helicobacter strains is the adaptive immune response. In ongoing studies employing $Rag2^{-/-}$ mice and wild-type mice on a BALB/c background, we have now shown[81] that infection with cholelithogenic helicobacter species causes nucleation of solid crystals from liquid crystals in lithogenic bile only when functional T and B immunocytes are present. Based on the near-absence of a mucin gel in the $Rag2^{-/-}$ mice, it is likely that the adaptive immune response stimulates excessive mucin production, creating a pronucleating gel matrix for phase separation of solid cholesterol monohydrate crystals leading to cholesterol gallstone formation. However, it may also relate to the possibility that fully 25% of all proteins identified in human gallstone bile function in the immune response[82] and many of these are proven to be pronucleating agents[31]. Hence, the more one investigates this complex sequence of molecular events in a common disease, the more pathobiological components appear to be involved. This scenario in cholelithogenesis is following a similar path which began three decades ago with the definition of the physical chemistry of bile[83] and shortly thereafter of the atherosclerotic plaque[84], and is expanding with many similarities to current concepts, particularly the putative roles of inflammation and immunity involved in the pathogenesis of human atherosclerosis[85].

Acknowledgements

This work was supported in part by NIH (US Public Health Service) Grants, R37 DK36588, R01 DK52911, and R01 DK73687.

References

1. Carey MC, Duane WC. Enterohepatic circulation. In: Arias IM, Boyer JL, Fausto N, Jakoby WB, Schachter DA, Shafritz DA, editors. The Liver: Biology and Pathobiology, 3rd edn. New York: Raven Press, 1994:719–67.
2. Carey MC. Enterohepatic circulation. Revista Gastroenterol Mex (Suppl. 1). 2000;65:56–60.
3. Smith RL. The Excretory Function of Bile. London: Chapman & Hall, 1973:16–34.
4. Paigen B, Carey MC. Gallstones. In: King RA, Rotter JI, Motulsky AG, editors. The Genetic Basis of Common Diseases, 2nd edn. New York: Oxford University Press, 2002: 298–335.
5. Moschetta A, Xu F, Hagey LR et al. A phylogenetic survey of biliary lipids in vertebrates. J Lipid Res. 2005;46:2221–32.
6. Small DM. A classification of biologic lipids based upon their interaction in aqueous systems. J Am Oil Chem Soc. 1968;45:108–19.
7. Neubrand MW, Laue TM, Carey MC. Bilirubin ditaurate, a natural conjugated bile pigment self-associates to limiting tetramers and binds with high-affinity to the hydroxy-studded α-faces of bile salt monomers and micelles. Biochemistry. 2006 (In revision).
8. Carey MC, Hernell O. Digestion and absorption of fat. Semin Gastrointest Dis. 1992;3: 189–208.
9. Hanninen ML. Sensitivity of *Helicobacter pylori* to different bile salts. Eur J Clin Microbiol Infect Dis. 1991;10:515–18.
10. Hylemon PB. Metabolism of bile acids in intestinal microflora. In: Danielsson H, Sjövall J, editors. Sterols and Bile Acids. Amsterdam: Elsevier, 1985:331–43.

11. Hylemon PB, Biochemistry and genetics of intestinal bile salt metabolism. In: Paumgartner G, Stiehl A, Gerok W, editors. Bile Acids as Therapeutic Agents. Dordrecht: Kluwer, 1991:1–11.
12. Kitahara M, Takamine F, Imamura T, Benno Y. Assignment of *Eubacterium* sp. VPI 12708 and related strains with high bile acid 7alpha-dehydroxylating activity to *Clostridium scindens* and proposal of *Clostridium hylemonae* sp. nov., isolated from human faeces. Int J Syst Evolut Microbiol. 2000;50:971–8.
13. Hofmann AF. Bile acids. In: Arias IM, Boyer JL, Fausto N, Jakoby WB, Schachter D, Schafritz DA, editors. The Liver: Biology and Pathobiology. New York: Raven Press, 1994: 677–718.
14. Russell DW. The enzymes, regulation, and genetics of bile acid synthesis. Annu Rev Biochem. 2003;72:137–74.
15. Meier PJ, Steiger B. Bile salt transporters. Annu Rev Physiol. 2002;64:635–61.
16. Hagey LR, Crombie DL, Espinosa E, Carey MC, Igimi H, Hofmann AF. Ursodeoxycholic acid in the Ursidae: biliary bile acids of bears, pandas, and related carnivores. J Lipid Res. 1993;34:1911–17.
17. Tint GS, Xu GR, Batta AK, Shefer S, Niemann W, Salen G. Ursodeoxycholic acid, chenodeoxycholic acid, and 7-ketolithocholic acid are primary bile acids of the guinea pig. J Lipid Res. 1990;31:1301–6.
18. Hay DW, Cahalane MJ, Timofeyeva N, Carey MC. Molecular species of lecithins in human gallbladder bile. J Lipid Res. 1993;34:759–68.
19. Cooper AD. Hepatic lipoprotein metabolism: recent molecular insights. Prog Liver Dis. 1995;13:173–200.
20. Mahley RW, Ji ZS. Remnant lipoprotein metabolism: key pathways involving cell-surface heparan sulfate proteoglycans and apolipoprotein E. J Lipid Res. 1999;40:1–16.
21. Vance JE, Vance DE. Phospholipid biosynthesis in mammalian cells. Biochem Cell Biol. 2004;82:113–28.
22. Sehayek E, Wang R, Ono JG et al. Localization of the PE methylation pathway and SR-BI to the canalicular membrane: evidence for apical PC biosynthesis that may promote biliary excretion of phospholipid and cholesterol. J Lipid Res. 2003;44:1605–13.
23. Alvaro D, Cantafora A, Attili AF et al. Relationships between bile salts hydrophilicity and phospholipid composition in bile of various animal species. Comp Biochem Physiol B. 1986;83:551–4.
24. Agellon LB, Walkey CJ, Vance DE, Kuipers F, Verkade HJ. The unique acyl chain specificity of biliary phosphatidylcholines in mice is independent of their biosynthetic origin in the liver. Hepatology. 1999;30:725–9.
25. Cohen DE. Hepatocellular transport and secretion of biliary lipids. Curr Opin Lipid. 1999;10:295–302.
26. Wu MK, Hyogo H, Yadav SK, Novikoff PM, Cohen DE. Impaired response of biliary lipid secretion to a lithogenic diet in phosphatidylcholine transfer protein-deficient mice. J Lipid Res. 2005;46:422–31.
27. Nibbering CP, Carey MC. Sphingomyelins of rat liver: biliary enrichment with molecular species containing 16:0 fatty acids as compared to canalicular-enriched plasma membranes. J Membr Biol. 1999;167:165–71.
28. Crawford JM, Möckel GM, Crawford AR et al. Imaging biliary lipid secretion in the rat: ultrastructural evidence for vesiculation of the hepatocyte canalicular membrane. J Lipid Res. 1995;36:2147–63.
29. Zanlungo S, Rigotti A, Nervi F. Hepatic cholesterol transport from plasma into bile: implications for gallstone disease. Curr Opin Lipid. 2004;15:279–86.
30. Groen AK, Oude Elferink RP. Lipid transport into bile and role in bile formation. Curr Drug Targets Immune Endocrinol Metabol Disord. 2005;5:131–5.
31. LaMont JT, Carey MC. Cholesterol gallstone formation. 2. Pathobiology and pathomechanics. Prog Liver Dis. 1992;10:165–91.
32. Robins SJ, Fasulo JM. High density lipoproteins, but not other lipoproteins, provide a vehicle for sterol transport to bile. J Clin Invest. 1997;99:380–4.
33. Robins SJ, Fasulo JM. Delineation of a novel hepatic route for the selective transfer of unesterified sterols from high-density lipoproteins to bile: studies using the perfused rat liver. Hepatology. 1999;29:1541–8.

34. Schwartz CC, Halloran LG, Vlahcevic ZR, Gregory DH, Swell L. Preferential utilization of free cholesterol from high-density lipoproteins for biliary cholesterol secretion in man. Science. 1978;200:62–4.
35. Schwartz CC, Berman M, Vlahcevic ZR, Halloran LG, Gregory DH, Swell L. Multicompartmental analysis of cholesterol metabolism in man. Characterization of the hepatic bile acid and biliary cholesterol precursor sites. J Clin Invest. 1978;61:408–23.
36. Schwartz CC, Vlahcevic ZR, Halloran LG, Gregory DH, Meek JB, Swell L. Evidence for the existence of definitive hepatic cholesterol precursor compartments for bile acids and biliary cholesterol in man. Gastroenterology. 1975;69:1379–82.
37. Schwartz CC, Vlahcevic ZR, Halloran LG, Swell L. An *in vivo* evaluation in man of the transfer of esterified cholesterol between lipoproteins and into the liver and bile. Biochim Biophys Acta. 1981;663:143–62.
38. Schwartz CC, Vlahcevic ZR, Halloran LG, Nisman R, Swell L. Evidence for a common hepatic cholesterol precursor site for cholic and chenodeoxycholic acid synthesis in man. Proc Soc Exp Biol Med. 1977;156:261–4.
39. Shamburek RD, Pentchev PG, Zech LA et al. Intracellular trafficking of the free cholesterol derived from LDL cholesteryl ester is defective *in vivo* in Niemann–Pick C disease: insights on normal metabolism of HDL and LDL gained from the NP-C mutation. J Lipid Res. 1997;38:2422–35.
40. Eriksson M, Berglund L, Rudling M, Henriksson P, Angelin B. Effects of estrogen on low density lipoprotein metabolism in males. Short-term and long-term studies during hormonal treatment of prostatic carcinoma. J Clin Invest. 1989;84:802–10.
41. Henriksson P, Einarsson K, Eriksson A, Kelter U, Angelin B. Estrogen-induced gallstone formation in males. Relation to changes in serum and biliary lipids during hormonal treatment of prostatic carcinoma. J Clin Invest. 1989;84:811–16.
42. Wittenburg H, Lyons MA, Paigen B, Carey MC. Mapping cholesterol gallstone susceptibility (*Lith*) genes in inbred mice. Dig Liver Dis. 2003;35(Suppl. 3):S2–7.
43. Paigen B, Carey MC. Gallstones. In: King RA, Rotter JI, Motulsky AG, editors. The Genetic Basis of Common Diseases, 2nd edn. New York: Oxford University Press, 2002: 298–335.
44. Lammert F, Carey MC, Paigen B. Chromosomal organization of candidate genes involved in cholesterol gallstone formation: a murine gallstone map. Gastroenterology. 2001;120: 221–38.
45. Lammert F, Sauerbruch T. Mechanisms of disease: the genetic epidemiology of gallbladder stones. Nat Clin Pract Gastroenterol Hepatol. 2005;2:423–33.
46. Lammert F, Matern S. The genetic background of cholesterol gallstone formation: an inventory of human lithogenic genes. Curr Drug Targets Immune Endocrinol Metab Disord. 2005;5:163–70.
47. Katsika D, Grjibovski A, Einarsson C, Lammert F, Lichtenstein P, Marschall HU. Genetic and environmental influences on symptomatic gallstone disease: a Swedish study of 43,141 twin pairs. Hepatology. 2005;41:1138–43.
48. Wang HH, Afdhal NH, Wang DQ. Estrogen receptor alpha, but not beta, plays a major role in 17beta-estradiol-induced murine cholesterol gallstones. Gastroenterology. 2004;127: 239–49.
49. Tran KQ, Graewin SJ, Swartz-Basile DA, Nakeeb A, Svatek CL, Pitt HA. Leptin-resistant obese mice have paradoxically low biliary cholesterol saturation. Surgery. 2003;134:372–7.
50. Hyogo H, Roy S, Cohen DE. Restoration of gallstone susceptibility by leptin in C57BL/6J ob/ob mice. J Lipid Res. 2003;44:1232–40.
51. Prigge WF, Ketover SR, Gebhard RL. Thyroid hormone is required for dietary fish oil to induce hypersecretion of biliary cholesterol in the rat. Lipids. 1995;30:833–8.
52. Andreini JP, Prigge WF, Ma C, Gebbard RL. Vesicles and mixed micelles in hypothyroid rat bile before and after thyroid hormone treatment: evidence for a vesicle transport system for biliary cholesterol secretion. J Lipid Res. 1994;35:1405–12.
53. Dubrac S, Parquet M, Blouquit Y et al. Insulin injections enhance cholesterol gallstone incidence by changing the biliary cholesterol saturation index and apo A-I concentration in hamsters fed a lithogenic diet. J Hepatol. 2001;35:550–7.
54. Vlahcevic ZR, Eggertsen G, Bjorkhem I, Hylemon PB. Regulation of sterol 12alpha-hydroxylase and cholic acid biosynthesis in the rat. Gastroenterology. 2000;118:599–607 [Erratum in Gastroenterology. 2000;119:280].

55. Cao WM, Murao K, Imachi H et al. Insulin-like growth factor-I regulation of hepatic scavenger receptor class BI. Endocrinology. 2004;145:5540–7.
56. Ishida H, Yamashita C, Kuruta Y, Yoshida Y, Noshiro M. Insulin is a dominant suppressor of sterol 12 alpha-hydroxylase P450 (CYP8B) expression in rat liver: possible role of insulin in circadian rhythm of CYP8B. J Biochem (Tokyo). 2000;127:57–64.
57. Jansen PL, Bosma PJ, Chowdhury JR. Molecular biology of bilirubin metabolism. Prog Liver Dis. 1995;13:125–50.
58. Handschin C, Meyer UA. Regulatory network of lipid-sensing nuclear receptors: roles for CAR, PXR, LXR, and FXR. Arch Biochem Biophys. 2005;433:387–96.
59. Wagner M, Halilbasic E, Marschall HU et al. CAR and PXR agonists stimulate hepatic bile acid and bilirubin detoxification and elimination pathways in mice. Hepatology. 2005; 42:420–30.
60. Fardel O, Jigorel E, Le Vee M, Payen L. Physiological, pharmacological and clinical features of the multidrug resistance protein 2. Biomed Pharmacother. 2005;59:104–14.
61. Trauner M, Boyer JL. Bile salt transporters: molecular characterization, function, and regulation. Physiol Rev. 2003;83:633–71.
62. Wolkoff AW, Cohen DE. Bile acid regulation of hepatic physiology: I. Hepatocyte transport of bile acids. Am J Physiol, Gastrointest Liver Physiol. 2003;284:G175–9.
63. Kullak-Ublick GA, Stieger B, Meier PJ. Enterohepatic bile salt transporters in normal physiology and liver disease. Gastroenterology. 2004;126:322–42.
64. Wang DQ, Zhang L, Wang HH. High cholesterol absorption efficiency and rapid biliary secretion of chylomicron remnant cholesterol enhance cholelithogenesis in gallstone-susceptible mice. Biochim Biophys Acta. 2005;1733:90–9.
65. Connelly MA, Williams DL. Scavenger receptor BI: a scavenger receptor with a mission to transport high density lipoprotein lipids. Curr Opin Lipid. 2004;15:287–95.
66. Green RM, Lo K, Sterritt C, Beier DR. Cloning and functional expression of a mouse liver organic cation transporter. Hepatology. 1999;29:1556–62.
67. Kulinski A, Vance DE, Vance JE. A choline-deficient diet in mice inhibits neither the CDP-choline pathway for phosphatidylcholine synthesis in hepatocytes nor apolipoprotein B secretion. J Biol Chem. 2004;279:23916–24.
68. Dawson PA. Intestinal bile acid transport: molecules, mechanism and malabsorption. In: Paumgartner G, Stiehl A, Gerok W, Keppler D, Leuschner, editors. Bile Acid in Cholestasis. Dordrecht: Kluwer, 1999:1–28.
69. Dawson PA, Hubbert M, Haywood J et al. The heteromeric organic solute transporter alpha-beta, (Ostalpha-Ostbeta), is an ileal basolateral bile acid transporter. J Biol Chem. 2005;280:6960–8.
70. Belinsky MG, Dawson PA, Shchaveleva I et al. Analysis of the in vivo functions of Mrp3. Mol Pharmacol. 2005;68:160–8.
71. Carey MC, Paigen B. Epidemiology of the American Indians' burden and its likely genetic origins. Hepatology. 2002;36:781–91.
72. Sandler RS, Everhart JE, Donowitz M et al. The burden of selected digestive diseases in the United States. Gastroenterology. 2002;122:1500–11.
73. Carey MC, Kwon RS, Maurer KJ, Fox JG. 'State of the Art' – Gallstone research in the post-genomic era. In: Adler G, Blum HE, Fuchs M, Stange EF, editors. Gallstones: Pathogenesis and Treatment. Dordrecht: Kluwer, 2004:207–24.
74. Wittenburg H, Lyons MA, Li R, Churchill GA, Carey MC, Paigen B. FXR and ABCG5/ABCG8 as determinants of cholesterol gallstone formation from quantitative trait locus mapping in mice. Gastroenterology. 2003;125:868–81.
75. Paigen B, Schork NJ, Svenson KL et al. Quantitative trait loci mapping for cholesterol gallstones in AKR/J and C57L/J strains of mice. Physiol Genom. 2000;4:59–65.
76. Erranz B, Miquel JF, Argraves WS, Barth JL, Pimentel F, Marzolo MP. Megalin and cubilin expression in gallbladder epithelium and regulation by bile acids. J Lipid Res. 2004; 45:2185–98.
77. Wang DQ, Schmitz F, Kopin AS, Carey MC. Targeted disruption of the murine cholecystokinin-1 receptor promotes intestinal cholesterol absorption and susceptibility to cholesterol cholelithiasis. J Clin Invest. 2004;114:521–8.
78. Thomas LA, Veysey MJ, Murphy GM et al. Octreotide induced prolongation of colonic transit increases faecal anaerobic bacteria, bile acid metabolising enzymes, and serum deoxycholic acid in patients with acromegaly. Gut. 2005;54:630–5.

79. Maurer KJ, Ihrig MM, Rogers AB et al. Identification of cholelithogenic enterohepatic helicobacter species and their role in murine cholesterol gallstone formation. Gastroenterology. 2005;128:1023–33.
80. Fox JG. The non-*H. pylori* helicobacters: their expanding role in gastrointestinal and systemic diseases. Gut. 2002;50:273–83.
81. Maurer KJ, Carey MC, Fox JG. The adaptive immune response appears critical in promoting cholesterol gallstone formation in a BALB/c murine model. Gastroenterology. 2006 (In press).
82. Zhou H, Chen B, Li RX et al. Large-scale identification of human biliary proteins from a cholesterol stone patient using a proteomic approach. Rapid Commun Mass Spectrom. 2005;19:3569–78.
83. Admirand WH, Small DM. The physicochemical basis of cholesterol gallstone formation in man. J Clin Invest. 1968;47:1043–52.
84. Small DM, Shipley GG. Physical–chemical basis of lipid deposition in atherosclerosis. Science. 1974;185:222–9.
85. Steinberg D. Atherogenesis in perspective: hypercholesterolemia and inflammation as partners in crime. Nat Med. 2002;8:1211–17.

2
Aetiology and pathogenesis of primary sclerosing cholangitis

J. ALLINA and J. A. ODIN

BACKGROUND

Primary sclerosing cholangitis (PSC) results from idiopathic, inflammatory, fibro-obliterative fibrosis of intrahepatic and extrahepatic bile ducts[1]. The diagnosis of PSC is based on characteristic biochemical, histological, and radiographic findings in the absence of any known causative agent[2]. Many patients present with abnormally elevated alkaline phosphatase levels without symptoms. Others present with cholangitis due to biliary strictures, while still others present with end-stage liver disease. In a fraction of cases involvement is limited to small, intrahepatic bile ducts. These individuals have a better long-term prognosis compared to those with involvement of large bile ducts[3,4]. Current treatments are ineffective in preventing cirrhosis and liver cancer in individuals with PSC. A better understanding of the aetiology and pathogenesis of PSC may lead to therapies to slow disease progression.

Clearly defined disease characteristics are needed to delineate the aetiology and pathogenesis of PSC. After ruling out causes of secondary sclerosing cholangitis, the differential diagnosis of PSC most often includes autoimmune hepatitis (AIH) and primary biliary cirrhosis (PBC). Certain clinical features of PSC are distinctive relative to PBC and AIH, such as greater frequency of affected men versus women, cholangiocarcinoma, and inflammatory bowel disease[2]. However, overlap syndromes of each of these diseases with PSC have been identified[5,6]. Overlap of PSC with AIH may be as high as 35% in children with PSC; the frequency appears to be lower in adults[7,8]. Juveniles and young adults with PSC presenting with overlapping features of AIH may respond to treatment with corticosteroids[7]. In contrast, only rarely are PBC and PSC diagnosed in the same patient. In a single individual, diagnostic features of AIH, PSC, and PBC were reported[9].

Besides autoimmune liver disease, PSC is associated with an increased prevalence of other immune-mediated diseases[10]. Approximately 70% of patients will also have inflammatory bowel disease and many have autoimmune thyroid disease. Conversely, the prevalence of PSC among those with ulcerative colitis and autoimmune thyroid disease is much lower. These diseases may be diagnosed before or after the diagnosis of PSC. Unlike treatment of these associated diseases, immunosuppressive agents in adult PSC patients have not been effective, albeit the studies may have been underpowered and too short to detect any benefit[11,12]. The association of PSC with inflammatory bowel disease is not universal and may vary geographically[2,13]. The variability in the phenotypes of individuals with PSC described above suggests that PSC does not have a single aetiology or pathogenesis.

The 'onion-skin' appearance of the fibro-obliterative bile duct destruction typifies PSC; however, the same lesion occurs in cases of secondary sclerosing cholangitis[1]. Secondary sclerosing cholangitis (SSC), caused by multiple known aetiologies, including environmental toxins, medications, and infectious agents, has a much more benign clinical course and is not associated with AIH, ulcerative colitis, autoimmune thyroid disease or cholangiocarcinoma[14]. Over time, bile duct lumens narrow to create strictures and cholestasis develops. Later stages may be characterized clinically by episodes of bacterial cholangitis and biliary cirrhosis. Other lesions are characteristic of PBC and AIH. The florid duct lesion of PBC shows an inflammatory granuloma surrounding intrahepatic bile ducts with invasion and distortion of the bile duct epithelial layer. Interface hepatitis with bridging necrosis typifies AIH. Often mixed or non-specific histological features are present and a diagnosis cannot be established by histology alone.

AETIOLOGY AND PATHOGENESIS

The long period between diagnosis and disease onset, as well as the low incidence of PSC (10–20 cases/100 000) make identifying aetiological agents more difficult[15]. The clinical course is unpredictable so that there is no good prognostic model to predict disease progression in asymptomatic individuals. With so little known about the onset and course of the disease, it is difficult to separate aetiological factors from those affecting disease progression. Examination of animal models of biliary disease and immune function in individuals with PSC have provided insight into the environmental and genetic factors that may play a role in the aetiology and pathogenesis of PSC.

Animal models

Several models reproduce the histological features of PSC (Table 1). Formalin and several other toxins directly damage cholangiocytes or induce ischaemia of cholangiocytes[16,17]. Mdr2$^{-/-}$ mice develop lesions similar to PSC[17]. Leakage of bile through disrupted tight junction appears to lead to a proinflammatory/ fibrotic cascade. However, genetic variation of the human homologue of Mdr2 (MDR3) does not appear to play a role in PSC[18]. Individuals with cystic fibrosis are homozygous for mutation of the cystic fibrosis transmembrane conductance regulator (CFTR), expressed in cholangiocytes as well as the lung, and many develop peribiliary fibrosis similar to PSC. However, an increased frequency of the common CFTR mutations is not found among those with

Table 1 Animal models

Model description	Peribiliary fibrosis	Auto-antibodies
1. Mdr2$^{-/-}$ knockout mice with bile leakage	+	−
2. CFTR$^{-/-}$ knockout mice with DSS-induced colitis.	+	−
3. Formalin injection in bile duct	+	−
4. Graft-versus-host disease	+	−
5. Bacterial overgrowth or LPS exposure in immunodeficient mice	+	−
6. 2,4,6-Trinitrobenzenesulphonic acid injection into a dilated bile duct	+	+
7. Oral alpha-naphthylisothiocyanate	+	−

PSC[19]. Colitis models including those in CFTR$^{-/-}$ mice and models of graft-versus-host disease (GVHD) may develop biliary inflammation[20,21]. The former model mimics the association between inflammatory bowel disease (IBD) and PSC. Murine bacterial overgrowth or LPS exposure in immunodeficient mice similarly may cause peribiliary inflammation[22,23]. These models confirm that the aetiology of sclerosing cholangitis is variable. Though none completely mimics all features of PSC, the models are useful in evaluating pathogenic features of PSC and response to treatments.

A rat model of fibrosing cholangitis induced by administration of the hapten reagent 2,4,6-trinitrobenzenesulphonic acid (TNBS) into a dilated bile duct develops immunological changes, including p-ANCA autoantibodies, as well as histological abnormalities consistent with PSC[24]. Biliary Mrp2 and Oatp1 transport protein. Replication of this model by additional groups would help validate the model. Cholangitis can also be induced in rats by low-dose oral administration of the biliary toxin alpha-naphthylisothiocyanate. Hepatic inflammation centreed on damaged bile ducts, significant bile duct proliferation, and progressive fibrosis develop in this model, but no autoantibodies are found[25].

Together, these models demonstrate potential roles for external toxins, abnormalities of cholangiocytes themselves, bile leakage, and bacterial components in the pathogenesis of PSC. Lastly, the development of peribiliary fibrosis in animal models is often strain-specific, indicating a role for genetic susceptibility in PSC also.

Environmental factors

Little epidemiological data is available regarding PSC[26]. A case–control study by Mitchell et al. demonstrated a decreased prevalence of PSC among former and current smokers, regardless of concomitant IBD, as well as among those with a history of appendectomy[27]. However, the risk of liver cancer is higher in those with PSC who smoke[28]. It is difficult to determine whether prevalence differences with regard to race, familial incidence, and geography are environmental or genetic in origin[15,26,27,29]. No monozygotic versus dizygotic twin studies have been performed in PSC to help discriminate between environmental and genetic influences.

In animal models exposure to a variety of toxins does induce peribiliary inflammation and fibrosis. In the TNBS animal model discussed above, autoantibodies, including p-ANCA, are induced along with transient fibrosis and inflammation. However, the natural history of known cases of SSC differs from that of PSC[14]. Additionally, no significant geographic clustering of PSC near toxic waste sites was observed, as opposed to cases of PBC[30]. These findings argue against the hypothesis that PSC is simply a collection of cases of SSC in which the toxic agents have escaped detection. Unidentified toxins probably play a limited role in the aetiology and pathogenesis of PSC.

Infection with Reovirus type 3 (Reo-3) has been postulated as a cause of cholestatic liver diseases[31]. Titres of anti-Reo-3 were significantly higher in PSC and PBC sera than in sera of those with other causes of chronic liver disease and healthy controls, but staining for Reo-3 viral markers and cultures of liver biopsy material for Reo-3 virus proved negative. Lastly, *Heliocobacter* species DNA can be found in the liver of those with PSC, suggesting a possible aetiological role. However, Boomkens et al. observed no significant difference between the incidence of *Helicobacter* spp.-specific DNA in PSC livers and a control group[32]. More extensive epidemiological studies are needed to idenify specific environmental risk factors in PSC.

Immune dysfunction

Several findings indicate that immune dysregulation, either primary or secondary, plays a significant role in PSC (Table 2)[33]. Autoantibodies are prevalent (e.g. p-ANCA) in PSC, though they are non-specific and non-pathogenic[34,35]. Several groups have reported the presence of serum autoantibodies against cholangiocytes in PSC, but the specific autoantigens have not been identified[36,37]. As noted above, PSC is closely associated with autoimmune disease and IBD. The latter may be due to aberrant homing of gut mucosa-derived CCR9[+] memory T cells to the liver due to expression of CCL25 in PSC livers[38,39]. Under normal conditions mucosal T cells circulate between the gut and the liver. In PSC, due to aberrant hepatic CCL25 expression, CCR9[+] memory T cells accumulate in liver. Increased expression of intercellular adhesion molecule 1 occurs on bile ducts[40]. If an appropriate antigen reaches the liver, activation of these memory cells may cause extensive inflammation.

Table 2 Immune dysregulation: aberrant immunological findings in PSC

A. Autoantibodies are prevalent (e.g. p-ANCA and ANA).
B. A majority of lymphocytes in the liver have a Th1 phenotype.
C. Up-regulation of MHC class II and co-stimulatory molecule expression on cholangiocytes.
D. Aberrant hepatic expression of the gut-specific chemokine CCL25.
E. Increased expression of intercellular adhesion molecule 1 on bile ducts.
F. Increased association with autoimmune diseases and IBD.

A Th1 cytokine milieu (e.g. TNF-α/IFN-γ) predominates in PSC[41]. TNF-α contributes to oxidative stress-related damage in the liver[33]. Cholangiocytes may regulate T cell responses via internal cytokine production and basolateral surface expression of MHC class II and co-stimulatory molecules (B7-2)[36,39,42–44]. Not all groups have obtained the same immunohistochemical staining results. In addition to causing bile duct strictures in PSC, fibrosis also increases retention of growth factors and proinflammatory cytokines. Growth factors and cytokines bound to the extracellular matrix induce proliferation of myofibroblasts and epithelial cells as well as chemotaxis and activation of inflammatory cells. Due to this positive feedback loop, fibrosis and inflammation may persist and progress even after removal of any aetiological agent.

Genetic susceptibility

PSC genetic studies are still in their infancy. There is a 100-fold increased prevalence in first-degree relatives of individuals known to have PSC[45]. Geographic differences also indicate a genetic basis. An abnormal prevalence of several genetic polymorphisms has been associated with PSC (Table 3). These associations have not been extensively validated and are not yet useful for screening or diagnostic purposes. Many of these genetic studies have focused on major histocompatibility complex (MHC) and inflammation-related genes due to the suspected role of aberrant immune function in the pathogenesis of PSC. Specific HLA class II (T cell recognition) and III (innate recognition) haplotypes may increase the odds ratio of developing PSC nearly 3-fold or reduce it up to 8-fold. HLADR4 may be protective[46]. Most HLA genes have yet to be studied for disease-related polymorphisms and additional HLA associations might yet be identified.

Table 3 Genetic factors: indications of a genetic basis for the aetiopathogenesis of PSC

A. 100-fold increased prevalence in first-degree relatives.
B. Geographic variation in prevalence.
C. HLA class II and III haplotypes associations.
D. Increased prevalence of TNF2 allele.
E. CFTR polymorphism associations are controversial.
F. No association with IL-1 and IL-10 promoter polymorphisms.

Based on its role in inflammation, TNF-α polymorphisms were investigated in individuals with PSC. Prevalence of the TNF2 allele was increased in PSC paitents[47]. Polymorphisms of other cytokines such as interleukins IL-1 and IL-10 do not appear to provide resistance to or increase susceptibility to PSC[47,48]. CFTR polymorphisms have been associated with PSC in some populations, but in a recent study the common CFTR mutations or variants were not associated with PSC[19]. Malfunction of MDR3, the human homologue of mouse MDR2, has been proposed as a PSC susceptibility factor given the development of biliary fibrosis in mdr2$^{-/-}$ mice, but no genetic association in those with PSC has been identified[18]. Likewise, no association with any bile salt

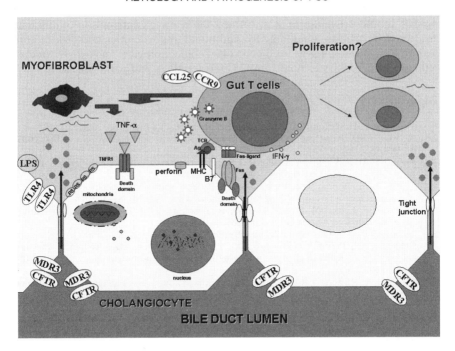

Figure 1 Primary sclerosing cholangitis. Fibro-obliterative destruction of the bile ducts occurs in response to unknown environmental and genetic factors. The homing of gut-derived T cells to the portal tract and immune-mediated apoptosis of cholangiocytes may be increased. Immune dysregulation appears to play a prominent role, but it may be secondary to the above factors. Animal models have suggested aberrant function of several different cholangiocyte receptors and tight junctions may also contribute to the pathogenesis of PSC

export pump (BSEP, ABCB11) polymorphism was discovered[18]. Many other transporters involved in bile production have yet to be examined. Tight junction proteins and Toll-like receptor genetic mutations or polymorphisms may also be involved based on animal models and observed immune dysregulation in PSC. Microarray analysis of cholangiocytes from PSC livers may aid in identifying unexpected genetic polymorphisms associated with PSC.

SUMMARY

The aetiology and pathogenesis of PSC remain poorly understood; however expanded research interest in this disease has led to several new hypotheses being investigated. In PSC the cholangiocyte appears to be the centre of a disordered fibro-inflammatory response to a combination of bacterial products, bile leakage, and possible unknown toxins (Figure 1). A constellation of cholangiocyte, fibroblast and immune cell susceptibility factors probably contribute to the initiation and persistence of PSC. Animal models should prove useful in discerning the relative contribution of different susceptibility factors. Undoubtedly, additional abnormalities and risk factors wait to be identified. Large, well-controlled epidemiological and genetic studies will also be necessary to finally unravel the aetiology and pathogenesis of PSC.

References

1. Lefkowitch JH. Histological assessment of cholestasis. Clin Liver Dis. 2004;8:27–40.
2. Rodriguez HJ, Bass NM. Primary sclerosing cholangitis. Semin Gastrointest Dis. 2003; 14:189–98.
3. Angulo P, Maor-Kendler Y, Lindor KD. Small-duct primary sclerosing cholangitis: a long-term follow-up study. Hepatology. 2002;35:1494–500.
4. Bjornsson E, Boberg KM, Cullen S et al. Patients with small duct primary sclerosing cholangitis have a favourable long term prognosis. Gut. 2002;51:731–5.
5. Schramm C, Lohse AW. Overlap syndromes of cholestatic liver diseases and auto-immune hepatitis. Clin Rev Allergy Immunol. 2005;28:105–14.
6. Beuers U, Rust C. Overlap syndromes. Semin Liver Dis. 2005;25:311–20.
7. Feldstein AE, Perrault J, El-Youssif M, Lindor KD, Freese DK, Angulo P. Primary sclerosing cholangitis in children: a long-term follow-up study. Hepatology. 2003;38:210–17.
8. Floreani A, Rizzotto ER, Ferrara F et al. Clinical course and outcome of autoimmune hepatitis/primary sclerosing cholangitis overlap syndrome. Am J Gastroenterol. 2005;100: 1516–22.
9. Kingham JG, Abbasi A. Co-existence of primary biliary cirrhosis and primary sclerosing cholangitis: a rare overlap syndrome put in perspective. Eur J Gastroenterol Hepatol. 2005; 17:1077–80.
10. Saarinen S, Olerup O, Broome U. Increased frequency of autoimmune diseases in patients with primary sclerosing cholangitis. Am J Gastroenterol. 2000;95:3195–9.
11. Mitchell SA, Chapman RW. The management of primary sclerosing cholangitis. Clin Liver Dis. 1998;2:353–72, x.
12. Talwalkar JA, Angulo P, Keach JC, Petz JL, Jorgensen RA, Lindor KD. Mycophenolate mofetil for the treatment of primary sclerosing cholangitis. Am J Gastroenterol. 2005;100: 308–12.
13. Okada H, Mizuno M, Yamamoto K, Tsuji T. Primary sclerosing cholangitis in Japanese patients: association with inflammatory bowel disease. Acta Med Okayama. 1996;50:227–35.
14. Gossard AA, Angulo P, Lindor KD. Secondary sclerosing cholangitis: a comparison to primary sclerosing cholangitis. Am J Gastroenterol. 2005;100:1330–3.
15. Bambha K, Kim WR, Talwalkar J et al. Incidence, clinical spectrum, and outcomes of primary sclerosing cholangitis in a United States community. Gastroenterology. 2003;125: 1364–9.
16. Bedossa P, Houry S, Bacci J, Martin E, Lemaigre G, Huguier M. A longitudinal study of histologic and immunohistologic changes in an experimental model of sclerosing cholangitis. Virchows Arch A Pathol Anat Histopathol. 1989;414:165–71.
17. Houry S, Languille O, Huguier M, Benhamou JP, Belghiti J, Msika S. Sclerosing cholangitis induced by formaldehyde solution injected into the biliary tree of rats. Arch Surg. 1990;125: 1059–61.
18. Pauli-Magnus C, Kerb R, Fattinger K et al. BSEP and MDR3 haplotype structure in healthy Caucasians, primary biliary cirrhosis and primary sclerosing cholangitis. Hepatology. 2004;39:779–91.
19. Gallegos-Orozco JF, CE Yurk, Wang N et al. Lack of association of common cystic fibrosis transmembrane conductance regulator gene mutations with primary sclerosing cholangitis. Am J Gastroenterol. 2005;100:874–8.
20. Nonomura A, Kono N, Minato H, Nakanuma Y. Diffuse biliary tract involvement mimicking primary sclerosing cholangitis in an experimental model of chronic graft-versus-host disease in mice. Pathol Int. 1998;48:421–7.

21. Blanco PG, Zaman MM, Junaidi O et al. Induction of colitis in cftr$^{-/-}$ mice results in bile duct injury. Am J Physiol Gastrointest Liver Physiol. 2004;287:G491–6.
22. Koga H, Sakisaka S, Yoshitake M et al. Abnormal accumulation in lipopolysaccharide in biliary epithelial cells of rats with self-filling blind loop. Int J Mol Med. 2002;9:621–6.
23. Lichtman SN, Keku J, Clark RL, Schwab JH, Sartor RB. Biliary tract disease in rats with experimental small bowel bacterial overgrowth. Hepatology. 1991;13:766–72.
24. Goetz M, Lehr HA, Neurath MF, Galle PR, Orth T. Long-term evaluation of a rat model of chronic cholangitis resembling human primary sclerosing cholangitis. Scand J Immunol. 2003;58:533–40.
25. Tjandra K, Sharkey KA, Swain MG. Progressive development of a Th1-type hepatic cytokine profile in rats with experimental cholangitis. Hepatology. 2000;31:280–90.
26. Feld JJ, Heathcote EJ. Epidemiology of autoimmune liver disease. J Gastroenterol Hepatol. 2003;18:1118–28.
27. Mitchell SA, Thyssen M, Orchard TR, Jewell DP, Fleming KA, Chapman RW. Cigarette smoking, appendectomy, and tonsillectomy as risk factors for the development of primary sclerosing cholangitis: a case–control study. Gut. 2002;51:567–73.
28. Bergquist A, Glaumann H, Persson B, Broome U. Risk factors and clinical presentation of hepatobiliary carcinoma in patients with primary sclerosing cholangitis: a case–control study. Hepatology. 1998;27:311–16.
29. Takikawa H. Recent status of primary sclerosing cholangitis in Japan. J Hepatobil Pancreat Surg. 1999;6:352–5.
30. Ala A, Stanca C, Bu-Ghanim M et al. Increased prevalence of primary biliary cirrhosis near superfund toxic waste sites. Hepatology. 2006;43:525–31.
31. Minuk GY, Rascanin N, Paul RW, Lee PW, Buchan K, Kelly JK. Reovirus type 3 infection in patients with primary biliary cirrhosis and primary sclerosing cholangitis. J Hepatol. 1987;5:8–13.
32. Boomkens SY, de Rave S, Pot RG et al. The role of *Helicobacter* spp. in the pathogenesis of primary biliary cirrhosis and primary sclerosing cholangitis. FEMS Immunol Med Microbiol. 2005;44:221–5.
33. Aoki CA, Bowlus CL, Gershwin ME. The immunobiology of primary sclerosing cholangitis. Autoimmun Rev. 2005;4:137–43.
34. Orth T, Kellner R, Diekmann O, Faust J, Meyer zum Buschenfelde KH, Mayet WJ. Identification and characterization of autoantibodies against catalase and alpha-enolase in patients with primary sclerosing cholangitis. Clin Exp Immunol. 1998;112:507–15.
35. Gur H, Shen G, Sutjita M et al. Autoantibody profile of primary sclerosing cholangitis. Pathobiology. 1995;63:76–82.
36. Xu B, Broome U, Ericzon BG, Sumitran-Holgersson S. High frequency of autoantibodies in patients with primary sclerosing cholangitis that bind biliary epithelial cells and induce expression of CD44 and production of interleukin 6. Gut. 2002;51:120–7.
37. Mandal A, Dasgupta A, Jeffers L et al. Autoantibodies in sclerosing cholangitis against a shared peptide in biliary and colon epithelium. Gastroenterology. 1994;106:185–92.
38. Eksteen B, Grant AJ, Miles A et al. Hepatic endothelial CCL25 mediates the recruitment of CCR9^{+} gut-homing lymphocytes to the liver in primary sclerosing cholangitis. J Exp Med. 2004;200:1511–17.
39. Ponsioen CY, Kuiper H, Ten Kate FJ, van Milligen de Wit M, van Deventer SJ, Tytgat GN. Immunohistochemical analysis of inflammation in primary sclerosing cholangitis. Eur J Gastroenterol Hepatol. 1999;11:769–74.
40. Adams DH, Hubscher SG, Shaw J et al. Increased expression of intercellular adhesion molecule 1 on bile ducts in primary biliary cirrhosis and primary sclerosing cholangitis. Hepatology. 1991;14:426–31.
41. Dienes HP, Lohse AW, Gerken G et al. Bile duct epithelia as target cells in primary biliary cirrhosis and primary sclerosing cholangitis. Virchows Arch. 1997;431:119–24.
42. Chapman RW, Kelly PM, Heryet A, Jewell DP, Fleming KA. Expression of HLA-DR antigens on bile duct epithelium in primary sclerosing cholangitis. Gut. 1988;29:422–7.
43. Tsuneyama K, Harada K, Yasoshima M, Kaji K, Gershwin ME, Nakanuma Y. Expression of co-stimulatory factor B7-2 on the intrahepatic bile ducts in primary biliary cirrhosis and primary sclerosing cholangitis: an immunohistochemical study. J Pathol. 1998;186:126–30.
44. Wu CT, Davis PA, Luketic VA, Gershwin ME. A review of the physiological and immunological functions of biliary epithelial cells: targets for primary biliary cirrhosis,

primary sclerosing cholangitis and drug-induced ductopenias. Clin Dev Immunol. 2004; 11:205–13.

45. Bergquist A, Lindberg G, Saarinen S, Broome U. Increased prevalence of primary sclerosing cholangitis among first-degree relatives. J Hepatol. 2005;42:252–6.
46. Czaja AJ, Santrach PJ, Breanndan Moore S. Shared genetic risk factors in autoimmune liver disease. Dig Dis Sci. 2001;46:140–7.
47. Mitchell SA, Grove J, Spurkland A et al. Association of the tumour necrosis factor alpha-308 but not the interleukin 10-627 promoter polymorphism with genetic susceptibility to primary sclerosing cholangitis. Gut. 2001;49:288–94.
48. Donaldson PT, Norris S, Constantini PK, Bernal W, Harrison P, Williams R. The interleukin-1 and interleukin-10 gene polymorphisms in primary sclerosing cholangitis: no associations with disease susceptibility/resistance. J Hepatol. 2000;32:882–6.
49. Martins EB, Graham AK, Chapman RW, Fleming KA. Elevation of gamma delta T lymphocytes in peripheral blood and livers of patients with primary sclerosing cholangitis and other autoimmune liver diseases. Hepatology. 1996;23:988–93.
50. Hashimoto E, Lindor KD, Homburger HA et al. Immunohistochemical characterization of hepatic lymphocytes in primary biliary cirrhosis in comparison with primary sclerosing cholangitis and autoimmune chronic active hepatitis. Mayo Clin Proc. 1993;68:1049–55.

3
Aetiology and pathogenesis of biliary cancer

K. N. LAZARIDIS

INTRODUCTION

Cholangiocarcinoma (CCA) is caused by malignant transformation of the epithelial cell that lines the bile ducts (i.e. cholangiocyte) and accounts for 10–15% of hepatobiliary neoplasms[1]. CCA is classified in two types based on its location along the biliary apparatus: intrahepatic and extrahepatic. Although these two entities have similar characteristics, each has discrete epidemiological and clinical features as well as probable independent aetiopathogenetic origins[1]. In this chapter, I discuss the epidemiology, classification, risk factors and pathogenesis of CCA. This knowledge should serve as the cornerstone for future studies in order to improve the prognosis, early detection and therapy of such a devastating disease[2].

EPIDEMIOLOGY

CCA is a rare neoplasm with approximately 5000 new cases diagnosed every year in the United States[3]. Nonetheless, in the past two decades its overall incidence has been increased[4]. About two-thirds of CCAs involve the extrahepatic bile ducts and the remaining one-third affect the intrahepatic biliary tree. It should be noted, however, that in several established registries, hilar CCAs, which involve the right and left hepatic ducts and their confluence, are classified as intrahepatic. In my view this is incorrect, and I consider these tumours extrahepatic.

Based on the Surveillance Epidemiology and End Results registries in the United States, the age-adjusted incidence rates of intrahepatic CCA increased from 0.32/100 000 in 1975–1979 to 0.85/100 000 in 1995–1999[4]. The increased incidence of intrahepatic CCA is probably real, and does not relate to earlier diagnosis of the disease. In contrast, the incidence of extrahepatic CCA decreased from 1.08/100 000 in 1979 to 0.82/100 000 in 1998[4]. However, the overall incidence of CCA is increasing because the raised incidence of intrahepatic CCA exceeds the small decrease in the incidence of extrahepatic CCA.

23

The incidence of intrahepatic CCA differs worldwide[4]. It is highest in northeast Thailand, probably because of the high prevalence of liver-fluke infestations in this population[4]. Recently there is also an observed shift in the average age of diagnosis of intrahepatic CCA from the 5th towards the 6th decade of life. In the United States the male to female ratio for intrahepatic CCA is about 1.5. Caucasians and African Americans have a comparable age-adjusted incidence, but in Asians the incidence is two times higher than that of Caucasians. However, the latter race group is the only one in which there is evidence of gradual increase in the age-adjusted incidence of intrahepatic CCA.

The mortality of intrahepatic CCA is also increasing across the world[5]; the percentage of intrahepatic CCA increased mortality was greater than the one observed for hepatocellular carcinoma. For example, in the United States, the age-adjusted mortality rate for intrahepatic CCA increased from 0.07/100 000 in 1973 to 0.69/100 000 in 1997[6]. To this end, the 5-year survival of patients with intrahepatic CCA remains disappointingly short, and practically without change over the past 20 years. This lack of improvement in survival occurs despite better diagnostic methods, employment of aggressive surgical approaches (i.e. hepatectomies) and promising new endoscopic modalities for palliative therapy (i.e. biliary stenting, photodynamic therapy).

On the other hand, the incidence of extrahepatic CCA is decreasing. In the United States the age-adjusted incidence has been reported to be 1.2/100 000 for men and 0.8/100 000 for women. Additionally, the age-adjusted mortality rates of extrahepatic CCA are declining in Western countries with the exception of Italy and Japan[5]. Moreover, in the United States, the age-adjusted mortality rates declined from 0.6/100 000 in 1979 to 0.3/100 000 in 1998[6]. There is also evidence of a slight improvement in the 5-year survival rates of extrahepatic CCA from 11.7% in 1973–1977 to 15.1% in 1983–1987[7].

CLASSIFICATION

CCA is a well-to-moderately differentiated tubular adenocarcinoma. It is a locally destructive tumour that forms glands with a prominent dense desmoplastic stroma. In addition to tubular adenocarcinoma other histological variants of CCA include papillary adenocarcinoma, signet-ring carcinoma, squamous cell or mucoepidermoid carcinoma and a lymphoepithelioma-like form.

CCA is classified into intrahepatic and extrahepatic (Figure 1). The extrahepatic variety is subdivided into: (a) hilar or Klatskin tumour; (b) middle tumours; and (c) distal tumours. Hilar tumours represent approximately 60% of all extrahepatic CCA (Figure 2) and are categorized into four different types according to Bismuth (Figure 3). Intrahepatic CCA grow and form mass lesions, which account for about one-third of bile duct tumours. Intrahepatic CCA may be solitary or multinodular, and can be misdiagnosed as hepatocellular carcinoma. They can present as a well-demarcated mass lesion or as a diffuse infiltrating neoplastic process.

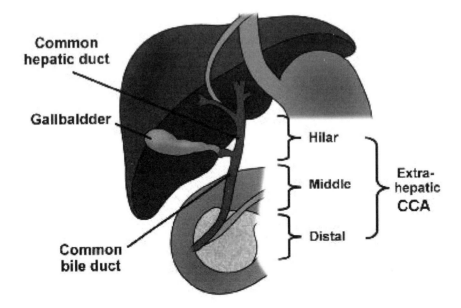

Figure 1 Classification of CCA. The term CCA refers to tumours involving the entire biliary tree (i.e. intrahepatic and extrahepatic). Intrahepatic CCA denotes malignancies affecting the intrahepatic bile ducts. Extrahepatic CCA are divided into hilar or Klatskin tumour, middle and distal tumours

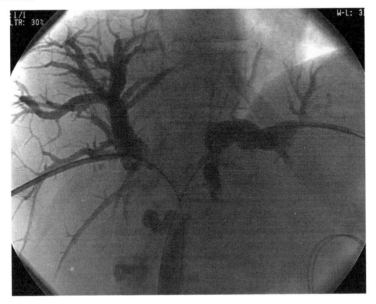

Figure 2 An endoscopic retrograde cholangiopancreatograph (ERCP) demonstrating a hilar CCA causing obstruction of the biliary bifurcation with extension into the left and the right hepatic ducts

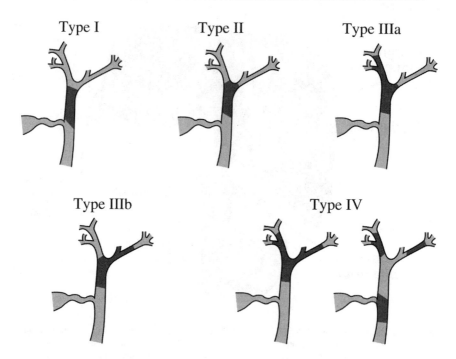

Figure 3 Bismuch classification of hilar CCA. Type I CCA affects the common hepatic duct; type II CCA involves the common hepatic duct and the confluence of the right and left hepatic ducts; type IIIa and IIIb CCA include the common hepatic duct and either the right or left hepatic duct, respectively; and type IV CCA involves the biliary confluence and extends to both right and left hepatic ducts or refers to multifocal bile duct tumours

RISK FACTORS

The majority of patients diagnosed with CCA have no known risk factor(s) (Table 1). As in many maladies, age more than 65 years old is a risk factor for developing CCA. In the eastern hemisphere, liver flukes, namely *Opisthorchis viverrini* and *Clonorchis sinensis*, are strongly associated with CCA. These worms inhabit the bile ducts in infected individuals who had ingesting undercooked fish. Contrary, in the western hemisphere, primary sclerosing cholangitis (PSC) is a known predisposing factor for CCA. The risk of developing CCA in a patient with PSC is approximately 1.5% annually after the diagnosis of the cholestatic liver disease[8]. Among the PSC patients who will develop CCA, about 30% will be found to have malignancy of the bile ducts within 2 years following the diagnosis of PSC[9,10]. Additionally, in patients with PSC the risk of developing CCA is not associated with the duration of the cholestatic liver disease[9].

Patients with Caroli's disease and choledochal cysts (i.e. congenital cystic dilation of bile ducts) have an increased lifetime risk for developing CCA. This

Table 1   CCA risk factors

Age (over 65 years)
Liver fluke infestation
   Opisthorchis viverrini
   Clonorchis sinensis
Primary sclerosing cholangitis (PSC)
Caroli's disease
Choledochal cysts
Bile duct adenoma and biliary papillomatosis
Chronic intraductal stones (i.e. hepatolithiasis)
Liver cirrhosis
Thorotrast
Surgical biliary–enteric drainage procedures
HIV
Hepatitis C
Diabetes mellitus
Smoking
Dioxin
Vinyl chloride

---

risk is ~ 10–20% and the median age of diagnosis is 34 years[11]. Hepatolithiasis (i.e. intrahepatic bile duct stones) is frequent in Asia, but rare in the Western world, and is associated with intrahepatic CCA[12]. Approximately 10% of patients with intrahepatic bile duct stones develop CCA. Finally, liver cirrhosis of any cause is a risk factor for CCA.

Thorotrast, a colloidal suspension of ^{232}ThO$_2$, had been linked to the development of CCA. Thorotrast emits alpha particles and was used as a contrast agent in radiology from the 1930s to the 1950s. It probably causes microsatellite instability and subsequently CCA via clonal expansion of bile duct cells and inactivation of the human MutL, *E. coli* Homolog 1 (MLH1)[13]. Recently it has been shown that surgical biliary–enteric drainage procedures are associated with the development of CCA[14]. This finding is important particularly when contemplating such surgical approaches in patients with PSC because the cholestatic disease itself increases the risk of CCA development.

Other risk factors that predispose to CCA include HIV infection, smoking, diabetes mellitus, hepatitis C virus infection and environmental exposure to agents such as dioxin and vinyl chloride[15]. Of interest, hepatitis B virus infection is not associated with CCA[15].

MOLECULAR PATHOGENESIS

Over the past 10 years there has been considerable scientific progress in understanding the pathogenesis of CCA. We now know that chronic biliary inflammation and cholestasis cause increased production of cytokines and reactive oxygen species, resulting in protracted cholangiocyte stresses and accrual of irreversible DNA damage[1]. Subsequently, biliary epithelia undergo malignant transformation by attaining molecular and cellular characteristics

Table 2 Molecular alterations of cholangiocyte leading to malignant transformation

Contribution in carcinogenesis	Molecular mechanisms	References
Autologous proliferation signalling	IL-6, gp80/gp130 up-regulation	Sugawara et al.[21]
	HGF/c-met up-regulation	Yokomuro et al.[18,19], Lai et al.[23], Aishima et al.[24]
	EGF/c-erbB-2	Aishima et al.[24], Ito et al.[26], Kiguchi et al.[28]
	COX-2 up-regulation	Chariyalertsak et al.[30], Endo et al.[31], Yoon et al.[51]
	k-ras mutations	Kang et al.[33], Tannapfel et al.[34], Tada et al.[35]
Loss of antigrowth signalling	p53 mutations	Kang et al.[33]
	p21/WAF mutations	Furubo et al.[63]
	Mdm-2 up-regulation	Furubo et al.[63]
	p16 ^{INK4} mutation	Tannapfel et al.[34]
Evasion of apoptosis	FLIP up-regulation	Que et al.[43]
	NO inhibition of caspases	Torok et al.[44]
	Bcl-2 up-regulation	Harnois et al.[64]
	Bcl-X_L up-regulation	Okaro et al.[65]
	Mcl-1 up-regulation	Yoon et al.[50]
	COX-2 up-regulation	Nzeako et al.[49]
Unlimited replicative potential	Telomerase expressed	Itoi et al.[54,55]
Angiogenesis	VEGF expressed	Benckert et al.[56]
Tissue invasiveness and metastasis	E-cadherin decreased	Ashida et al.[66]
	α-catetin and β-catetin decreased	Ashida et al.[66]
	Matrix metalloproteinase (MMP) up-regulation	Terada et al.[58]
	Human aspartyl (asparaginyl) β-hydroxylase expression	Lavaissiere et al.[59], Ince et al.[60], Maeda et al.[61]
	WISPv1 expression	Tanaka et al.[62]

(Modified from Berthiaume EP et al. Molecular pathogenesis of cholangiocarcinoma. Semin Liver Dis. 2004;24:127–37)

they lack otherwise in normal conditions. The molecular alterations of cholangiocytes which contribute to carcinogenesis of bile ducts represent a complex process of interrelated events. An overview of the proposed pathways is shown in Table 2. However, we should keep in mind that the experimental studies that describe the molecular pathogenesis of CCA in humans were performed in specimens derived from patients with intrahepatic CCA; to collect samples from these tumours is easier compared to extrahepatic CCA. For instance, hilar CCA are highly desmoplastic and therefore obtaining adequate tissue for studies is very challenging, if not impossible. Thus, it remains indeterminate whether the reported molecular pathways of intrahepatic CCA are pertinent to extrahepatic ones.

In health, cholangiocytes retain tissue homeostasis despite exposure to exogenous or endogenous signals. However, during chronic biliary inflammation, local interleukin 6 (IL-6) and hepatocyte growth factor (HGF) production increases due to activation of stellate cells. IL-6 is a powerful mitogen that causes cholangiocyte proliferation by binding to its plasma membrane receptor and forming the active heterodimer, gp80/gp130[16–19]. Subsequently, the latter activates cellular transcription through the mitogen-activated protein kinase (MAPK)/(signal transducer and activator of transcription) STAT pathway[20]. Malignant but not normal cholangiocytes also produce high levels of IL-6[21] and over-express the gp80/gp130 heterodimer. Hepatocyte growth factor (HGF) also promotes cholangiocyte growth via its plasma-membrane receptor, c-met[16,22]. In addition, CCA cells attain the capability to produce HGF and up-regulate its c-met receptor[18,23,24]. Therefore, via the IL-6 and HGF pathways, malignant bile duct cells maintain autologous proliferating mechanisms. Another pathway that contributes in cholangiocarcinogenesis is the epidermal growth factor (EGF) and its receptor (EGFR)[25,26]. Interaction of EGF with EGFR leads to activation of the MAPK pathway[27]. The c-erb-B2/ protein, a homologue of the EGFR, is a tyrosine kinase which is activated in CCA[24]. To this extent constitutive expression of c-erb-B2 in gallbladder epithelium leads to adenocarcinoma[28].

Cyclooxygenase-2 (COX-2), an isoform that catalyses the formation of prostaglandins from arachidonic acid[29], is also involved in the pathogenesis of CCA. COX-2 is over-expressed in malignant, but not normal, cholangiocytes[30,31]. The complex and interrelated processes of carcinogenesis in bile ducts is indicated by the fact that IL-6, HGF and EGF stimulate COX-2 expression in cholangiocytes[28,32]. Nonetheless, the exact mechanism by which COX-2 causes CCA is uncertain, but probably involves inhibition of apoptotic pathways.

K-ras plays a critical role in the mitogenic signals to cells. Mutations of this gene have been detected in 20–100% of biopsy-proven CCA[33,34]. K-ras mutations have also been associated with hilar CCA and periductal tumour extension[33,35]. Further verification of these observations is needed because, if proven reliable, detection of K-ras mutations could be incorporated in the clinical management of patients at high risk for developing CCA. For example, PSC patients with specific mutations of K-ras may benefit from aggressive surveillance protocols for detection of CCA, development of chemopreventive strategies, or early orthotopic liver transplantation.

Critical pathways, which inhibit cell proliferation. are usually lost during the development of cholangiocarcinogenesis. For example, loss of heterozygosity for the tumour suppressor gene p53 is frequent in CCA[36]. The p53 gene directs the cellular machinery of cell cycle and apoptosis. Specifically, p53 regulates the p21/WAF1 (wild-type p53 activated fragment 1) protein which binds to the cell division kinase (CDK) 4:cyclin D complex (Figure 4). To this end, p53 causes negative feedback of the CDK4:cyclin D complex, therefore averting phosphorylation of Rb, and as a result release of the E2F transcription factor (Figure 4). Consequently, the E2F molecule controls the transcription of multiple cellular proteins important in the S phase of the cell cycle[37,38]. Moreover, p53 can induce apoptosis by promoting Bax insertion in the mitochondrial membrane and stimulating mitochondrial depolarization and subsequently apoptosis. Additionally, inactivation of the p14/mdm/p53

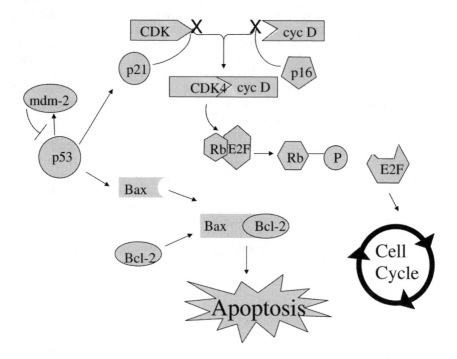

Figure 4 The molecular pathways of p53. p53 regulates both cholangiocyte cell cycle and apoptosis; p53 controls the cell division kinase (CDK)4:cyclin D complex via the p21/WAF1 protein which binds to the latter. As a result, p53 causes negative feedback of the CDK4:cyclin D complex, therefore averting phosphorylation of Rb leading to release of the E2F transcription factor. Subsequently, E2F regulates the transcription of multiple proteins in the S phase of the cell cycle. p53 can also induce apoptosis by promoting Bax insertion into the mitochondrial membrane stimulating mitochondrial depolarization resulting in apoptosis. The p16 protein also inhibits the CDK4:cyclin D complex. (Modified from Berthiaume EP et al. Molecular pathogenesis of cholangiocarcinoma. Semin Liver Dis. 2004;24:127–37)

pathway and p16, a tumour-suppressor gene, via a variety of molecular mechanisms, has been described in CCA and in PSC-associated CCA[39,40]. For instance, p16 is frequently inactivated in PSC-associated CCA via point mutations of its promoter[41].

Apoptosis (i.e. programmed cell death) is a pivotal cellular mechanism that controls tissue homeostasis. Lack of apoptosis may lead to aberrant cell proliferation and subsequently to carcinogenesis. Apoptosis could function as a protective mechanism to eliminate biliary cells transformed to a malignant phenotype. Thus, loss of the protective act of apoptosis in biliary epithelia may result in the development of CCA. Cholangiocytes express the Fas receptor on plasma membrane[32] and respond to FAS ligand stimulation with apoptosis. Nevertheless, in a CCA cell line there was diminished responsiveness of the Fas/FAS ligand due to alteration of the FLIP (flice inhibitory protein)[42]. FLIP inhibits activation of pro-caspase 8 causing diminished signalling of the Fas/FAS ligand pathway[43]. Ligand activation of the Fas/TRAIL(tumour necrosis factor (TNF)-related apoptosis inducing ligand)/TNF receptor family or release of cytochrome c by mitochondria causes activation of caspases resulting in DNA fragmentation and cell destruction[42]. Moreover, cholangiocytes under the effect of nitric oxide (NO) display inhibition of both caspase 3 and 9, probably via nitrosylation, and become relatively resistant to apoptosis[44]. Overall, it is the balance of pro- and anti-apoptotic signals in the cholangiocyte that guide the depolarization of the mitochondrial membrane releasing cytochrome-c into the cytosol and then the activation of caspases.

Studies have also shown that biliary inflammation up-regulates the inducible nitric oxide synthase (iNOs) leading to NO production. Among its other effects, NO production causes oxidative DNA damage and inhibition of DNA repair enzymes[45,46]. Moreover, iNOS-mediated carcinogenesis is induced by the COX-2 and Notch-1 pathways[47,48]. Of interest, COX-2 induced by inflammation is anti-apoptotic. Up-regulation of COX-2 inhibits Fas/FAS ligand-induced apoptosis by increasing expression of the inhibitory protein myeloid cell leukaemia-1 (Mcl-1)[49]. Of interest, bile acids which are usually elevated in CCA have a positive effect on the expression of Mcl-1 protein via inhibition of proteosome degradation[50]. Besides bile acids, inflammatory mediators up-regulate Mcl-1; as a result, potential malignant cholangiocytes are averted from apoptosis. In addition to biliary inflammation as a precipitant of cholangiocarcinogenesis, CCA demonstrate an inherent tropism for bile. To this end, bile acids have been reported to trans-activate the EGFR and to promote the expression of COX-2 in cholangiocytes[50,51].

CCA have the ability of continued growth. In this process progressive telomere shortening may be contributory. Telomeres, long stretches of repeat sequences, are present at the end of chromosomes and involved in DNA synthesis. After multiple cell cycles, telomere shortening causes chromosomal instability which renders cells incompetent to divide[52]. In CCA, preservation of telomere shortening due to overexpression of the human telomerase reverse transcriptase (hTERT) permits these tumours to sustain chromosomal replication and to maintain eternal proliferation[53]. Detectable hTERT activity and increased expression of its mRNA have been reported in intrahepatic CCA[54,55].

Many malignancies promote angiogenesis to ensure an adequate blood supply for feeding the constantly dividing tumour cells. CCAs have a high vascular supply and the intrahepatic ones express the vascular endothelial growth factor (VEGF)[56]. Moreover, in a CCA cell line the increased expression of VEGF was dependent on transforming growth factor beta (TGF-β) stimulation[56]. A feature of many neoplastic tumours is invasiveness of the surrounding tissues and metastasis. Mutations or deletions of E-cadherin, a cell surface protein involved in cellular adhesion, cause diminished cell adhesiveness facilitating tissue invasion and metastasis. To this extent, intrahepatic CCAs with reduced expression of E-cadherin demonstrate advanced tumour histological stage[57]. The clinical invasiveness of CCA is also associated with up-regulation of matrix metalloproteinases (MMP)[58]. Moreover, a protein involved in tumour invasion, the human aspartyl (asparaginyl) β-hydroxylase (HAAH), is also expressed in both hepatocellular carcinoma and CCA[59]. Expression of HAAH in transfected cell lines was associated with anchorage-independent growth and tumour development in nude mice[60]. Of interest, CCA cell lines are reported to overexpress HAAH[61]. Other molecules that are postulated to participate in the pathogenesis of CCA include WISP1v (WNT1-inducible signaling pathway protein 1), a protein associated with the connective tissue growth factor family[62].

The list of proposed molecular pathways involved in the pathobiology of CCA is increasing. The interactions of these paths lead to the initiation and subsequently development of clinically apparent disease. Likely clusters of these and other yet unknown molecules and modules are relevant to the induction, progression and advancement of CCA and its subtypes (i.e. intrahepatic vs extrahepatic).

SUMMARY

CCA is an insidious disease associated with high mortality. The incidence of intrahepatic CCA is increasing across the world, although the aetiology of this observation is unclear. Our knowledge of CCA pathogenesis is improving but early diagnosis and curative therapies remain limited. We need to invest on more basic research and clinical studies in order to elucidate the pathobiology of this devastating disease.

References

1. Gores GJ. Cholangiocarcinoma: current concepts and insights. Hepatology. 2003;37:961–9.
2. Khan SA, Davidson BR, Goldin R et al. Guidelines for the diagnosis and treatment of cholangiocarcinoma: consensus document. Gut. 2002;51(Suppl. 6:1–9.
3. Jemal A, Murray T, Samuels A, Ghafoor A, Ward E, Thun MJ. Cancer statistics, 2003. CA Cancer J Clin. 2003;53:5–26.
4. Shaib YH, Davila JA, McGlynn K, El-Serag HB. Rising incidence of intrahepatic cholangiocarcinoma in the United States: a true increase? J Hepatol. 2004;40:472–7.
5. Khan SA, Taylor-Robinson SD, Toledano MB, Beck A, Elliott P, Thomas HC. Changing international trends in mortality rates for liver, biliary and pancreatic tumours. J Hepatol. 2002;37:806–13.

6. Patel T. Increasing incidence and mortality of primary intrahepatic cholangiocarcinoma in the United States. Hepatology. 2001;33:1353–7.

7. Carriaga MT, Henson DE. Liver, gallbladder, extrahepatic bile ducts, and pancreas. Cancer. 1995;75(Suppl. 1):171–90.

8. Bergquist A, Broome U. Hepatobiliary and extra-hepatic malignancies in primary sclerosing cholangitis. Best Pract Res Clin Gastroenterol. 2001;15:643–56.

9. Broome U, Olsson R, Loof L et al. Natural history and prognostic factors in 305 Swedish patients with primary sclerosing cholangitis. Gut. 1996;38:610–15.

10. Rosen CB, Nagorney DM, Wiesner RH, Coffey RJ Jr, LaRusso NF. Cholangiocarcinoma complicating primary sclerosing cholangitis. Ann Surg. 1991;213:21–5.

11. Simeone DM. Gallbladder and Biliary Tree: Anatomy and Structural Anomalies. Philadelphia: Lippincott, Williams & Wilkins, 1999.

12. Chen MF, Jan YY, Wang CS et al. A reappraisal of cholangiocarcinoma in a patient with hepatolithiasis. Cancer. 1993;71:2461–5.

13. Liu D, Momoi H, Li L, Ishikawa Y, Fukumoto M. Microsatellite instability in thorotrast-induced human intrahepatic cholangiocarcinoma. Int J Cancer. 2002;102:366–71.

14. Tocchi A, Mazzoni G, Liotta G, Lepre L, Cassini D, Miccini M. Late development of bile duct cancer in patients who had biliary-enteric drainage for benign disease: a follow-up study of more than 1000 patients. Ann Surg. 2001;234:210–14.

15. Shaib YH, El-Serag HB, Davila JA, Morgan R, McGlynn KA. Risk factors of intrahepatic cholangiocarcinoma in the United States: a case–control study. Gastroenterology. 2005; 128:620–6.

16. Matsumoto K, Fujii H, Michalopoulos G, Fung JJ, Demetris AJ. Human biliary epithelial cells secrete and respond to cytokines and hepatocyte growth factors *in vitro*: interleukin-6, hepatocyte growth factor and epidermal growth factor promote DNA synthesis *in vitro*. Hepatology. 1994;20:376–82.

17. Park J, Tadlock L, Gores GJ, Patel T. Inhibition of interleukin 6-mediated mitogen-activated protein kinase activation attenuates growth of a cholangiocarcinoma cell line. Hepatology. 1999;30:1128–33.

18. Yokomuro S, Tsuji H, Lunz JG 3rd et al. Growth control of human biliary epithelial cells by interleukin 6, hepatocyte growth factor, transforming growth factor beta1, and activin A: comparison of a cholangiocarcinoma cell line with primary cultures of non-neoplastic biliary epithelial cells. Hepatology. 2000;32:26–35.

19. Yokomuro S, Lunz JG, Sakamoto T, Ezure T, Murase N, Demetris AJ. The effect of interleukin-6 (IL-6)/gp130 signalling on biliary epithelial cell growth, *in vitro*. Cytokine. 2000;12:727–30.

20. Heinrich PC, Behrmann I, Haan S, Hermanns HM, Muller-Newen G, Schaper F. Principles of interleukin (IL)-6-type cytokine signalling and its regulation. Biochem J. 2003;15:1–20.

21. Sugawara H, Yasoshima M, Katayanagi K et al. Relationship between interleukin-6 and proliferation and differentiation in cholangiocarcinoma. Histopathology. 1998;33:145–53.

22. Boccaccio C, Gaudino G, Gambarotta G, Galimi F, Comoglio PM. Hepatocyte growth factor (HGF) receptor expression is inducible and is part of the delayed-early response to HGF. J Biol Chem. 1994;269:12845–51.

23. Lai GH, Radaeva S, Nakamura T, Sirica AE. Unique epithelial cell production of hepatocyte growth factor/scatter factor by putative precancerous intestinal metaplasias and associated 'intestinal-type' biliary cancer chemically induced in rat liver. Hepatology. 2000;31:1257–65.

24. Aishima SI, Taguchi KI, Sugimachi K, Shimada M, Tsuneyoshi M. c-erbB-2 and c-Met expression relates to cholangiocarcinogenesis and progression of intrahepatic cholangiocarcinoma. Histopathology. 2002;40:269–78.

25. Harada K, Terada T, Nakanuma Y. Detection of transforming growth factor-alpha protein and messenger RNA in hepatobiliary diseases by immunohistochemical and *in situ* hybridization techniques. Hum Pathol. 1996;27:787–92.

26. Ito Y, Takeda T, Sasaki Y et al. Expression and clinical significance of the erbB family in intrahepatic cholangiocellular carcinoma. Pathol Res Pract. 2001;197:95–100.

27. Schlessinger J. Ligand-induced, receptor-mediated dimerization and activation of EGF receptor. Cell. 2002;110:669–72.

28. Kiguchi K, Carbajal S, Chan K et al. Constitutive expression of ErbB-2 in gallbladder epithelium results in development of adenocarcinoma. Cancer Res. 2001;61:6971–6.
29. Williams CS, Mann M, DuBois RN. The role of cyclooxygenases in inflammation, cancer, and development. Oncogene. 1999;18:7908–16.
30. Chariyalertsak CS, Sirikulchayanonta V, Mayer D et al. Aberrant cyclooxygenase isoenzyme expression in human intrahepatic cholangiocarcinoma. Gut. 2001;48:80–6.
31. Endo K, Yoon BI, Pairojkul C, Demetris AJ, Sirica AE. ERBB-2 overexpression and cyclooxygenase-2 up-regulation in human cholangiocarcinoma and risk conditions. Hepatology. 2002;36:439–50.
32. Shimonishi T, Isse K, Shibata F et al. Up-regulation of fas ligand at early stages and down-regulation of Fas at progressed stages of intrahepatic cholangiocarcinoma reflect evasion from immune surveillance. Hepatology. 2000;32:761–9.
33. Kang YK, Kim WH, Lee HW, Lee HK, Kim YI. Mutation of p53 and K-ras, and loss of heterozygosity of APC in intrahepatic cholangiocarcinoma. Lab Invest. 1999;79:477–83.
34. Tannapfel A, Benicke M, Katalinic A et al. Frequency of p16-INK4A alterations and k-ras mutations in intrahepatic cholangiocarcinoma of the liver. Gut. 2000;47:721–7.
35. Tada M, Omata M, Ohto M. High incidence of ras gene mutation in intrahepatic cholangiocarcinoma. Cancer. 1992;69:1115–18.
36. Isa T, Tomita S, Nakachi A et al. Analysis of microsatellite instability, K-ras gene mutation and p53 protein overexpression in intrahepatic cholangiocarcinoma. Hepatogastroenterology. 2002;49:604–8.
37. Evan GI, Vousden KH. Proliferation, cell cycle and apoptosis in cancer. Nature. 2001;411:342–8.
38. Levine AJ. p53, the cellular gatekeeper for growth and division. Cell. 1997;88:323–31.
39. Cong WM, Bakker A, Swalsky PA et al. Multiple genetic alterations involved in the tumorigenesis of human cholangiocarcinoma: a molecular genetic and clinicopathological study. J Cancer Res Clin Oncol. 2001;127:187–92.
40. Ahrendt SA, Eisenberger CF, Yip L et al. Chromosome 9p21 loss and p16 inactivation in primary sclerosing cholangitis-associated cholangiocarcinoma. J Surg Res. 1999;84:88–93.
41. Taniai M, Higuchi H, Burgart LJ, Gores GJ. p16INK4a promoter mutations are frequent in primary sclerosing cholangitis (PSC) and PSC-associated cholangiocarcinoma. Gastroenterology. 2002;123:1090–8.
42. Hengartner MO. The biochemistry of apoptosis. Nature. 2000;407:770–6.
43. Que FG, Phan VA, Phan VH et al. Cholangiocarcinomas express Fas ligand and disable the Fas receptor. Hepatology. 1999;30:1398–404.
44. Torok NJ, Higuchi H, Bronk S, Gores GJ. Nitric oxide inhibits apoptosis downstream of cytochrome C release by nitrosylating caspase 9. Cancer Res. 2002;62:1648–53.
45. Jaiswal M, LaRusso NF, Burgart LJ, Gores GJ. Inflammatory cytokines induce DNA damage and inhibit DNA repair in cholangiocarcinoma cells by a nitric oxide-dependent mechanism. Cancer Res. 2000;60:184–90.
46. Jaiswal M, LaRusso NF, Shapiro RA, Billiar TR, Gores GJ. Nitric oxide-mediated inhibition of DNA repair potentiates oxidative DNA damage in cholangiocytes. Gastroenterology. 2001;120:190–9.
47. Ishimura N, Bronk S, Gores G. Inducible nitric oxide synthase upregulates cycloogenase-2 in mouse cholangiocytes promoting cell growth. Am J Physiol Gastrointest Liver Physiol. 2004;287:G88–95.
48. Ishimura N, Bronk S, Gores G. Inducible nitric oxide synthase up-regulates Notch-1 in mouse cholangiocytes: implications for carcinogenesis. Gastroenterology. 2005;128:1354–68.
49. Nzeako UC, Guicciardi ME, Yoon JH, Bronk SF, Gores GJ. COX-2 inhibits Fas-mediated apoptosis in cholangiocarcinoma cells. Hepatology. 2002;35:552–9.
50. Yoon JH, Werneburg NW, Higuchi H et al. Bile acids inhibit Mcl-1 protein turnover via an epidermal growth factor receptor/Raf-1-dependent mechanism. Cancer Res. 2002;62:6500–5.
51. Yoon JH, Higuchi H, Werneburg NW, Kaufmann SH, Gores GJ. Bile acids induce cyclooxygenase-2 expression via the epidermal growth factor receptor in a human cholangiocarcinoma cell line. Gastroenterology. 2002;122:985–93.
52. Buys CH. Telomeres, telomerase, and cancer. N Engl J Med. 2000;342:1282–3.

53. Shay JW, Bacchetti S. A survey of telomerase activity in human cancer. Eur J Cancer. 1997; 33:787–91.
54. Itoi T, Shinohara Y, Takeda K et al. Detection of telomerase activity in biopsy specimens for diagnosis of biliary tract cancers. Gastrointest Endosc. 2000;52:380–6.
55. Itoi T, Shinohara Y, Takeda K et al. Detection of telomerase reverse transcriptase mRNA in biopsy specimens and bile for diagnosis of biliary tract cancers. Int J Mol Med. 2001;7:281–7.
56. Benckert C, Jonas S, Cramer T et al. Transforming growth factor beta 1 stimulates vascular endothelial growth factor gene transcription in human cholangiocellular carcinoma cells. Cancer Res. 2003;63:1083–92.
57. Endo K, Ashida K, Miyake N, Terada T. E-cadherin gene mutations in human intrahepatic cholangiocarcinoma. J Pathol. 2001;193:310–17.
58. Terada T, Okada Y, Nakanuma Y. Expression of immunoreactive matrix metallo-proteinases and tissue inhibitors of matrix metalloproteinases in human normal livers and primary liver tumors. Hepatology. 1996;23:1341–4.
59. Lavaissiere L, Jia S, Nishiyama M et al. Overexpression of human aspartyl(asparaginyl) beta-hydroxylase in hepatocellular carcinoma and cholangiocarcinoma. J Clin Invest. 1996; 98:1313–23.
60. Ince N, de la Monte SM, Wands JR. Overexpression of human aspartyl (asparaginyl) beta-hydroxylase is associated with malignant transformation. Cancer Res. 2000;60:1261–6.
61. Maeda T, Sepe P, Lahousse S et al. Antisense oligodeoxynucleotides directed against aspartyl (asparaginyl) beta-hydroxylase suppress migration of cholangiocarcinoma cells. J Hepatol. 2003;38:615–22.
62. Tanaka S, Sugimachi K, Kameyama T et al. Human WISP1v, a member of the CCN family, is associated with invasive cholangiocarcinoma. Hepatology. 2003;37:1122–9.
63. Furubo S, Harada K, Shimonishi T, Katayanagi K, Tsui W, Nakanuma Y. Protein expression and genetic alterations of p53 and ras in intrahepatic cholangiocarcinoma. Histopathology. 1999;35:230–40.
64. Harnois DM, Que FG, Celli A, LaRusso NF, Gores GJ. Bcl-2 is over-expressed and alters the threshold for apoptosis in a cholangiocarcinoma cell line. Hepatology. 1997;26:884–90.
65. Okaro AC, Deery AR, Hutchins RR, Davidson BR. The expression of antiapoptotic proteins Bcl-2, Bcl-X(L), and Mcl-1 in benign, dysplastic, and malignant biliary epithelium. J Clin Pathol. 2001;54:927–32.
66. Ashida K, Terada T, Kitamura Y, Kaibara N. Expression of E-cadherin, alpha-catenin, beta-catenin, and CD44 (standard and variant isoforms) in human cholangiocarcinoma: an immunohistochemical study. Hepatology. 1998;27:974–82.

4
Primary sclerosing cholangitis: diagnosis, surveillance and timing of interventions

A. STIEHL and D. ROST

CLINICS

Primary sclerosing cholangitis (PSC) is chraracterized by progressive fibrosing inflammation of the bile ducts leading to cholestasis and finally to cirrhosis of the liver[1-3]. The disease is diagnosed by endoscopic retrograde cholangiography (ERC) which shows the typical perl like picture with multiple bile duct stenoses. Alternatively, magnetic resonance cholangiography (MRC) detects PSC with a specificity and sensitivity of approximately 90%. Unspecific symptoms are fatigue and pruritus[1-3].

There are no specific symptoms and no specific laboratory parameters. Of the laboratory tests alkaline phosphatase (AP) and gamma glutamyl transferase (GGT) are more markedly elevated than the serum transaminases. Serum bilirubin increases only in advanced stages of the disease. The disease is frequently associated with ulcerative colitis[1-4].

For adequate surveillance and treatment it appears most important to detect the disease as early as possible. Patients with inflammatory bowel disease who have an elevated alkaline phosphatase have an 80% chance of contracting PSC. Therefore, performing an ERC, or with somewhat less sensitivity and specificity a MRC, in such patients, will allow recognition of the disease in the majority of patients.

A specific complication represents the high incidence of cholangiocarcinoma and colonic carcinomas and, according to a recent study, also pancreatic carcinomas[5]. Another problem represents the frequent formation of dominant stenoses which are often associated with bacterial cholangitis[6].

MEDICAL TREATMENT

With the exception of one study[7], in all other studies with sufficient dosage, ursodeoxycholic acid (UDCA) led to significant improvement of AP, GGT, alanine transaminase, aspartate transaminase and in part also of serum bilirubin[8–12]. High doses of UDCA (20 mg/kg) led to a significant improvement in liver histology, whereas lower doses were less effective[11]. High doses may be needed since in patients with cholestasis the absorption of UDCA may be reduced[13]. In the majority of patients the optimal dose appears to be between 22 and 25 mg/kg[14]. The efficacy of high-dose UDCA has been confirmed by others[12], but a further randomized study with high-dose UDCA found no significant effect[7]. The discrepancies between the different studies are difficult to understand, but one major point may be the compliance problem in placebo-controlled studies over a period of years. It seems possible that the patients who do not know whether they take an effective drug or a placebo are not compliant over such long periods, and intermittently do not take the drug/placebo.

Treatment of PSC patients with immunosuppressive, anti-inflammatory or antifibrotic agents was not very successful. Patients with an overlap syndrome with autoimmune hepatitis need additional immunosuppressive treatment with corticosteroids and/or azathioprine.

ENDOSCOPIC TREATMENT

A problem in the treatment of patients with PSC is the development of dominant stenoses which occlude the major bile ducts and which cannot be expected to be treated efficiently by medical treatment[15] and need endoscopic intervention[15–22]. When dominant stenoses of the larger bile ducts are detected by ERCP early endoscopic intervention with dilation of the duct is mandatory. In most cases a single dilation is not sufficient, and repeated dilations are necessary until the duct remains open[15,22]. In general, after successful opening of the duct, one endoscopic intervention per year is necessary to keep a dominant stenosis open[15,22].

Intermittent stenting has also been used[15–22], but the stents tend to occlude early due to the inflammatory material shed from the bile ducts. Moreover, in a controlled study additional stenting was of no benefit in patients undergoing balloon dilation[20]. Since occlusion of the stent leads to bacterial infection of the proximal biliary tree, the routine exchange of stents after 3 months is insufficient, and may lead to bacterial cholangitis. Therefore, in dominant stenoses, the stents in some medical centres are removed or replaced early, i.e. within 2 weeks. In our hands dilation is by far the more effective form of endoscopic treatment.

In many patients with dominant stenoses, yearly endoscopic controls help to prevent the complete occlusion of the duct which makes reopening very difficult if not impossible. In some centres MRC is used as primary step in identifying dominant stenoses. However, up to now, despite much progress in unclear difficult cases, the sensitivity and specificity of MRC in detecting dominant stenoses is still not as good as that of ERC.

In the surveillance of patients with PSC endoscopic controls should be performed whenever clinical or biochemical parameters indicate that cholestasis is increasing as the consequence of a dominant stenosis. The delay in the endoscopic relief of biliary obstruction may lead to bacterial cholangitis which is often difficult to eradicate. It is obvious that any medical treatment including UDCA will have little or no effect on liver histology when dominant stenoses are present and are not treated by endoscopic means.

ROLE OF ANTIBIOTICS

It seems to be very important that all endoscopic procedures are performed under antibiotic prophylaxis, since bacterial cholangitis is a possible complication of endoscopic procedures[23]. Dominant stenoses are associated with bacterial cholangitis in half of the patients[6]. Studies on the long-term treatment of patients with bacterial cholangitis with antibiotics do not exist. Whether the beneficial effect of metronidazole on laboratory parameters and liver histology reported recently[24], is related to its antibiotic potency, is unclear at present.

BILE DUCT CARCINOMA

An unresolved problem in the surveillance and treatment of patients with PSC is the development of bile duct carcinomas[1–3,5]. To date it is very difficult to detect cholangiocarcinomas at an early stage. Brush-border cytology of dominant strictures is insufficiently sensitive[25]. Tumour markers CEA and CA 19-9 are neither sensitive nor specific[26]. The imaging methods (CT, NMR) do not allow detection of early carcinomas, and results with positron emission tomography[27] need further confirmation in larger trials. When the carcinoma has developed the prognosis in general is very poor.

Most bile duct carcinomas are detected within the first year after diagnosis of the disease with a subsequent annual incidence rate of 1.5%. In a study in which 305 PSC patients were followed over a median follow-up time of 63 months, a bile duct carcinoma was observed in 8% of patients, and 44% of these were asymptomatic at the time of diagnosis of PSC[3]. In 37% of patients with bile duct carcinoma this diagnosis was made within 1 year after detection of PSC, and as a consequence it seems possible that the patients already had a bile duct carcinoma when the PSC was recognized. The high incidence of bile duct carcinomas in the first year after diagnosis has recently been confirmed[28]. No factors were found which would allow the identification of patients who will later develop a bile duct carcinoma.

A bile duct carcinoma rate of 8%[3] appears much lower than that observed by others[29]. In patients with endstage disease who were considered for transplantation, 30% had bile duct carcinomas[3]. Very high rates of bile duct carcinomas have repeatedly been reported in studies coming from transplantation centres[3,29], and it appears that they reflect very selected patient groups.

In a controlled study 0/52 of patients with PSC on UDCA developed a bile duct carcinoma in comparison to 3/53 patients in the placebo group (Table 1)[10]. In a further placebo-controlled study 3/97 of the patients on UDCA had a bile duct carcinoma in comparison to 4/101 in the control group[7]. Since two of the three carcinomas in the UDCA group were detected within 5 months after the start of the study it appears likely that in the UDCA

Table 1 Bile duct carcinomas in PSC treated with ursodeoxycholic acid

	Lindor[10]	Olsson[7]
UDCA	0/53	3*/97
Placebo	3/52	4/101

*2/3 diagnosed within 5 months after randomization probably had the tumour at entry into study.

group only 1/97 developed the tumour. Thus, in both placebo-controlled studies a lower rate of hepatobiliary carcinomas of patients on UDCA compared to placebo was observed, but the difference was not significant. In a prospective study over 15 years, of 106 patients treated with UDCA, only 3 (2.8%) developed a bile duct carcinoma, supporting the concept that the incidence of bile duct carcinomas may be reduced after treatment with UDCA[22].

In a recent study of 225 patients listed for liver transplantation hepatobiliary malignancies developed in 20% of patients. UDCA treatment was associated with a significantly decreased incidence of hepatobiliary cancer[30]. It seems possible that the reduced inflammation around the bile ducts observed after UDCA treatment[8,9,11] may reduce the incidence of bile duct carcinomas.

COLONIC CARCINOMA

Colorectal carcinoma occurs more frequently in patients with chronic inflammatory bowel disease than in the normal population. Risk factors are involvement of the whole colon and long duration of the disease. Recently it has been shown that PSC represents an independent risk factor for the development of colonic carcinoma[31]. In a study in which 40 patients with PSC and colitis were matched with 40 patients of the same age, comparable colitis and comparable duration of disease, the absolute cumulative risk of developing colorectal dysplasia or carcinoma in patients with PSC was almost five times higher than in patients without PSC. The study also indicates that patients with PSC and colitis who develop colonic dysplasia or carcinoma are at a high risk of developing cholangiocarcinoma. It is evident that patients with PSC and colitis need colonoscopic surveillance at short intervals. We recommend a yearly colonoscopy in patients with colitis and PSC.

In animal experiments bile acids have cocarcinogenic effects in the development of colonic adenocarcinomas, and UDCA may prevent this cocarcinogenic effect[32]. After oral administration of UDCA to patients with ileostomy at the end of the ileum, of a single oral dose of 500 mg UDCA 59% were excreted from the ileostomy[33]. Thus, due to its poor absorption in the upper small intestine, substantial amounts of UDCA enter the colon where it is bacterially degraded. As a consequence the effect of UDCA on the incidence of colonic dysplasias, adenomatous polyps and carcinomas is of much interest.

In two placebo-controlled trials on the effect of UDCA on liver disease in PSC the incidence of dysplasias and carcinomas has been evaluated (Figure 1).

In the first study, in which 59 patients were included, the incidence of dysplasias and carcinomas in the UDCA group was 32% and in the control group it was 72%[34], the difference being significant. In a second placebo-controlled study with 52 patients, of 29 patients in the UDCA group only 10% had dysplasias or carcinomas, whereas in the placebo group of 23 patients, 35% developed dysplasias or carcinomas[35] ($p < 0.05$). Thus, in two controlled trials in patients with ulcerative colitis and PSC, UDCA significantly reduced the incidence of colonic dysplasias and carcinomas.

Colonic dysplasias or carcinomas, %

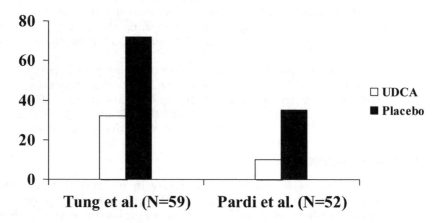

Figure 1 Effect of ursodeoxycholic acid treatment on dysplasias and carcinomas in patients with PSC and colitis (from refs 34 and 35). Ursodeoxycholic acid treatment significantly reduced the frequency of colonic dysplasias and carcinomas

EFFECT OF TREATMENT ON SURVIVAL

PSC is a progressive disease, and survival of such patients is reduced. Survival is better in asymptomatic patients than in symptomatic patients. In a prospective non-randomized study performed in our institution, in which 65 patients were treated with UDCA and, whenever necessary, by additional endoscopic dilations the actuarial Kaplan–Meier estimate of survival after treatment with UDCA and dilation of major duct stenoses was significantly improved compared to the predicted survival ($p < 0.001$)[13]. The data were confirmed after extension of this study to 106 patients and prolongation for up to 13 years[22].

The need for endoscopic treatment of dominant stenoses has been confirmed in a multicentre study in which 63 patient were included. Actuarial survival compared with predicted survival was significantly improved after treatment[21].

LIVER TRANSPLANTATION

In endstage disease liver transplantation represents the treatment of choice. The 5-year survival rate after liver transplantation for PSC is approximately 72% (European Transplant Registry). In view of the fact that the incidence of bile duct carcinomas is much lower than the lethality after transplantation, it appears unjustified to recommend prophylactic liver transplantation in precirrhotic stages of the disease in order to prevent the development of bile duct carcinomas.

CONCLUSION

We conclude that PSC may be treated conservatively by UDCA with good treatment results and prolongation of survival free of liver transplantation only when patients who develop major duct stenoses are recognized early and are additionally treated by endoscopic means. Patients with PSC have a high neoplastic potential. There is good evidence that the incidence of colonic dysplasias and carcinomas may be reduced by treatment with UDCA. There are some indications that UDCA treatment may lead to a reduction of dysplasias and carcinomas of the bile ducts. These findings await further confirmation. In endstage disease liver transplantation is indicated.

References

1. Chapman RW, Arborgh BA, Rhodes JM et al. Primary sclerosing cholangitis – a review of its clinical features, cholangiography and hepatic histology. Gut. 1980;21:870–7.
2. Wiesner RH, Grambsch PM, Dickson ER et al. Natural history, prognostic factors, and survival analysis. Hepatology. 1989;10:430–6.
3. Broome U, Olson R, Lööf L et al. Natural history and prognostic factors in 305 Swedish patients with primary sclerosing cholangitis. Gut. 1996;38:610–15.
4. Olsson R, Danielsson A, Järnebrot G et al. Prevalence of primary sclerosing cholangitis in patients with ulcerative colitis. Gastroenterology. 1991;100:1319–23.
5. Bergquist A, Ekbom A, Olsson R et al. Hepatic and extrahepatic malignancies in primary sclerosing cholangitis. J Hepatol. 2002;36:321–7.
6. Pohl J, Ring A, Stremmel W, Stiehl A. The role of dominant stenoses in bacterial infections of bile ducts in primary sclerosing cholangitis. Eur J Gastroenterol Hepatol. 2006;18:69–74.
7. Olsson R, Boberg KM, Schaffalisky de Muckadell O et al. High-dose ursodeoxycholic acid in primary sclersosing cholangitis. A five year multicenter randomised study. Gastroenterology. (In press)
8. Stiehl A, Walker S, Stiehl L et al. Effects of ursodeoxycholic acid on liver and bile duct disease in primary sclerosing cholangitis. A 3 year pilot study with a placebo-controlled study period. J Hepatol. 1994;20:57–64.
9. Beuers U, Spengler U, Kruis W et al. Ursodeoxycholic acid for treatment of primary sclerosing cholangitis: a placebo controlled trial. Hepatology. 1992;16:707–14.
10. Lindor KD and the Mayo PSC/UDCA Study Group. Ursodiol for the treatment of primary sclerosing cholangitis. N Engl J Med. 1997;336:691–5.
11. Mitchell SA, Bansi D, Hunt N et al. A preliminary trial of high dose ursodeoxycholic acid in primary sclerosing cholangitis. Gastroenterology. 2001;121:900–7.
12. Harnois DM, Angulo P, Jorgensen RA, LaRusso NF, Lindor KD. High-dose ursodeoxycholic acid as therapy for patients with primary sclerosing cholangitis. Am J Gastroenterol. 2001;96:1558–62.
13. Sauer P, Benz C, Rudolph G et al. Influence of cholestasis on absorption of ursodeoxycholic acid. Dig Dis Sci. 1999;44:817–22.

14. Rost D, Rudolph G, Kloeters-Plachky P, Stiehl A. Effect of high-dose ursodeoxycholic acid on its biliary enrichment in primary sclerosing cholangitis. Hepatology. 2004;40:693–8.
15. Stiehl A, Rudolph G, Sauer P et al. Efficacy of ursodeoxycholic acid and endoscopic dilation of major duct stenoses in primary sclerosing cholangitis. An 8-year prospective study. J Hepatol. 1997;26:560–6.
16. Grijm R, Huibregtse K, Bartelsman J et al. Therapeutic investigations in primary sclerosing cholangitis. Dig Dis Sci. 1986;31:792–8.
17. Johnson GK, Geenen JE, Venu RP, Hogan WJ. Endoscopic treatment of biliary duct strictures in sclerosing cholangitis: Follow up assessment of a new therapeutic approach. Gastrointest Endosc. 1987;33:9–12.
18. Lee JG, Schutz SM, England RE, Leung JW, Cotton PB. Endoscopic therapy of sclerosing cholangitis. Hepatology. 1995;21:661–7.
19. van Milligen AWM, van Bracht J, Rauws EAJ et al. Endoscopic stent therapy for dominant extrahepatic bile duct strictures in primary sclerosing cholangitis. Gastrointest Endosc. 1006;44:293–9.
20. Kaya M, Petersen BT, Angulo, P et al. Balloon dilatation compared to stenting of dominant strictures in primary sclerosing cholangitis. Am J Gastroenterol. 2001;96:1059–66.
21. Baluyut AR, Sherman S, Lehman GA, Hoen H, Chalasani N. Impact of endoscopic therapy on the survival of patients with primary sclerosing cholangitis. Gastrointest Endosc. 2001;53:308–12.
22. Stiehl A, Rudolph G, Klöters-Plachky P et al. Development of bile duct stenoses in patients with primary sclerosing cholangitis treated with ursodeoxycholic acid. Outcome after endoscopic treatment. J Hepatol. 2002;36:151–6.
23. Olsson R, Björnsson E, Bäckman L et al. Bile duct bacterial isolates in primary sclerosing cholangitis: a study of explanted livers. J Hepatol. 1998;28:426–32.
24. Färkkilä M, Karvonen AL, Nurmi H et al. Metronidazole and ursodeoxycholic acid for primary sclerosing cholangitis: a randomized placebo-controlled trial. Hepatology. 2004; 40:1379–86.
25. Ponsionen C IJ, Vrouenraets SME, van Milligen AWM et al. Value of brush border cytology for dominant strictures in primary sclerosing cholangitis. Endoscopy. 1999;31:305–9.
26. Hultcrantz R, Olsson R, Danielsson A et al. A three year prospective study on serum tumor markers used for detecting cholangiocarcinoma in patients with primary sclerosing cholangitis. J Hepatol. 1999;30:669–73.
27. Keiding S, Rasmussen HH, Gee A et al. Detection of cholangiocarcinoma in primary sclerosing cholangitis by positron emission tomography. Hepatology. 1998;28:700–6.
28. Burak K, Angulo P, Pasha TM et al. Incidence and risk factors for cholangiocarcinoma in primary sclerosing cholangitis. Am J Gastroenterol. 2004;99:523–6.
29. Nashan B, Schlitt HJ, Tusch G et al. Biliary malignancies in primary sclerosing cholangitis: timing of liver transplantation. Hepatology. 1996;23:1105–11.
30. Brandsaeter B, Isoniemi H, Broome U et al. Liver transplantation for primary sclerosing cholangitis; predictors and consequences of hepatobiliary malignancy. J Hepatol. 2004;40: 815–22.
31. Broome U, Löfberg R, Veress B, Erikson LS: Primary sclerosing cholangitis and ulcerative colitis: evidence for increased neoplastic potential. Hepatology. 1995;22:1404–8.
32. Earnest DL, Holubec H, Wali RK et al. Chemoprevention of azomethane-induced colonic carcinogenesis by supplemental dietary ursodeoxycholic acid. Cancer Res. 1994;54:5071–4.
33. Stiehl A, Raedsch R, Rudolph G. Ileal excretion of bile acids: comparison with biliary bile composition and effect of ursodeoxycholic acid treatment. Gastroenterology. 1988;94: 1201–6.
34. Tung BY, Emond MJ, Haggitt RC et al. Ursodiol use is associated with lower prevalence of colonic neoplasia in patients with ulcerative colitis and primary sclerosing cholangitis. Ann Intern Med. 2001;134:89–95.
35. Pardi DS, Loftus EV, Kremers WK et al. Ursodeoxycholic acid as a chemoprotective agent in patients with ulcerative colitis and primary sclerosing cholangitis. Gastroenterology. 2003;124:889–93.

5
Surgical treatment of central bile duct carcinoma

P. NEUHAUS and S. JONAS

HISTORY

In 1964 Gerald Klatskin, from New Haven, Connecticut, published an article on adenocarcinoma of the hepatic duct bifurcation in the porta hepatis[1]. He described the tumour as 'unusual with distinctive clinical pathological features'. Soon these later so-called Klatskin tumours attracted broad interest. They were treated with resection or with transplantation, but in most cases only with stenting. The prognosis of the tumours without operation was poor; patients died from infection and other complications. With operation, and also with successful stenting in selected cases, patient survival could be improved. Transplant surgeons also looked at the possibility of curing the disease with liver transplantation. A radical surgical approach resulted in 5-year survival rates of up to 30%, and transplantation results with a 30% 5-year survival were not regarded as optimal for these patients.

Because the location in the bile duct bifurcation and the extension into the liver lobes was important for surgery, Bismuth and Corlett divided Klatskin tumours into three types: type I below the bifurcation, type II in the bifurcation and type III extending into the right or left hepatic duct. Type IV was the so-called inoperable case with extensions into the segmental ducts (Figure 1). Three pathoanatomical types were distinguished (Figure 2): the papillary or protruding type (5%), the nodular type in the bile duct wall (15%) and the sclerosing or infiltrating type (80%), where it was especially cholangiographically, but also during surgery, very difficult to assess the margins of the tumour (Figure 3).

Surgery consisted of excision of the extrahepatic bile duct portion extending as far as possible into the liver. Sometimes five or six orifices of bile ducts in the liver were left present after resection and had to be carefully anastomosed to the Roux-Y loop for biliary drainage. The 5-year survival was poor with only a handful of patients surviving more than five years. Recurrence of the tumour was common and occurred locally in 75%, indicating that resection had been incomplete in most cases (Figure 4).

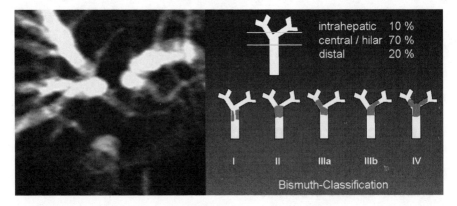

Figure 1 Classification of central bile duct carcinomas according to Bismuth and Corlett

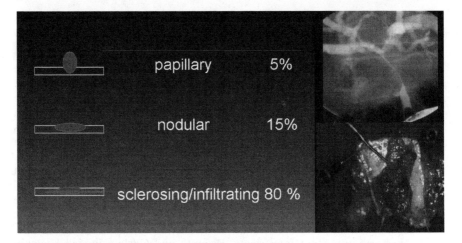

Figure 2 Macroscopic growth pattern of hilar cholangiocarcinomas

RESULTS OF SURGICAL RESECTION OF CENTRAL BILE DUCT TUMOURS

The only significant prognostic parameter in all series published between 1990 and 2000 was the resectability and the resection status (R0–R1/2) on histopathological examination[3–5]. Grading and staging, as well as lymph node involvement, were significant prognostic parameters in some but not in all the series (Table 1).

In 2001 Jarnagin and colleagues published their results of 80 resected patients, comprising 18 extrahepatic bile duct resections and 62 resections of the bile duct in combination with the right or left liver[6]. Sixty-two of the 80 (78%) resections were R0 resections. In this group of R0 resections the combination of bile duct and liver resection was the only independent

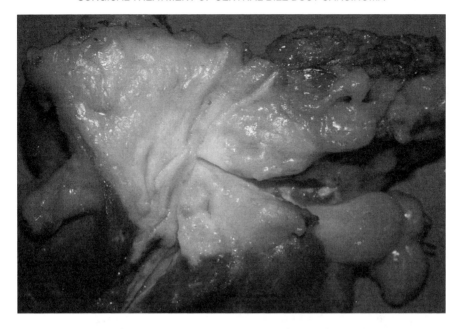

Figure 3 Sclerosing type of hilar cholangiocarcinoma with unclear surgical margins

			Primary recurrence
	Liver	62 %	
	Resection line	42 %	**76 %**
	Regional lymph nodes	20 %	
	Peritoneum	16 %	
	Lungs	71 %	
	Bones	31 %	**24 %**
	Skin/Subcutis	7 %	

Figure 4 Recurrence pattern after local resection of hilar cholangiocarcinomas

significant prognostic parameter. After a follow-up of more than five years only nine patients were alive. All were patients with liver resections; none of the patients with extrahepatic bile duct resection alone had survived.

At the same time Nimura and colleagues from Nagoya University in Japan published their experience with 142 patients: 108 patients (76%) were R0 resected[7]. Of these, only eight were extrahepatic bile duct resections alone, but 100 were combinations of liver and bile duct resections. As in the series of

Table 1   Prognostic parameters: multivariate analyses

Reference	n	Resectability	Histopathological grading	UICC stage
Reding et al., 1991	307	+	–	
Su et al., 1996[4]	49	+	+	–
Pichlmayr et al., 1996	125	+	–	+
Miyazaki et al., 1998	76	+	–	–
Kosuge et al., 1999	65	+	+	–
Jarnagin et al., 2001[6]	80	+	+	–

Table 2   Resection for hilar cholangiocarcinoma

	Hilar resection alone		Additional liver resection	
	n (R0%)	5 year-survival	n (R0%)	5 year-survival
Lillemore et al., 2000	94 (–)	11%	15 (–)	10%
Tabata et al., 2000	22 (–)	20%	53 (–)	24%
Gazzaniga et al., 2000	20 (–)	0%	17 (–)	25%
Miyazaki et al., 1998	11 (45%)	0%	65 (75%)	27%
Lee et al., 2000	17 (24%)	0%	111 (77%)	24%
Nimura et al., 2000[7]	14 (57%)	16%	128 (78%)	26%
Berlin results 2004	20 (25%)	0%	107 (68%)*	24%

*w/o right trisectionectomy and portal vein resection.

Jarnagin, the 5-year survival of patients with bile duct resection alone was almost zero (only one patient survived $5\frac{1}{2}$ years). The 5-year survival of the patients with combined rejection was 26%, which is in the range of the published series from Japan, Europe and the United States in the years 1990–2000. Our own results with 127 standard operations – this means either bile duct resection alone ($n = 20$) or a combination of bile duct resection and standard hepatectomy (107 patients) – are in line with the international literature with 24% 5-year survival (Table 2).

INCREASED RESECTABILITY OF THE TUMOURS

During retrospective analysis of our resection results we found in 1995 that patients with extrahepatic bile duct resection, extended right hepatectomy and resection of the portal vein bifurcation had a significantly better 5-year survival prognosis than patients who had liver resection and bile duct resection alone[8]. In most of these cases with portal vein resection histologically the wall of the portal vein was not involved, but only attached to the tumour by inflammatory changes. Clearly these resections had been done for possible infiltration of the portal vein bifurcation. They had been deemed to be necessary in order to make the patient resectable. With the resection of the right liver also the right hepatic artery, which runs in close proximity between bile duct bifurcation and portal vein, was resected, while in hilar resection alone the right hepatic artery must quite often be dissected out of the tumour tissue.

INCREASED RADICALITY OF RESECTION

The next step was to increase not only the resectability of the bile duct tumour, but also the radicality of this resection by routinely performing a right hemihepatectomy, possibly together with the bile duct, right hepatic artery and the portal vein bifurcation. The better results of this increased radicality in surgical treatment went along with close adherence to the principles of oncological surgery[9].

PRINCIPLES OF ONCOLOGICAL SURGERY IN BILE DUCT CANCER SURGERY

The principles of oncological surgery demand achieving as wide as possible tumour-free margins, en-bloc excision of all tumour-adherent tissue and avoiding dissection near the tumour. Since the tumour is typically located a little to the right side of the portal vein bifurcation, and on top of the right hepatic artery, this field should not be dissected.

For example, nobody would dissect a rectal carcinoma inside the fascia or even take biopsies from outside. The operative solution for Klatskin tumours was to excise all the lymph nodes along the hepatic arteries down to the aorta, then dissect the proper hepatic artery and divide the right hepatic artery at the left side of the hepatoduodenal ligament. Subsequent dissection of the left hepatic artery could be done 2–3 cm away from the tumour up into the umbilical fissure.

With retraction of the artery to the left side, the left portal vein could be identified and dissected in the umbilical fissure for about 1 cm in length. Then the common hepatic bile duct was transected at the head of the pancreas and a frozen section for tumour infiltrates was obtained. Now the portal vein stem could be dissected for about 2–3 cm, leaving the tumour area completely untouched. Portal vein and left portal vein branch were then clamped and divided. The portal vein stem could then be anastomosed with little tension directly to the left portal vein branch. The vena cava was completely freed from the liver, the right liver vein was divided and then the liver parenchyma was divided 1 cm right to the falciforme ligament. So the resection included segments I, IV, V, VI, VII and VIII of the liver, the extrahepatic bile duct system, the portal vein bifurcation and the lymph nodes (Figure 5).

With this operation more than 50% 5-year survival figures were achieved. A higher resection rate, a higher radicality (R0 resection rate) and a higher survival rate are convincing arguments for the new surgical approach to central bile duct cancers.

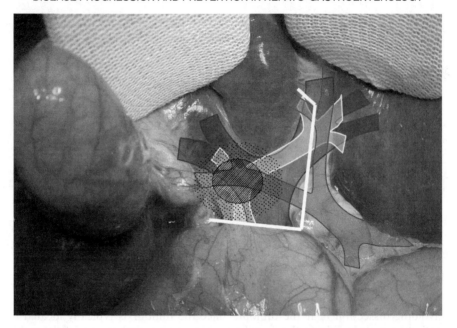

Figure 5 Radical resection with no-touch technique of hilar cholangio-carcinoma: en-bloc resection of bile duct, right hepatic artery, portal vein, bifurcation and right liver

PREVENTION OF MORBIDITY AND MORTALITY

Unfortunately, with this 75–80% liver resection in sometimes severely cholestatic livers, a high morbidity and mortality (10–12%) were associated. One way to increase the remaining liver volume was embolization of the right vascular system[10]. This could be done either by arterial embolization, known from chemoembolization of HCC tumours, or by percutaneous transhepatic portal vein embolization, which produces much better hypotrophy of the remaining left lobe than arterial embolization. Together with embolization, selective decompression of the left biliary system was achieved with either endoscopic stenting to the left side or percutaneous transhepatic biliary drainage with radiologically placed catheters (Figure 6). Complication rate and mortality has thus been reduced, but is of course still considerably higher than with less radical surgical methods. This on the other hand is outweighed by the higher long-term survival.

Of course not all bile duct cancers can be dissected with this method. Sometimes the tumour is predominantly located in the left portion of the bile duct system and the left liver is already atrophied. In this case only a left resection can be performed. In other cases liver function is borderline, the patient is old or significant co-morbidity prevents extended operations, and therefore in these cases extrahepatic bile duct resection is still a good option for palliation.

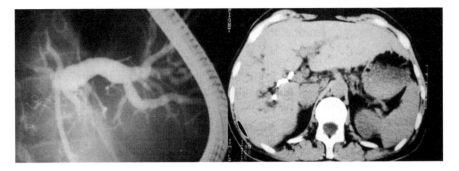

Figure 6 Biliary decompression of the left side and vascular embolization of the right liver lobe increase liver cell mass and function of remaining left lobe

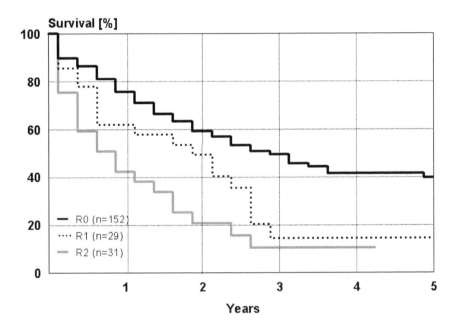

Figure 7 Survival after resection of hilar cholangiocarcinoma according to radicality

RESULTS OF THE NEW CONCEPT IN BERLIN

Including perioperative mortality and R1/R2 resections, we have achieved a 24% 5-year survival in Berlin. If we analyse only R0 resections our survival after 5 years is 40%; but even R2-resected patients had a better palliation then with stenting, because 31 patients had a 1-year and 2-year survival of 40% and 20% respectively. For R1-resected patients, the 1- and 2-year survival was 60% and 50% (Figure 7).

Other influencing factors in our series, apart from radicality, were lymph node involvement, grading, lymphangiosis carcinomatosa and perineural infiltration[11]. But none of these negative prognostic factors, when present, was associated with a zero 5-year survival. Therefore the rule remains that resectability is the most important factor for patients with central bile duct cancer. Interesting in this regard is also the finding of the Japanese group of Nimura and Kitagawa from Nagoya[12]. They found 53% positive lymph nodes in 110 patients and a 5-year survival rate of 31% and 15% in lymph node-negative or regionally positive patients.

None of the patients survived for more than 5 years if the para-aortic lymph nodes were macroscopically suspect and histologically positive. If these routinely removed para-aortic lymph nodes were macroscopically normal and only microscopically positive, then survival of these patients was 29%, as good as in the LN-negative patients. Similar results have been found in Berlin in our patients with extended resections including liver resection, bile duct resection, resection of portal vein bifurcation and lymphadenectomy.

LIVER TRANSPLANTATION FOR CENTRAL BILE DUCT CANCER

Liver transplantation for cholangiocellular carcinoma and bile duct cancer has been abandoned worlwide because of the poor survival data. According to the European liver transplant registry, 5-year and 10-year survival for both cancers is 30% and 18% (Figure 8). This is of course not worse than the resection data for this subgroup of surgically irresectable patients. Only the shortage of

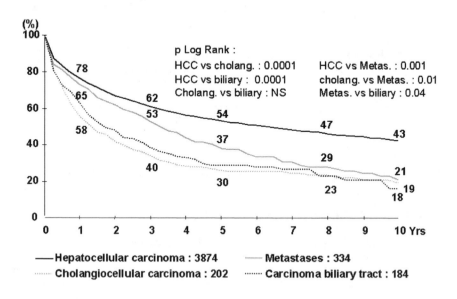

Figure 8 Survival of patients with cholangiocarcinoma after liver transplantation (ELTR data)

organs prevents the use of liver transplantation for those bile duct cancer patients, who otherwise at present have no other curative chance. The possibility now of living donor liver transplantation opens a new chapter in the treatment of inoperable bile duct cancer with liver transplantation, since an individual donor would be available only for this individual patient, but not for other patients with better prognosis.

A remarkable series of liver transplantation with a new protocol of neoadjuvant chemoradiation has been published by the Mayo Clinic[13]. It included external beam irradiation (4500 cGy) and bolus 5-FU therapy (3×500 mg/m^2 per day) for patients with unresectable cholangiocellular carcinoma and no intrahepatic or extrahepatic known metastasis. The patients received a transcatheter irradiation with Iridium (2000 cGy and 5-FU chemotherapy with 225 mg/m^2 per day. The patients were then thoroughly explored by laparotomy for metastasis and received further chemotherapy with 5-FU until they were transplanted.

Fifty-six patients were included in the protocol, eight died during the irradiation protocol due to progression of the tumour or other causes, 14 were excluded due to metastasis after laparotomy and 34 were listed for transplantation. Of these 34 patients, 28 received a liver transplant and showed a survival of 82% after 5 years. Only four patients died due to recurrence[14]. Although from the 56 patients only 21 (38%) survived 5 years, this protocol shows a promising new approach to treat patients who otherwise have no option.

CONCLUSIONS

It may be concluded that a significant long-term survival in patients suffering from hilar cholangiocarcinoma is an exception after limited resection, as for instance extrahepatic or hilar resections alone. It has been shown that resectability and radicality are the most important prognostic parameters for the patient. Both increase with principal hepatic resections when compared to extrahepatic bile duct resection alone. In addition the rules of surgical oncology (wide tumour-free margins, no-touch techniques) are best adhered to by right trisectionectomy with en-bloc resection of the portal vein and hepatic artery. An increased postoperative risk after liver resection appears justified when considering the long-term results, all the more as this risk has generally decreased in some centres over recent years.

Liver transplantation, which was for a long time excluded from the therapy of central bile duct cancer, may again become an option for selected patients, especially when used in conjunction with modern adjuvant and neoadjuvant therapeutic approaches.

References

1. Klatskin G. Adenocarcinoma of the hepatic duct at its bifurcation within the porta hepatis. Am J Med. 1965;38:241–56.
2. Mittal B, Deutsch M, Iwatsuki S. Primary cancers of the extrahepatic biliary passages. Int J Radiat Oncol Biol Phys. 1985;11:849–55.

3. Klempnauer J, Ridder GJ, von Wasielewski R, Werner M, Weimann A, Pichlmayr R. Resectional surgery of hilar cholangiocarcinoma: a multivariate analysis of prognostic factors. J Clin Oncol. 1997;15:947–54.
4. Su CH, Tsay SH, Wu CC et al. Factors influencing postoperative morbidity, mortality, and survival after resection for hilar cholangiocarcinoma. Ann Surg. 1996;223:384–94.
5. Nimura Y, Kamiya J, Nagino M et al. Aggressive surgical treatment of hilar cholangiocarcinoma. J Hepatobil Pancreat Surg. 1998;5:52–61.
6. Jarnagin WR, Fong Y, DeMatteo RP et al. Staging, resectability, and outcome in 225 patients with hilar cholangiocarcinoma. Ann Surg. 2001;234:507–17.
7. Nimura Y, Kamiya J, Kondo S et al. Aggressive preoperative management and extended surgery for hilar cholangiocarcinoma: Nagoya experience. J Hepatobil Pancreat Surg. 2000;7:155–62.
8. Jonas S, Bechstein WO, Kling N, Neuhaus P. Extent of resection in surgical therapy of central bile duct carcinomas. Langenbecks Arch Chir Suppl Kongressbd. 1997;114:1075–7.
9. Neuhaus P, Jonas S, Bechstein WO et al. Extended resections for hilar cholangiocarcinoma. Ann Surg. 1999;230:808–18.
10. Hanninen EL, Pech M, Jonas S et al. Magnetic resonance imaging including magnetic resonance cholangiopancreatography for tumor localization and therapy planning in malignant hilar obstructions. Acta Radiol. 2005;46:462–70.
11. Bhuiya MR, Nimura Y, Kamiya J et al. Clinicopathologic studies on perineural invasion of bile duct carcinoma. Ann Surg. 1992;215:344–9.
12. Kitagawa Y, Nagino M, Kamiya J et al. Lymph node metastasis from hilar cholangiocarcinoma: audit of 110 patients who underwent regional and paraaortic node dissection. Ann Surg. 2001;233:385–92.
13. De Vreede I, Steers JL, Burch PA et al. Prolonged disease-free survival after orthotopic liver transplantation plus adjuvant chemoirradiation for cholangiocarcinoma. Liver Transplant. 2000;6:309–16.
14. Heimbach JK, Gores GJ, Haddock MG et al. Liver transplantation for unresectable perihilar cholangiocarcinoma. Semin Liver Dis. 2004;24:201–7.

6
Special Lecture: Genetic epidemiology and future developments in the treatment of cholecystolithiasis

F. LAMMERT and T. SAUERBRUCH

INTRODUCTION

Gallstones represent a serious burden for our healthcare systems: 10–20% of Europeans and Americans carry gallbladder stones, and the prevalence of gallstone disease is rising as a result of longer life expectancy[1]. Many gallstones are silent, but symptoms and complications ensue in around 25% of cases, necessitating surgical removal of the gallbladder, usually by laparoscopic cholecystectomy[1]. Each year an estimated 700 000 cholecystectomies are performed in the US[2], and 174 000 in Germany[3]. Cholelithiasis incurs annual medical expenses of $6.5 billion in the US and is currently the second most expensive digestive disease, exceeded only by reflux disease[4].

Mortality rates following cholecystectomy range from less than 0.1% in clinical studies[5] to 0.7% (as documented for all cholecystectomies performed in Germany in 2004)[3], and in the US about 3000 deaths (0.12% of all deaths) per year are attributed to complications of cholelithiasis and gallbladder disease[2]. However, non-surgical approaches, including gallstone dissolution by ursodeoxycholic acid and extracorporeal shockwave lithotripsy, have more and more lost their impact on therapy and are performed only for non-complicated symptomatic cholecystolithiasis in a very small number of selected patients[1,6]. The high risk of stone recurrence is the major drawback of extracorporeal shock wave lithotripsy of gallbladder stones (43% after 5 years)[7].

MOLECULAR PATHOGENESIS

Bile formation enables the removal of excess cholesterol, either directly or after catabolism to bile salts, and it is a key function of the liver. Bile is an aqueous solution of lipids, with bile salts (67% wt/vol), phospholipids (22%) and cholesterol (4%) representing the three main lipid species[8]. Hepatocytes express specific ATP-binding-cassette transport proteins – known as ABC transporters – for each of these three lipids at the canalicular membrane domain. The ABCB11 transporter is the bile salt export pump, ABCB4 is the transporter for the major biliary phospholipid phosphatidylcholine, and ABCG5 and ABCG8 form obligate heterodimers for biliary cholesterol secretion[9].

Figure 1 illustrates that on biliary secretion, phosphatidylcholine and cholesterol form metastable unilamellar vesicles, which are converted into mixed micelles during their passage through the biliary tree[8]. These micelles solubilize hydrophobic molecules such as cholesterol. The composition of hepatic bile is further modified by the bicarbonate-rich and chloride-rich secretions of cholangiocytes, which are associated with a net influx of water into bile through aquaporin channels. An important chloride channel in cholangiocytes is the cystic fibrosis transmembrane conductance regulator (CFTR or ABCC7), the gene for which is mutated in cystic fibrosis.

More than 70% of gallstones consist mainly of cholesterol and are formed within the gallbladder[1]. Three key mechanisms contribute to the formation of cholesterol gallbladder stones[8,10]: cholesterol supersaturation of bile, gallbladder hypomotility, and destabilization of bile by kinetic protein factors. Cholesterol-supersaturated bile contains more cholesterol than can be solubilized by mixed micelles (cholesterol saturation index > 1). It generates multilamellar vesicles (liquid crystals), whose fusion and aggregation precede the formation of solid cholesterol crystals (Figure 1). As illustrated in the classic triangular phase diagram[11], solid crystals occur in bile at high relative bile salt and low phospholipid concentrations and at cholesterol:phospholipid ratios > 1[8].

An excess of biliary cholesterol can result from hypersecretion of cholesterol, or from hyposecretion of phospholipids (or bile salts). Cholesterol hypersecretion might be caused by increased hepatic uptake or synthesis of cholesterol, decreased hepatic synthesis of bile salts, or decreased hepatic synthesis of cholesteryl esters for incorporation in VLDL. In humans, most cholesterol present in gallstones is of dietary origin, consistent with the observation that hepatic biosynthesis contributes less than 20% to biliary cholesterol[1]. The hepatic uptake of cholesterol is mediated by the scavenger receptor B1 for HDL, which contributes most of the biliary cholesterol under physiological conditions, and the apolipoprotein (Apo) B/E receptor for LDL and the LDL-receptor-related protein for chylomicron remnants, which carry

---

Figure 1 (opposite) Cholesterol gallstone formation. Schematic illustration of hepatobiliary lipid transporters, cholesterol carriers in bile, and cholesterol saturation index (CSI). The biliary lipids (cholesterol, phosphatidylcholine, bile salts) are secreted by hepatic ATP-dependent transport proteins (ABC transporters). The ABCG5/ABCG8 heterodimer represents the cholesterol transporter. On biliary secretion, bile salts form micelles, whereas phosphatidyl-choline and cholesterol are contained in metastable unilamellar vesicles, which are converted into mixed micelles during their passage through the biliary tree. Cholesterol-supersaturated gallbladder bile contains more cholesterol than can be solubilized by mixed micelles (CSI > 1). It generates multilamellar vesicles (liquid crystals), whose fusion and aggregation precede the nucleation of solid cholesterol crystals. Mucins secreted by the gallbladder form the matrix for the formation of crystal aggregates and gallstones

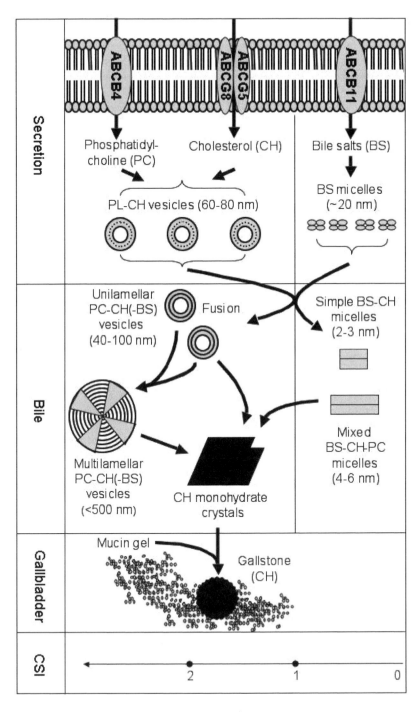

exogenous cholesterol from the intestine to the liver. The inverse correlation between serum HDL levels and gallstones suggests that cholesterol cholelithiasis is associated with an induced reverse cholesterol transport and hepatic catabolism of HDL[1]. The rate-limiting enzymes of hepatic cholesterol and bile salt synthesis are 3-hydroxy-3-methylglutaryl-coenzyme A reductase and cholesterol 7α-hydroxylase (CYP7A1), respectively. These enzymes are regulated by the sterol-regulatory-element-binding protein (SREBP) and nuclear receptor (NR) signalling pathways[12]. Studies in knockout and transgenic mice have demonstrated that many of the genes involved in hepatic cholesterol metabolism affect cholesterol gallstone formation *in vivo*[12,13], but with a few exceptions, variants of these genes have yet to be studied in patients with gallstones.

Stasis of bile in the gallbladder favours stone formation, as indicated by stone formation during pregnancy, rapid weight loss, or total parenteral nutrition. Postprandial gallbladder volumes are increased and gallbladder emptying in response to cholecystokinin is impaired in patients with gallstones[10], probably as a result of absorption of cholesterol from supersaturated bile by the gallbladder wall. Excess cholesterol in smooth-muscle cells stiffens sarcolemmal membranes and decouples the G-protein-mediated signal transduction that usually ensues when cholecystokinin binds to its receptor, thereby paralysing gallbladder contractile function[14].

Nucleation and growth of cholesterol crystals in model biles *in vitro* are modulated by promoter and inhibitor proteins, which interact with vesicles and solid crystals, respectively.[10] However, only gallbladder mucin – the main component of biliary sludge – has been shown to promote stone formation *in vivo* in experimental models[15]. Mucin is a mixture of sparingly soluble high-molecular-weight mucous glycoproteins that are secreted by biliary epithelial cells. Emerging evidence indicates that enterohepatic bacteria[16] and bacterial biofilms promote cholesterol crystallization, as well as the formation of sludge and gallstones (Figure 1).

A small proportion of gallbladder stones are black pigment stones. These consist predominantly of polymerized calcium bilirubinate, which precipitates if the ionic product of calcium and unconjugated bilirubin exceeds its solubility product, and polymerizes slowly in biliary sludge. Haemolytic anaemias or ineffective erythropoiesis are the most conspicuous sources of excess unconjugated bilirubin. Another recently highlighted[17] pathway involves severe ileal disease or resection, which causes spillage of bile salts into the colon and promotes solubilization and absorption of unconjugated bilirubin that results in increased enterohepatic cycling and biliary secretion of bilirubin[18].

TWIN AND FAMILY STUDIES

A large study in Swedish twins provided strong evidence for a role of genetic factors in gallstone pathogenesis[19]. The Swedish Twin Registry was linked with the inpatient-discharge and causes-of-death registries for symptomatic gallstone disease and gallstone surgery-related diagnoses in 43 141 twin pairs.

Concordance rates were significantly higher in monozygotic compared with dizygotic twins for both genders, with greater differences in younger twin cohorts. However, the rather low concordance between monozygotic twins indicated that environmental factors are also important. Genetic factors accounted for 25% (95% confidence interval (CI) 9–40%), shared environmental effects (e.g. diet in childhood) for 13% (CI 1–25%), and individual environmental effects for 62% (CI 56–68%) of the phenotypic variation among twins, as estimated by structural equation modelling, which is a general approach for the analysis of variance and correlations[19].

To investigate biliary lipid compositions in twins, 35 male pairs were randomly selected from the Finnish Twin Cohort[20]. Serum levels of methylsterols, which reflect hepatic cholesterol synthesis, and biliary concentrations of deoxycholate, which stimulates biliary cholesterol secretion, showed significant correlations in monozygotic but not dizygotic twins[20]. These findings are consistent with the concept that genetic factors determine biliary lipid secretion.

Several ultrasound surveys have documented that gallstones are two to four times more common in first-degree relatives of gallstone patients compared with age-matched stone-free controls[1]. Duggirala et al.[21] used variance component analysis in 32 Mexican–American families to assess the genetic determinants of symptomatic gallladder disease. After adjusting for potentially confounding effects of age, leptin, and total and HDL cholesterol levels, heritability for gallbladder disease was high ($44 \pm 18\%$). Another variance component analysis in 358 families in Wisconsin, each of which contained at least two obese siblings, determined that the heritability of symptomatic gallstones is $29 \pm 14\%$[22], which is similar to the figure obtained in the Swedish twin study[19].

EPIDEMIOLOGICAL STUDIES: AT-RISK POPULATIONS AND ENVIRONMENTAL FACTORS

As determined by cross-sectional ultrasound surveys, prevalence rates of gallbladder stones show remarkable geographic variations. Gallbladder stones are common in most European countries, as well as in North and South America, but the prevalence is low in Asia and Africa[1]. Environmental factors are likely to contribute to these marked differences. Data from several large epidemiological studies in the US, Europe, China and Japan implicate chronic overnutrition with refined carbohydrates and triglycerides as well as depletion of dietary fibre as potential triggers for cholesterol gallstone formation[23–26]. Gallstone disease phenotypes are likely to result from the complex interaction of genetic factors, high-carbohydrate, high-fat and low-fibre diets and other not fully defined environmental factors including low physical activity (Table 1)[23,27]. This hypothesis is supported by the profound increases of cholesterol gallstone prevalence rates in Native Americans, postwar European countries and current urban centres in East Asia, all of which were associated with the introduction of high-caloric 'Westernized' diets[1,28].

Table 1   Predisposing environmental factors for symptomatic gallstones (examples)

High-caloric diet, high glycaemic load[25,26]
Low-fibre diet[24]
Physical inactivity[23,27]
Abdominal adiposity (metabolic syndrome)[69,70]
Oestrogens[72]

However, a cholesterol-rich diet induces lithogenic bile only in gallstone carriers but not in stone-free controls[29], consistent with intestinal cholesterol absorption and/or biliary cholesterol secretion being in part under genetic control[30]. Such genetic factors are likely to contribute to the extraordinarily high prevalence of gallstones in American Indian populations both in North and South America. A recent ultrasound survey in 13 American Indian tribes in Arizona, Oklahoma, and South and North Dakota[31] found cumulative stone prevalence rates of 64% in American Indian women and 30% in men, even though their total caloric intake is comparable to that of white Americans. It has been speculated that the wide distribution of genes conferring gallstone susceptibility in American Indians might be related to 'thrifty' genes that conferred survival advantages when Paleo-Indians migrated to the Americas during the last Great Ice Age (20 000–10 000 years ago)[28]. This speculation is driven by the epidemiological associations of gallstones with obesity and type 2 diabetes mellitus, both of which might be caused by 'thrifty' genes[1,28]. The main pathophysiological link appears to be biliary hypersecretion of cholesterol owing to persistently increased cholesterol synthesis in obese and hyperinsulinaemic patients[1].

In the Third National Health and Nutrition Examination Survey, the highest age-standardized gallstone prevalence was seen in Mexican American women (27%), followed by white (17%) and African American women (14%)[32]. This 'admixture hypothesis' is supported by a study from Chile[33], which assessed the degree of admixture by mitochondrial DNA (mtDNA) in Mapuche Indians, Easter Island Maoris, and Hispanics. The prevalence of gallstone disease was highest (35%) in Mapuches, who migrated from North America (100% American Indian mtDNA), intermediate (27%) in Hispanics (88% American Indian mtDNA), and still 21% in Maoris, who originate from Polynesia (0% American Indian mtDNA) and in whom obesity appears to be a major factor causing gallstones[33].

MONOGENIC CHOLELITHIASIS: PROTOTYPES IN HUMANS

Despite accumulating evidence that gallstone formation is genetically determined in humans, direct confirmation of the role of individual genes in human gallstone disease is sparse. In specific subgroups of patients with gallstones, monogenic predisposition has been ascribed to mutations in the genes that encode the ABC transporters for phosphatidylcholine (*ABCB4*) or bile salts (*ABCB11*)[34], and *CYP7A1*[35].

The first evidence that a single gene defect causes gallstone formation in a defined subgroup – young patients with a symptomatic and recurring form of choleithiasis – was provided by Rosmorduc et al.[36]. These findings prompted a mutation search in the *ABCB4* gene, and point mutations were identified in 18 out of 32 patients (56%)[36]. The key clinical characteristics are age at onset of symptoms <40 years, the presence of both cholesterol gallbladder stones and intrahepatic sludge or microlithiasis, and the recurrence of biliary symptoms after cholecystectomy. The pathophysiological basis of this syndrome is consisent with the spontaneous occurrence of cholesterol crystals and gallstones in *Abcb4* knockout mice and the crystallization of transient cholesterol intermediates in phospholipid-poor model as well as human biles[37].

In contrast to ABCB4 deficieny, sitosterolaemia, which is caused by lost or low function of the cholesterol transporter ABCG5/G8, seems to confer resistance to cholesterol gallstone disease, at least patients secrete less cholesterol into bile[38], but might actually present with pigment stones (G. Salen, personal communication).

Single gene mutations causing haemolytic anaemias (hereditary spherocytosis, *ANK1*, *EPB42*, *SPTA1*, *SPTB*, *SLC4A1*; sickle cell disease, *HBB*; thalassaemia major and intermedia, *HBB*; and erythrocyte enzyme deficiencies, *AK1*, *G6PD*, *GPI*, *GSR*, *PGK1*, *PKLR*, *TPI1*) and thus increased biliary bilirubin concentrations are well documented (for gene abbreviations see OMIM database at http://www.ncbi.nlm.nih.gov/entrez). In addition to these gene defects, where black pigment stones are to be expected, there are also genes that predispose to increased enterohepatic cycling of bilirubin, another recently emphasized cause of pigment stone formation[17]. Such a gene defect that is associated with pigment stone formation is cystic fibrosis. Gallstone prevalence in cystic fibrosis is 10–30% compared with <5% in age-matched controls, but biliary cholesterol saturation does not differ between patients with and without gallstones[39]. Experimental findings in mice with mutations in the *CFTR* gene indicate that enterohepatic cycling, as well as biliary secretion and deconjugation of bilirubin, is increased in cystic fibrosis[40].

POLYGENIC CHOLELITHIASIS: GENOME ANALYSIS IN INBRED MICE

In humans the identification of lithogenic genes is hampered by the multifactorial pathogenesis of gallstones, so crossbreeding experiments in inbred mouse strains that differ in genetic susceptibility to cholesterol gallstone formation have been used to identify the genetic factors that contribute to gallstone formation. The mouse model is based on a lithogenic diet that contains 10% fat, 1% cholesterol and 0.5% cholic acid, which promotes intestinal absorption and biliary secretion of cholesterol[41]. Using quantitative trait locus analysis[13,41–44] and association mapping[45], more than 20 murine gene loci for gallstone susceptibility (*Lith* genes) and several candidate genes (ABC transporters, NRs, mucins) have been identified (for update see http://pga.jax.org/qtl). The characterization of lithogenic genes in knockout and transgenic mice and the identification of many gallstone-susceptibility loci in inbred mice provides the basis for studies of the corresponding genes in patients with gallstones. The transfer of findings from mouse genetics to the bedside might lead to new strategies for individual risk assessment and reveal molecular targets for the development of new strategies for prevention and medical therapies.

A recent study[16] suggested that chronic enterohepatic infection with *Helicobacter* spp. predisposes to cholesterol gallstone formation in mice fed the lithogenic diet. Thus, the gallstone-prone strains could well be first genetically susceptible to chronic infection, and as a secondary event, more prone to develop gallstones. This would imply that genes determining the immune response to enterohepatic infection might represent candidate gallstone genes. However, detailed analyses of human gallstone genes have yet to be performed to assess whether this concept also applies to gallstone patients.

ASSOCIATION STUDIES IN HUMANS: LIPOPROTEIN METABOLISM AND GALLSTONES

Association studies are widely used to assess common genetic variants in complex traits, and *APOE* polymorphisms have been extensively investigated in human gallstone disease. ApoE is the high-affinity ligand for the hepatic LDL receptor and the LDL receptor-related protein. There are three common codominant *APOE* alleles (ε2, ε3 and ε4), and the six resulting ApoE isoforms (E2/E2, E3/E3, E4/E4, E2/E3, E2/E4, E3/E4) can be distinguished by isoelectric focusing. These isoforms cause differences in receptor-binding affinities and clearance rates of circulating lipoproteins.

Presence of the ε4 allele has been associated with conditions such as coronary heart disease and Alzheimer's disease, and Bertomeu et al.[46] showed that the ε4 allele is also associated with cholelithiasis. The ApoE2 isoform, by contrast, was found less frequently in women with gallstones than in controls[47]. Other studies failed to confirm the association between gallstones and ApoE isoforms[48–52]. Different ethnicities and the inclusion of younger control probands might explain some of the discrepancies, since the ε4 allele frequency is low in Asian populations and decreases with age. However, other studies showed a higher ε4 allele frequency in patients with cholesterol stones than in patients with pigment stones[53], and a higher stone recurrence rate after extracorporeal shockwave lithotripsy in ε4 carriers[54]. In addition upon challenge with a high-cholesterol diet, *Apoe* knockout mice show a markedly lower frequency of gallstones than wild-type controls[55]. The association between gallstones and *APOE* could be due to increased hepatic cholesterol uptake via chylomicrons in patients carrying the isoform ApoE4[1,46]. Alternatively, biliary ApoE might have a role in the destabilization of bile[46,48].

ApoB functions as a ligand for receptor-mediated endocytosis of LDL. *APOB* gene polymorphisms have been associated with other complex diseases, such as coronary heart disease and type 2 diabetes mellitus. Significant associations between a common polymorphism in exon 26 and cholesterol gallstone prevalence, as well as increased total cholesterol, LDL cholesterol and ApoB concentrations in serum, have been detected in two Chinese

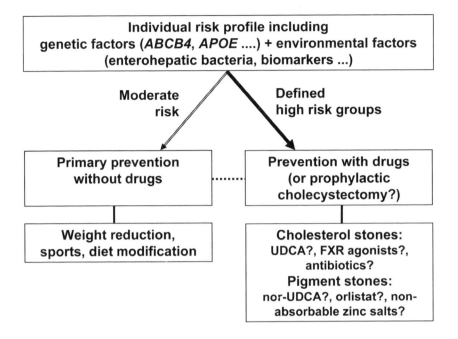

Figure 2 Future developments in gallstone prevention. Clinical stratification in moderate- and high-risk groups and specific strategies for primary prevention according to the individual genetic and environmental risk profile. Abbreviations: *ABCB4* = ATP-binding cassette transporter B4 gene; *APOE* = apolipoprotein E gene; FXR = farnesoid X receptor (bile salt sensor); UDCA = ursodeoxycholic acid

studies[52,56]. The lipid profile is not typical for cholesterol stone patients, and the association could not be detected in a Finnish population[57] and a study from India[58]. However, the Finnish study[57] found an association between stone prevalence and a common polymorphism of the cholesteryl ester transfer protein, which shifts cholesteryl esters and phospholipids from HDL to triglyceride-rich lipoproteins in exchange for triglycerides. This transfer lowers HDL cholesterol and increases VLDL triglyceride levels, a lipid pattern that is associated with an increased risk of gallbladder stones[1].

FUTURE STRATEGIES FOR TREATMENT AND PREVENTION

The epidemiological, family and twin studies in humans, as well as the genetic studies in mice, have demonstrated that cholelithiasis is a complex disease caused by genetic and environmental factors. Figure 2 illustrates that, in the future, individual risk profiling might allow the identification of moderate- and high-risk groups of patients. These risk profiles are likely to include both genetic factors (e.g. *ABCB4* mutations)[36] and environmental factors. Potential environmental factors are dietary components (Table 1), enterohepatic bacteria[16], or specific biomarkers that represent surrogate markers of lithogenic alterations in lipoprotein or bile salt metabolism[20]. Primary preventive measures for individuals with moderate risk include weight reduction, lifestyle, and diet modifications (Figure 2). In contrast, high-risk patients might be offered specific drugs for prevention or even prophylactic cholecystectomy, recently shown to be a safe procedure in the treatment of patients under 50 years of age with asymptomatic gallstones[59].

Besides ursodeoxycholic acid[60], NR agonists that selectively induce ABC transporters[12] or antibiotics to eradicate enterohepatic *Helicobacter* spp.[16] could be anti-lithogenic drugs preventing the formation of cholesterol gallstones. With respect to pigment stones, non-toxic drugs for the treatment of hyperbilirubinbilia have to be developed. Past attempts to decrease the extensive enterohepatic circulation of unconjugated bilirubin include the administration of agents that either trap unconjugated bilirubin in the intestine by absorption to non-absorbable solids, e.g. activated charcoal or cholestyramine[61,62], or form insoluble bilirubinate salts with calcium[63,64] or zinc[65,66]. Recently bilirubin-lowering effects without increase of serum zinc concentrations to toxic levels have been reported in hyperbilirubinaemic rats fed zinc methacrylate[67]. In addition, the lipase inhibitor orlistat, which increases intestinal and faecal fat contents, has been shown to enhance faecal bilirubin excretion and to decrease serum bilirubin levels in Gunn rats[64], albeit this is no reasonable option for patients with malabsorption, and efficacy in humans has yet to be investigated. Of note, nor-ursodeoxycholic acid, the C23-synthetic homologue of ursodeoxycholic acid without the C-24 methylene group of the side chain[68], has recently been shown to induce bicarbonate rich choleresis and to reduce bilirubin precipitation in bile of mouse cystic fibrosis models[40].

In the future, whole-genome association studies in gallstone patients are likely to identify the whole set of common lithogenic genes. Since the disease phenotype results from the manifestation of genetic susceptibility factors under the influence of environmental triggers, discovery of lithogenic genes would open avenues to control the influence of environmental challenges. This might lead to the design of new interventions, which extend our currently limited strategies for prevention and therapy of this exceptionally prevalent digestive disease.

Acknowledgements

The authors' experimental work relating to the gallstone formation has been supported by research grants from the Deutsche Forschungsgemeinschaft and the Ministry of Science and Research of North-Rhine-Westphalia. This contribution is based on and updated from our review published in Nat Clin Pract Gastroenterol Hepatol. 2005;2:423–33, which contains additional tables of epidemiological and genetic association studies in gallstone disease with primary references not cited here due to space limitations.

References

1. Lammert F, Sauerbruch T. Mechanisms of disease: the genetic epidemiology of gallbladder stones. Nat Clin Pract Gastroenterol Hepatol. 2005;2:423–33.
2. Liver Diseases Subcommittee of the Digestive Diseases Interagency Coordinating Committee. Gallbladder and biliary disease. In: US Department of Health and Human Services, National Institutes of Health. Action Plan for Liver Disease Research. Bethesda, 2004:144–50.
3. BQS Bundesgeschäftsstelle Qualitätssicherung. Cholezystektomie. In: Qualität sichtbar machen. BQS-Qualitätsreport 2004. Düsseldorf, 2004:22–34.
4. Sandler RS, Everhart JE, Donowitz M et al. The burden of selected digestive diseases in the United States. Gastroenterology. 2002;122:1500–11.
5. The Southern Surgeons Club. A prospective analysis of 1518 laparoscopic cholecystectomies. N Engl J Med. 1991;324:1073–8.
6. Paumgartner G, Sauter GH. Extracorporeal shockwave lithotripsy of gallstones: 20th anniversary of the first treatment. Eur J Gastroenterol Hepatol. 2005;17:525–7.
7. Rabenstein T, Radespiel-Tröger M, Höpfner L et al. Ten years experience with piezoelectric extracorporeal shockwave lithotripsy of gallbladder stones. Eur J Gastreonterol Hepatol. 2005;17:629–39.
8. Carey MC, LaMont JT. Cholesterol gallstone formation. 1. Physical-chemistry of bile and biliary lipid secretion. Prog Liver Dis. 1992;10:136–63.
9. Small DM. Role of ABC transporters in secretion of cholesterol from liver into bile. Proc Natl Acad Sci USA. 2003;100:4–6.
10. Paumgartner G, Sauerbruch T. Gallstones: pathogenesis. Lancet. 1991;338:1117–21.
11. Admirand WH, Small DM. The physicochemical basis of cholesterol gallstone formation in man. J Clin Invest. 1968;47:1045–52.
12. Moschetta A, Bookout AL, Mangelsdorf DJ. Prevention of cholesterol gallstone diseases by FXR agonists in a mouse model. Nat Med. 2004;10:1352–8.
13. Lammert F, Carey MC, Paigen B. Chromosomal organization of candidate genes involved in cholesterol gallstone formation: a murine gallstone map. Gastroenterology. 2001;120:221–38.
14. Wang DQ-H, Schmitz F, Kopin AS, Carey MC. Targeted disruption of the murine cholecystokinin-1 receptor promotes intestinal cholesterol absorption and susceptibility to cholesterol cholelithiasis. J Clin Invest. 2004;114:521–8.
15. Wang HH, Afdhal NH, Gendler SJ, Wang DQ-H. Targeted disruption of the murine mucin gene 1 decreases susceptibility to cholesterol gallstone formation. J Lipid Res. 2004;45:438–47.
16. Maurer KJ, Ihrig MM, Rodghers AB et al. Identification of cholelithogenic enterohepatic *Helicobacter* species and their role in murine cholesterol gallstone formation. Gastroenterology. 2005;128:1023–33.
17. Vitek L, Carey MC. Enterohepatic cycling of bilirubin as a cause of 'black' pigment gallstones in adult life. Eur J Clin Invest. 2003;33:799–810.
18. Brink MA, Slors JF, Keulemans YC et al. Enterohepatic cycling of bilirubin: a putative mechanism for pigment gallstone formation in ileal Crohn's disease. Gastroenterology. 1999;116:1420–7.
19. Katsika D, Grjibovski A, Einarsson C, Lammert F, Lichtenstein P, Marschall HU. Genetic and environmental influences on symptomatic gallstone disease: a Swedish study of 43,141 twin pairs. Hepatology. 2005;41:1138–43.
20. Kesäniemi YA, Koskenvuo M, Vuoristo M, Miettinen TA. Biliary lipid composition in monozygotic and dizygotic pairs of twins. Gut. 1989;30:1750–6.
21. Duggirala R, Mitchell BD, Blangero J, Stern MP. Genetic determinants of variation in gallbladder disease in the Mexican–American population. Genet Epidemiol. 1999;16:191–204.
22. Nakeeb A, Comuzzie AG, Martin L et al. Gallstones: genetics versus environment. Ann Surg. 2002;235:842–9.
23. Leitzmann MF, Rimm EB, Willett WC et al. Recreational physical activity and the risk of cholecystectomy in women. N Engl J Med. 1999;341:777–84.
24. Tsai CJ, Leitzmann MF, Willett WC, Giovannucci EL. Long-term intake of dietary fiber and decreased risk of cholecystectomy in women. Am J Gastroenterol. 2004;99:1364–70.

25. Tsai CJ, Leitzmann MF, Willett WC, Giovannucci EL. Dietary carbohydrates and glycaemic load and the incidence of symptomatic gall stone disease in men. Gut. 2005;54: 823–8.

26. Tsai CJ, Leitzmann MF, Willett WC, Giovannucci EL. Glycemic load, glycemic index, and carbohydrate intake in relation to risk of cholecystectomy in women. Gastroenterology. 2005;129:105–12.

27. Leitzmann MF, Giovannucci EL, Rimm EB et al. The relation of physical activity to risk for symptomatic gallstone disease in men. Ann Intern Med. 1998;128:417–25.

28. Carey MC, Paigen B. Epidemiology of the American Indians' burden and its likely genetic origins. Hepatology. 2002;36:781–91.

29. Kern F. Effects of dietary cholesterol on cholesterol and bile acid homeostasis in patients with cholesterol gallstones. J Clin Invest. 1994;93:1186–94.

30. Lammert F, Wang DQ-H. New insights into the genetic regulation of intestinal cholesterol absorption. Gastroenterology. 2005;129:718–34.

31. Everhart JE, Yeh F, Lee ET et al. Prevalence of gallbladder disease in American Indian populations: findings from the Strong Heart Study. Hepatology. 2002;35:1507–12.

32. Everhart JE, Khare M, Hill M, Maurer KR. Prevalence and ethnic differences in gallbladder disease in the Unites States. Gastroenterology. 1999;117:632–9.

33. Miquel JF, Covarrubias C, Villaroel L et al. Genetic epidemiology of cholesterol cholelithiasis among Chilean Hispanics, Amerindians, and Maoris. Gastroenterology. 1998;115:937–46.

34. Van Mil SW, van der Woerd WL, van der Brugge G et al. Benign recurrent intrahepatic cholestasis type 2 is caused by mutations in ABCB11. Gastroenterology. 2004;127:379–84.

35. Pullinger CR, Eng C, Salen G et al. Human cholesterol 7α-hydroxylase (*CYP7A1*) deficiency has a hypercholesterolemic phenotype. J Clin Invest. 2002;110:109–17.

36. Rosmorduc O, Hermelin B, Boelle PY, Parc R, Taboury J, Poupon R. *ABCB4* gene mutation-associated cholelithiasis in adults. Gastroenterology. 2003;125:452–9.

37. Weihs D, Schmidt J, Goldiner I et al. Biliary cholesterol crystallization characterized by single-crystal cryogenic electron diffraction. J Lipid Res. 2005;46:942–8.

38. Salen G, Nicolau G, Shefer S, Mosbach EH. Hepatic cholesterol metabolism in patients with gallstones. Gastroenterology. 1975;69:676–84.

39. Angelico M, Gandin C, Canuzzi P et al. Gallstones in cystic fibrosis: a critical reappraisal. Hepatology. 1991;14:768–75.

40. Broderick AL, Wittenburg H, Lyons MA, Stechell KD, Hofmann AF, Carey MC. Cystic fibrosis transmembrane conductance regulator gene mutations cause 'black' pigment gallstone formation: new insights from mouse models and implications for therapeutic interventions in cystic fibrosis. In: Adler G, Blum HE, Fuchs M, Stange EF, editors. Gallstone Pathogenesis and Treatment. Dordrecht: Kluwer Academic Publishers, 2004: 24–7.

41. Wang DQ-H, Lammert F, Cohen DE, Paigen B, Carey MC. Cholic acid aids absorption, biliary secretion, and phase transitions of cholesterol in murine cholelithogenesis. Am J Physiol. 1999;276:G751–60.

42. Lammert F, Wang DQ-H, Wittenburg H et al. *Lith* genes control mucin accumulation, cholesterol crystallization, and gallstone formation in A/J and AKR/J inbred mice. Hepatology. 2002;36:1145–54.

43. Wittenburg H, Lyons MA, Li R, Churchill GA, Carey MC, Paigen B. FXR and ABCG5/ABCG8 as determinants of cholesterol gallstone formation from quantitative trait locus mapping in mice. Gastroenterology. 2003;125:868–81.

44. Lyons MA, Wittenburg H, Li R et al. *Lith6*: a new QTL for cholesterol gallstones from an intercross of CAST/Ei and DBA/2J inbred mouse strains. J Lipid Res. 2003;44:1763–71.

45. Pletcher MT, McClurg P, Batalov S et al. Use of a dense single nucleotide polymorphism map for in silico mapping in the mouse. PLoS Biol. 2004;2:e393.

46. Bertomeu A, Ros E, Zambon D et al. Apolipoprotein E polymorphism and gallstones. Gastroenterology. 1996;111:1603–10.

47. Niemi M, Kervinen K, Rantala A et al. The role of apolipoprotein E and glucose intolerance in gallstone disease in middle aged subjects. Gut. 1999;44:557–62.

48. Juvonen T, Kervinen K, Kairaluoma MI, Lajunen LH, Kesäniemi YA. Gallstone cholesterol content is related to apolipoprotein E polymorphism. Gastroenterology. 1993; 104:1806–13.

49. Rollán A, Loyola G, Covarrubias C, Giancaspero R, Acevedo K, Nervi F. Apolipoprotein E polymorphism in patients with acute pancreatitis. Pancreas. 1994;9:349–53.

50. Lin QY, Du JP, Zhang MY et al. Effect of apolipoprotein E gene Hha I restricting fragment length polymorphism on serum lipids in cholecystolithiasis. World J Gastroenterol. 1999;5: 228–30.

51. Hasegawa K, Terada S, Kubota K et al. Effect of apolipoprotein E polymorphism on bile lipid composition and the formation of cholesterol gallstone. Am J Gastroenterol. 2003;98: 1605–9.

52. Jiang ZY, Han TQ, Suo GJ et al. Polymorphisms at cholesterol 7α-hydroxylase, apolipoproteins B and E and low density lipoprotein receptor genes in patients with gallbladder stone disease. World J Gastroenterol. 2004;10:1508–12.

53. Van Erpecum KJ, Portincasa P, Dohlu MH, van Berge Henegouwen GP, Jüngst D. Biliary pronucleating proteins and apolipoprotein E in cholesterol and pigment stone patients. J Hepatol. 2003;39:7–11.

54. Venneman NG, van Berge-Henegouwen GP, Portincasa P et al. Absence of apolipoprotein E4 genotype, good gallbladder motility and presence of solitary stones delay rather than prevent gallstone recurrence after extracorporeal shock wave lithotripsy. J Hepatol. 2001; 35:10–16.

55. Amigo L, Quinones V, Mardones P et al. Impaired biliary cholesterol secretion and decreased gallstone formation in apolipoprotein E-deficient mice fed a high-cholesterol diet. Gastroenterology. 2000;118:772–9.

56. Han T, Jiang Z, Suo G, Zhang S. Apolipoprotein B-100 gene Xba I polymorphism and cholesterol gallstone disease. Clin Genet. 2000;57:304–8.

57. Juvonen T, Savolainen MJ, Kairaluoma MI, Lajunen LH, Humphries SE, Kesäniemi YA. Polymorphisms at the apoB, apoA-I, and cholesteryl ester transfer protein gene loci in patients with gallbladder disease. J Lipid Res. 1995;36:804–12.

58. Singh MK, Pandey UB, Ghoshal UC et al. Apolipoprotein B-100 XbaI gene polymorphism in gallbladder cancer. Hum Genet. 2004;114:280–3.

59. Coelho JC, Vizzoto AO, Salvalaggio PR, Tolazzi AR. Laparoscopic cholecystectomy to treat patients with asymptomatic gallstones. Dig Surg. 2000;17:344–7.

60. Shiffman ML, Kaplan GD, Brinkman-Kaplan V, Vickers EF. Prophylaxis against gallstone formation with ursodeoxycholic acid in patients participatimg in a very-low-calorie diet program. Ann Intern Med. 1995;122:899–905.

61. Amitai Y, Regev M, Arad I, Peleg O, Boehnert M. Treatment of neonatal hyper-bilirubinemia with repetitive oral activated charcoal as an adjunct to phototherapy. J Perinat Med. 1993;21:189–94.

62. Nicolopoulos D, Hadjigeorgiou E, Malamitsi A, Kalpoyannis N, Karli I, Papadakis D. Combined treatment of neonatal jaundice with cholestyramine and phototherapy. J Pediatr. 1978;93:684–8.

63. Van der Veere CN, Schoemaker B, Bakker C, van der Meer R, Jansen PL, Oude Elferink RP. Influence of dietary calcium phosphate on the disposition of bilirubin in rats with unconjugated hyperbilirubinemia. Hepatology. 1996;24:620–6.

64. Hafkamp AM, Havinga R, Sinaasappel M, Verkade HJ. Effective oral treatment of unconjugated hyperbilirubinemia in Gunn rats. Hepatology. 2005;41:526–34.

65. Méndez-Sánchez N, Roldan-Valadez E, Flores MA, Cardenas-Vazquez R, Uribe M. Zinc salts precipitate unconjugated bilirubin in vitro and inhibit enterohepatic cycling of bilirubin in hamsters. Eur J Clin Invest. 2001;31:773–80.

66. Méndez-Sánchez N, Martinez M, Gonzalez V, Roldan-Valadez E, Flores MA, Uribe M. Zinc sulfate inhibits the enterohepatic cycling of unconjugated bilirubin in subjects with Gilbert's syndrome. Ann Hepatol. 2002;1:40–3.

67. Vitek L, Muchova L, Zelenka J, Zadinova M, Malina J. The effect of zinc salts on serum bilirubin levels in hyperbilirubinemic rats. J Pediatr Gastroenterol Nutr. 2005;40:135–40.

68. Hofmann AF, Zakko SF, Lira M et al. Novel biotransformation and physiological properties of norursodeoxycholic acid in humans. Hepatology. 2005;42:1391–8.

69. Maclure KM, Hayes KC, Colditz GA, Stampfer MJ, Speizer FE, Willett WC. Weight, diet, and the risk of symptomatic gallstones in middle-aged women. N Engl J Med. 1989;321: 563–9.

70. Shiffman ML, Sugerman HJ, Kellum JM, Moore EW. Changes in gallbladder bile composition following gallstone formation and weight reduction. Gastroenterology. 1992; 103:214–21.
71. Thornton JR, Heaton KW, Macfarlane DG. A relation between high-density-lipoprotein cholesterol and bile cholesterol saturation. Br Med J. 1981;283:1352–4.
72. Cirillo DJ, Wallace RB, Rodabough RJ et al. Effect of estrogen therapy on gallbladder disease. J Am Med Asoc. 2005;293:330–9.

7
Special Lecture: Future perspectives in the treatment of biliary tumour disease: a multidisciplinary approach

F. BERR, R. HUBER, J. HAUSS and H. WITZIGMANN

INTRODUCTION

Malignant biliary tumours comprise gallbladder cancer (GBC), intrahepatic cholangio-carcinoma (not covered here) and extrahepatic bile duct cancer (BDC) which involves the bile duct bifurcation (65% perihilar tumours), distal duct (20%) or the duct diffusely (15%). About 80% of gallbladder and bile duct neoplasms are well or moderately differentiated adenocarcinomas of the papillary or diffusely infiltrating type (1:4) often with strong desmoplastic reaction of the stroma tissue[1-4]. When the diagnosis is made, only 30–50% of cases show lymph node metastases, and 10–20% distant metastases (liver, peritoneum)[3,4]. However, the majority (about 80%) of patients are diagnosed in a tumour stage precluding curative resection, i.e. with bilobar involvement of segmental bile ducts, bilateral vascular involvement or metastases[4,5]. Non-resectable tumours lead to complex stenoses of the hilar bile ducts and in about 10–20% of cases to tumour infiltration and stenosis of the duodenum[4,5]. The tumour spread favours local extension along the biliary tree leading to refractory mechanical cholestasis, secondary bacterial cholangitis and liver failure.

Overall survival for patients with gallbladder or bile duct cancer is poor, because most tumours are diagnosed in an advanced stage. The minority (20–30%) is curatively resectable and long-term survival after curative resection ranges between 20% and 40%, and below 20% in pN1-positive tumours[6-13]. Nevertheless, resection will remain the only option to improve cure, provided the tumours are diagnosed earlier and/or down-staged/sized with neoadjuvant therapy. This requires interdisciplinary teams of gastroenterologists, hepatobiliary surgeons and radio-oncologists.

DIAGNOSIS

Biliary cancers present with cholestasis in about 90% of cases and with persistent epigastric pain in the remainder. The majority of GBC belong to the diffusely infiltrating type and are not recognized before spread to the bile duct causes cholestasis or to nerve sheaths causes pain; some early carcinomas are removed incidentally by cholecystecomy for other indications[6]. Early use of magnetic resonance cholangiopancreaticography (in a maximum intensified projection technique) for rising cholestatic serum enzymes – well before the onset of jaundice – might increase the detection rate of curatively resectable BDC. Nowadays, multi-array computerized axial tomography (CAT) scans show much higher resolution than in recent years, and this will improve the detection rate of hilar tumours and enlarged lymph nodes. The definite diagnosis is made by forceps biopsies or brush cytology from biliary tree strictures during endoscopic retrograde cholangiography[14,15], or alternatively with linear-array endosonography-targeted biopsies[15]. The diagnostic sensitivity is around 75% and 60%, respectively. Positron emission tomography using 18-fluorodeoxy-glucose (FDG-PET) has a high predictive value for the detection of the primary tumour and distant metastases, but not regional lymph node metastases[16]. Recent advances in [18]C-deoxyglucose-positron emission tomography–computerized tomography scans (PET-CT) will allow PET-CT-targeted biopsies during surveillance of high-risk conditions such as primary sclerosing cholangitis, ulcerative colitis, and especially the combination of the two diseases.

CLINICAL STAGING

Clinical staging has improved considerably over the past decade and is now used for planning oncosurgical en-bloc resection of hilar bile duct cancers as well as for categorizing the response to antineoplastic treatment according to WHO definitions based on the largest perpendicular diameters of primary tumour and metastases[10,13]. The response/non-response to local tumour ablation is assessed with ERC findings (including biopsies) according to reopening or occlusion of hepatic and segmental bile ducts and negative or positive tumour histology[13]. Tumour extension along the bile ducts according to bismuth type 1–4[17] and T category[18] are staged with intraluminal ultrasound during ERC using a 15 MHz miniprobe transducer, and with MRI in the HASTE technique using paramagnetic ferrous oxides as hepatic signal enhancers[13]. Furthermore, the clinical N category should be classified in addition by CT scan and gastroduodenal endosonography with a 12 MHz transducer[14,15]. Exploration of BDC with ERC or ultrasound minitransducer must be followed by bilateral hepatic duct drainage[13,19].

SURGICAL RESECTION

If the tumour is detected at an early stage, this is the only curative approach to the treatment of patients with GBC or BDC. Cholecystectomy is curative for early cancer of the gallbladder (stage 0 or 1a) incidentally removed and detected during histological work-up of the specimen[6]. More advanced tumour stages require resection of the gallbladder bed including a 3 cm margin of liver tissue, or a partial hepatectomy of segments IVa and V combined with lymphadenectomy in the ligamentum hepatoduodenale[6–8]. Positive lymph nodes in the ligamentum heptoduodenale decrease the chance of 5-year survival after curative resection to 20–50%; positive coeliac nodes preclude curative resection[8]. Traditional resection of perihilar BDC often combined with hemihepatectomy, has not improved the long-term survival rate[4,9,12,13], but extended en-bloc resections of the tumour including the adjacent portal vein and hemihepatectomy in the no-touch technique yielded significantly higher rates of long-term survival, between 50% and 60% at 5 years[10,11]. Nevertheless, the rate of overall survival at 5 years after curative resection is between 40% and 50%[10–13]. Liver transplantation of non-resectable perihilar tumours offers some chance (30–35%) of long-term survival[20]; however, BDC has not been accepted as an established indication for liver transplantation. Neoadjuvant protocols followed by liver transplantation[21,22] or tumour resection including partial hepatectomy[23] have been tested in pilot studies in order to improve survival after curative resection.

NEOADJUVANT PROTOCOLS

Pilot studies have tried downstaging of hilar bile duct tumours classified as non-resectable. The MAYO group treated unresectable stage I/II perihilar cholangiocarcinoma with neoadjuvant external beam irradiation, 192-iridium-brachytherapy and 5-fluorouracil and/or oral capecitabine prior to liver transplantation (OLT). OLT was achieved in 28/56 patients and long-term survival after OLT in 22 of them[22]. Our own group used local photodynamic therapy of the tumour stenoses and adjacent bile ducts for down-sizing of unresectable perihilar cholangiocarcinoma in seven patients. Curative resection (R0), including one liver transplantation, was achieved in all of them without serious complications[23], and 5-year survival in five of seven. These approaches, including living donor-related liver transplantation, must be further studied in prospective multicentre trials for locally confined, unresectable bile duct tumours.

BILIARY DRAINAGE

In a randomized trial, endoscopic insertion of a 10-French Teflon stent matched the technical success rate of open surgery with biliodigestive anastomosis (95% vs 94%) and showed similar median survival time (21 vs 26 weeks), but less complications (11% vs 29%) and procedure-related mortality (3% vs 14%); the median patency interval of the Teflon stents was 4.5 months[24]. In another randomized trial, self-expandable metal stents provided longer median patency intervals (9 vs 4.1 months) than 10-French plastic stents, but the median survival time was similar (5.8 vs 4.8 months)[25]. The preferred palliative treatment for distal extrahepatic cholangiocarcinoma is endoscopic or percutaneous insertion of a biliary endoprosthesis[26]. Self-expandable metal stents may be preferred in patients with an estimated prognosis of about 6 months[26].

LOCAL ABLATIVE TUMOUR THERAPY

The majority of perihilar BDC remain locally confined for several years, but cause lethal complications by local spread of the tumour. The palliative effect of local tumour ablation has been investigated with brachytherapy and with photodynamic therapy (PDT). Brachytherapy with 192-iridium (dose of 25 Gy at 1 cm distance) alone did not extend median survival time (4.3–5 months)[27,28], but when combined with external beam radiotherapy (EBRT) (30 Gy) resulted in median survival times in the range of 10–10.5 months[29,30]. Four highly selected series of brachytherapy and EBRT ($\pm$ 5-fluorouracil) resulted in median survival times of 11.6–4.5 months, but this was complicated by cholangitis in 50% to 92% of patients[31–34]. PDT using haematoporphyrin derivatives and photoactivation with red laser light (630 nm) via ERC access shows local tumour response, control of cholestasis, improved quality of life, and no serious adverse effects[35–40]. PDT combined with endoprosthesis insertion has resulted in median survival times in the range of 11.5–14.4 months in two prospective pilot trials[36,37] and in a randomized study[41]. The randomized trial comparing standard endoprosthesis treatment vs PDT plus endoprosthesis insertion, showed prolonged survival time with PDT (14.5 vs 3.5 months)[41]. The tumoricidal tissue penetration of the PDT procedure reaches 4 mm depth in bile duct cancers, whereas tumour tissues located deeper in the tissue are not affected by PDT[23]. The PDT procedure should be modified for a tumoricidal tissue penetration of 8–10 mm, e.g by use of laser light of 650–750 nm wavelength and an appropriate photosensitizer. PDT with temoporfin (Foscan®) yielded 10 mm tumoricidal tissue penetration in pancreatic cancer[42] and is currently being evaluated in a pilot study for PDT of BDC.

DUODENAL STENOSIS

Duodenal stenosis by tumour infiltration is observed in 10–17% of patients with BDC[29,37]. Rapid weight loss, symptoms of gastric outlet obstruction and/ or gastro-oesophageal reflux should alert one to the presence of duodenal stenosis. Typically, a short stenosis is located just distal to the duodenal bulb. It can be relieved with laparoscopic gastroenterostomy[43] or endoscopic insertion of a large-bore self-expanding metal stent (Wallstent enteral®, Boston Scientific Inc.)[44,45]. The functional restitution of gastric emptying is satisfactory after endoprosthesis insertion in most patients with cholangiocarcinoma-related duodenal stenosis[45].

RADIOCHEMOTHERAPY AND SYSTEMIC CHEMOTHERAPY

These are not yet evidence-based procedures for biliary tract cancers[46]. Phase II trials indicated poor responsiveness to external beam radiotherapy, but moderate responsiveness to 5-FU- or gemcitabine-based radiochemotherapy and to chemotherapy in particular with 5-FU or capecitabine, gemcitabine and cisplatin or oxaliplatin[46–51]. Improved biliary drainage, including local tumour ablation with photodynamic therapy, palliates against mechanical cholestasis and cholangitis and patients become suitable candidates for antitumour therapies including radiochemotherapy and combination chemotherapy. Prospective multicentre trials are under way to define the responsiveness of biliary tract cancers to radiochemotherapy and combination chemotherapy, and furthermore to combinations including targeted therapies (www. clinicaltrials.com). Growing knowledge of the relevant oncogenic pathways in biliary tract cancers will lead to targeted therapies[52]. In a human cholangiocarcinoma model, a novel tyrokinase inhibitor against erb-B1, erbB-2 and VEGF-R has shown 68% growth reduction of cholangiocarcinomas transplanted to SCID mice[53]. Thus biliary cancers will become better treatable within the next 10 years.

SUMMARY

Curative treatment for GBC as well as BDC is en-bloc R0 resection. Only the minority of tumours is curatively resectable at the time of diagnosis. Promising neoadjuvant protocols are under way for preoperative downstaging of BDC by combined radio-/chemotherapy modalities prior to liver transplantation[21] or to achieve down-sizing of tumours and purging of tumour margins prior to curative resection[23]. The mainstay of palliative treatment is satisfactory biliary drainage by endoprosthesis insertion and local tumour ablation with porfimer-PDT, in order to avoid cholestasis and cholangitis. This treatment provides better quality of life, a lower risk of tumour complications, and prolonged survival time[35], and renders patients eligible for radiochemotherapy or combination chemotherapy protocols. Better therapeutic options are expected from targeted systemic therapies and from a new generation of photosensitizers that will increase tumoricidal penetration for local tumour therapy.

References

1. Lazaridis KN, Gores G. Cholangiocarcinoma (review). Gastroenterology. 2005;128:1655–67.
2. Henson DE, Albores-Saavedra J, Corle D. Carcinoma of the extrahepatic bile ducts. Histologic types, stage of disease, grade and survival rates. Cancer. 1992;70:1498–501.
3. Klatskin G. Adenocarcinoma of the hepatic duct at its bifurcation within the porta hepatis. An unusual tumor with distinctive clinical and pathological features. Am J Med. 1965;38: 241–56.
4. de Groen PC, Gores GJ, LaRusso NF et al. Biliary tract cancers (review). N Engl J Med. 1999;341:1368–78.
5. Berr F, Neuhaus P, Jonas S. Tumoren der Gallenwege. In: Domschke W, Hohenberger W, Meinertz T, Possinger K, Reinhardt T, Tölle R, editors. Therapiehandbuch. Munich: Urban & Schwarzenberg, 2004:H11:1–5.

6. Cubertafond P, Gainant A, Cucchiaro G et al. Surgical treatment of 724 carcinomas of the gallbladder. Results of the French Surgical Association survey. Ann Surg. 1994;219:275–80.
7. Onoyma H, Yamamoto M, Tseng A et al. Extended cholecystectomy for carcinoma of the gallbladder. World J Surg. 1995;19:758–63.
8. Kondo S, Nimura Y, Hayakawa N et al. Regional and paraortic lymphadenectomy in radical surgery for advanced gallbladder carcinoma. Br J Surg. 2000;87:418–22.
9. Launois B, Terblanche J, Lachal M et al. Proximal bile duct cancer: high resectability rate and 5-year survival. Ann Surg. 1999;230:266–75.
10. Neuhaus P, Jonas S, Bechstein WO et al. Extended resections for hilar cholangiocarcinoma. Ann Surg. 1999;230:808–19.
11. Kosuge T, Yamamoto J, Shimada K et al. Improved surgical results for hilar cholangiocarcinoma with procedures including major hepatic resection. Ann Surg. 1999; 230:663–71.
12. Jarnagin WR, Fong Y, DeMatteo RP et al. Staging, resectability, and outcome in 225 patients with hilar cholangiocarcinoma. Ann Surg. 2001;234:567–79.
13. Witzigmann H, Berr F, Ringel U et al. Surgical and palliative management and outcome in 184 patients with hilar cholangiocarcinoma – palliative photodynamic therapy plus stenting is comparable to R1/R2 resection. Ann Surg. 2006;244 (In press).
14. Domagk D, Poremba C, Dietl KH et al. Endoscopic transpapillary biopsies and intraductal sonography in the diagnostics of bile duct strictures: a prospective study. Gut. 2002;51:240–4.
15. Rösch T, Hofrichter K, Frimberger E et al. ERCP or EUS for tissue diagnosis of biliary strictures? A prospective comparative study. Gastrointest Endosc. 2004;60:390–6.
16. Kluge R, Schmidt F, Caca K et al. Positron emission tomography with [18-F]fluoro-2-deoxy-D-glucose for diagnosis and staging of bile duct cancer. Hepatology. 2001;33:1029–35.
17. Bismuth H, Nakache R, Diamond T. Management strategies in resection for hilar cholangiocarcinoma. Ann Surg. 1992;215:31–8.
18. Sobin LH, Wittekind Ch, editors. UICC: TNM Classification of Malignant Tumors, 5th edn. New York: Wiley-Liss, 1997:81–3.
19. Chang WH, Kortan P, Haber GB. Outcome in patients with bifurcation tumors who undergo unilateral versus bilateral hepatic duct drainage. Gastrointest Endosc. 1998;47:354–62.
20. Robles R, Figueras J, Turrión VS et al. Spanish experience in liver transplantation for hilar and peripheral cholangiocarcinoma. Ann Surg. 2004;239:265–71.
21. Heimbach JK, Gores GJ, Haddock MG et al. Liver transplantation for unresectable perihilar cholangiocarcinoma. Semin Liver Dis. 2004;24:201–7.
22. Rea DJ, Heimbach JK, Rosen CB. Liver transplantation with neoadjuvant chemoradiation is more effective than resection for hilar cholangiocarcinoma. Ann Surg. 2005;242:451–61.
23. Wiedmann M, Caca K, Berr F et al. Neoadjuvant photodynamic therapy as a new approach to treating hilar cholangiocarcinoma. Cancer. 2003;97:2783–90.
24. Smith AC, Dowsett JF, Russell RCG et al. Randomised trial of endoscopic stenting versus surgical bypass in malignant low bile duct obstruction. Lancet. 1994;344:1655–60.
25. Davids PHP, Groen AK, Rauws EAJ, Tytgat GNJ, Huibregtse K. Randomised trial of self-expanding metal stents versus polythylene stents for distal malignant biliary obstruction. Lancet. 1992;340:1488–92.
26. Levy MJ, Baron TH, Gostout CJ et al. Palliation of malignant extrahepatic biliary obstruction with plastic versus expandable metal stents: an evidence-based approach. Clin Gastroenterol Hepatol. 2004;2:273–85.
27. Molt P, Hopfan S, Watson R, Botet JF, Brennan MF. Intraluminal radiation therapy in the management of malignant biliary obstruction. Cancer. 1986;57:536–44.
28. Kamada T, Saitou H, Takamura A et al. The role of radiotherapy in the management of extrahepatic bile duct cancer: an analysis of 145 consecutive patients treated with intraluminal and/or external beam radiotherapy. Int J Radiation Oncol Biol Phys. 1996; 34:767–74.
29. Bowling TE, Galbraith SM, Hatfield ARW et al. A retrospective comparison of endoscopic stenting alone with stenting and radiotherapy in non-resectable cholangiocarcinoma. Gut. 1996;39:852–5.

30. Ede RJ, Williams SJ, Hatfield ARW et al. Endoscopic management of inoperable cholangiocarcinoma using iridium-192. Br J Surg. 1989;76:867–9.
31. Tsujino K, Landry JC, Smith RG et al. Definitive radiation therapy for extrahepatic bile duct carcinoma. Radiology. 1995;196:275–80.
32. Kuvshinoff BW, Armstrong JG, Fong Y et al. Palliation of irresectable hilar cholangiocarcinoma with biliary drainage and radiotherapy. Br J Surg. 1995;82:1522–5.
33. Eschelman DJ, Shapiro MJ, Bonn J et al. Malignant biliary obstruction: long-term experience with Gianturco stents and combined-modality radiation therapy. Radiology. 1996;200:717–24.
34. Foo ML, Gunderson LL, Bender CE et al. External radiation therapy and transcatheter iridium in the treatment of extrahepatic bile duct carcinoma. Int Radiation Oncol Biol Phys. 1997;39:929–35.
35. Berr F. Photodynamic therapy for cholangiocarcinoma. Semin Liver Dis. 2004;24:177–87.
36. Ortner MA, Liebetruth J, Schreiber S et al. Photodynamic therapy of nonresectable cholangiocarcinoma. Gastroenterology. 1998;114:536–42.
37. Berr F, Wiedmann M, Tannapfel A et al. Photodynamic therapy for advanced bile duct cancer: evidence for improved palliation and extended survival. Hepatology. 2000;31:291–8.
38. Rumalla A, Baron T, Wang K et al. Endoscopic application of photodynamic therapy for cholangiocarcinoma. Gastrointest Endosc. 2001;53:500–4.
39. Zoepf T, Jakobs R, Arnold JC et al. Photodynamic therapy for palliation of nonresectable bile duct cancer – preliminary results with a new diode laser system. Am J Gastroenterol. 2001;96:2093–7.
40. Dumoulin FL, Gerhardt T, Fuchs S et al. Phase II study of photodynamic therapy and metal stent as palliative treatment for nonresectable hilar cholangiocarcinoma. Gastrointest Endosc. 2003;57:860–7.
41. Ortner MAE, Caca K, Berr F et al. Successful photodynamic therapy for nonresectable cholangiocarcinoma: a randomized prospective study. Gastroenterology. 2003;125:1355–63.
42. Bown SG, Rogowska AZ, Whitelaw DE et al. Photodynamic therapy for cancer of the pancreas. Gut. 2002;50:549–57.
43. Brune IB, Feussner H, Neuhaus H, Classen M, Siewert JR. Laparoscopic gastrojejunostomy and endoscopic biliary stent placement for palliation of incurable gastric outlet obstruction with cholestasis. Surg Endosc. 1997;11:834–7.
44. de Baere T, Harry G, Ducreux M et al. Self-expanding metallic stents as palliative treatment for malignant gastroduodenal stenosis. Am J Roentgenol. 1997;169:1079–83.
45. Schiefke I, Zabel-Langhenning A, Wiedmann M et al. Self-expandable metallic stents for malignant duodenal obstruction caused by biliary tract cancer. Gastrointest Endosc. 2003;58:213–19.
46. Khan SA, Davidson BR, Goldin R et al. Guidelines for the diagnosis and treatment of cholangiocarcinoma: consensus document. Gut. 2002;51(Suppl. 6):VI1–9.
47. McMasters KM, Tuttle TM, Leach SD et al. Neoadjuvant Chemoradiation for extrahepatic cholangiocarcinoma. Am J Surg. 1997;174:605-609.
48. de Aretxabala X, Roa I, Burgos L et al. Preoperative chemoradiotherapy in the treatment of gallbladder cancer. Ann Surg. 1999;65:241–6.
49. Ducreux M, Rougier P, Fandi A et al. Effective treatment of advanced biliary tract carcinoma using 5-fluorouracil continuous infusion with cisplatin. Ann Oncol. 1998;9:653–6.
50. Sanz-Altamira PM, Ferrante K, Jenkins RL, Lewis WD, Huberman MS, Stuart KE. A phase-II trial of 5-fluorouracil, leucovorin, and carboplatin in patients with unresectable biliary tree carcinoma. Cancer. 1998;82:2321–5.
51. André T, Tournigand C, Rosmorduc O et al. Gemcitabine combined with Oxaliplatin (GEMOX) in advanced biliary tract adenocarcinoma: a GERCOR study. Ann Oncol. 2004;15:1339–43.
52. Sirica AE. Cholangiocarcinoma: molecular targeting strategies for chemoprevention and therapy. Hepatology. 2005;41:5–15.
53. Wiedmann M, Faisthammel J, Blüthner T et al. Der Tyrosinkinase-Inhibitor NVP-AEE788: ein neuer Ansatz bei der Therapie von Tumoren der Gallenwege (Abstrakt). Z Gastroenterol. 2006;44:108.

Pancreatic carcinoma

Chair: W.E. SCHMIDT and B. WIEDENMANN

8
Genetics of chronic pancreatitis and pancreatic carcinoma

P. SIMON, F. U. WEISS, J. MAYERLE, M. KRAFT and M. M. LERCH

INTRODUCTION

A wide range of mutations and polymorphisms in a variety of genes that relate to pancreatic function, and to the regulation of inflammation and carcinogenesis, appear to be important in the development of pancreatitis and pancreatic carcinoma. These gene mutations are likely to determine each individual's susceptibility for the development of pancreatic disease, the severity of the disease or the disease progression. While some mutations that are associated with a high disease penetrance lead to early disease onset and severe disease phenotypes, others may function in combination with additional genetic changes, defects or environmental cofactors such as toxins and risk factors such as alcohol and tobacco. The identification of such environmental and genetic cofactors, and the elucidation of their interaction, is important for the understanding of the pathophysiology of chronic pancreatitis and pancreatic carcinoma.

CHRONIC PANCREATITIS

Pancreatitis is an inflammatory disease which is initiated by events that cause acinar cell injury, the release of prematurely activated digestive enzymes, subsequent tissue and endothelial damage and the development of a potentially lethal inflammatory response[1].

Chronic pancreatitis (CP) is clinically characterized by acinar cell degeneration and fibrosis that may lead to destruction of exocrine and endocrine organ function and results in maldigestion and diabetes mellitus. Several underlying conditions appear to play a role in the pathogenesis of chronic pancreatitis. Recent progress in molecular techniques has intensified the search for genetic changes that play a role in the onset and progression of inflammation. A number of human inborn genetic varieties have been found to be associated with the development of chronic pancreatitis.

HEREDITARY PANCREATITIS

In 1952 a hereditary predisposition to chronic pancreatitis that is independent of additional environmental factors was reported in a number of families by Comfort and Steinberg[2]. Hereditary pancreatitis (HP) is an autosomal dominant disorder with a clinical manifestation that is indistinguishable from other aetiological varieties of pancreatitis. In affected patients, HP begins with recurrent attacks of acute pancreatitis that usually start in childhood, but the age of onset of the disease can vary and can sometimes be delayed until late in adulthood. The severity of disease ranges from mild to complicated cases with progression to pancreatic necrosis and organ failure. Recurrent attacks of pancreatitis frequently progress to chronic disease at an early age and are associated with a significant lifetime risk for the development of pancreatic cancer. Although hereditary pancreatitis is not a very common disease, and to date only several hundred families have been identified worldwide, the studies addressing the onset of hereditary pancreatitis have permitted some recent breakthroughs in understanding the pathophysiology of acute and chronic pancreatitis in general.

CATIONIC TRYPSINOGEN

In 1996 a mutation in the cationic trypsinogen gene on chromosome 7 in families with hereditary pancreatitis was reported, and this was an early success in the effort to understand the pathophysiology of acute and chronic pancreatitis on a molecular level[3]. This mutation leads to a substitution of the amino acid arginine (R) to histidine (H) at position 122 and is the most common mutation in the cationic trypsinogen gene in patients with HP. A pathophysiological mechanism through which carriers of the R122H mutation develop pancreatitis has been proposed in that this amino acid substitution leads to a gain of trypsin function by either a more rapid or more efficient intracellular trypsinogen activation, or by an impaired inactivation and autolysis, once the trypsin is enzymatically activated. In either case the result would be an extended trypsinogen activity that may initiate an autodigestive process within the acinar cell. The trypsin crystal structure[4] and recent biochemical data[5] are consistent with the hypothesis that R122 represents the trypsin autolysis site which may become disrupted by a R122H mutation. This mutation affects an important failsafe mechanism against premature activation or 'over'-activation' of trypsin within the pancreas, and enhances or prolongs the trypsin protease function. Recently three groups independently reported families with an arginine–cystein exchange mutation affecting the same codon 122 (R122C)[6–8]. Interestingly, R122C trypsinogen appears to differ from the R122H mutant by a greatly reduced autoactivation and an increased resistance to autolysis. Activation of recombinantly expressed R122C mutant human trypsinogen by cathepsin-B was also greatly reduced, which is presumably due to a misfolding caused by disulphide mismatches. If this protein misfolding reflects the 'in vivo' situation, a dramatic loss of cellular trypsin activity should be observed, and this raises the fundamental question whether a gain or a loss of trypsin function is crucial for the triggering mechanism in HP. Despite the remaining uncertainty about the molecular events that precede the induction of pancreatitis, it its remarkable that two different mutations, as well as a silent polymorphism, have been found at the same codon 122 of cationic trypsinogen. This arginine 122 therefore appears to represent a key site for the biochemical properties of trypsin and the events that determine the onset of pancreatitis. Support for a fundamental role of the arginine 122 in the disease process and its 'hot-spot' function comes from the recent discovery of a spontaneous *'de novo'* R122H mutation at this site[9]. Without knowing the frequency of such spontaneous mutations the finding suggests that the diagnosis of hereditary pancreatitis – as defined by a genetic predisposition – must be considered even in the complete absence of a familial history for pancreatitis.

Another disease-relevant trypsinogen mutation leading to a substitution of asparagine by isoleucine at position 29 (N29I) has been suggested to result in a conformational change of the trypsin molecule that prevents proteolytic accession of its autolysis site and therefore renders trypsin more resistant to inactivation. Crystallographic data confirm that N29 is in short proximity to R122H on the protein surface, and the main support for this hypothesis comes from *in-vitro* studies of recombinant rat cationic trypsinogen[10]. However, enhanced autoactivation at pH 5.0 has also been reported[5], suggesting an alternative explanation for an increased trypsin function. A comparison of clinical data from R122H and N29I-HP patients suggests that both have a fairly similar clinical course[11].

Furthermore, a mutation in the signal peptide cleavage site has been found associated with chronic pancreatitis[12]. A substitution of valine by alanine at position 16 (A16V) is presumed to interfere with the intracellular processing of trypsinogen, but the pathophysiological mechanisms remains unclear. It has been assumed that A16V may disturb the segregation of trypsinogen from lysosomal cathepsin-B. As a result the colocalized hydrolase cathepsin-B could activate trypsinogen more readily. A16V appears to be a relatively frequent mutation, whose penetrance seems lower than that of the mutations described above.

Other rare mutations have been identified within the trypsinogen activation peptide (D22G, K23R)[13] which is cleaved from the N-terminus of trypsinogen during its proteolytic activation to trypsin. The pathophysiological mechanism suggested here would be an increased autoactivation of trypsinogen leading to elevated trypsin levels that may initiate pancreatitis.

Further trypsinogen variants L104P, R116C and C139F[14] have been described in a mutational screening of patients with non-alcoholic chronic pancreatitis. However, to date these mutations have been reported only in single individuals, and therefore their relevance to the pathogenesis of pancreatitis remains open.

The discovery of not only one single mutation, but of at least five independently acting mutations in the cationic trypsinogen gene is evidence for a genetic heterogeneity in HP.

PANCREATIC SECRETORY TRYPSIN INHIBITOR (SPINK-1)

The pancreatic secretory trypsin inhibitor gene (PSTI), a 59 amino acid long Kazal type 1 serine protease inhibitor (SPINK-1), is synthesized in acinar cells as a 79 amino acid single-chain polypeptide precursor, that is subsequently processed to the mature peptide and that is secreted into pancreatic ducts. It is regarded as a first-line defence system that is capable of inhibiting up to 20% of total trypsin activity which may result from accidental premature activation of trypsinogen to trypsin within acinar cells. Initial studies on the role of PSTI mutations in CP patients reported that some of these patients had a point mutation in exon 3 of the PSTI gene that leads to the substitution of an asparagine by serine at position 34 (N34S).

Analysis of intronic sequences showed that the N34S mutation is in complete linkage disequilibrium with four additional sequence variants: IVS1-37TC, IVS2+268AG, IVS3-604GA and IVS3-69insTTTT. In a number of studies further mutations and polymorphisms have been detected in PSTI which also include a methionine to threonine exchange that destroys the start codon of PSTI (1MT). These are a leucine to proline exchange in codon 14 (L14P), an aspartate to glutamine exchange in codon 50 (D50E) and a proline to serine exchange in codon 55 (P55). Few studies have reported the frequencies of these mutations and they seem to be fairly low in comparison to the N34S mutation. Most studies have therefore apparently restricted their analysis to this most frequent N34S mutation. N34S is found at a low abundance of 0.4–2.5% in the normal healthy population but is much more common among selected groups of CP patients. Due to inconsistent selection criteria different groups reported N34S mutations in 6%, 19%, 26% or even 86% of alcoholic, hereditary or familial idiopathic pancreatitis patient groups[15–19]. The prevalence of the N34S mutation appears to be increased in pancreatitis, but does not follow a clear Mendelian inheritance pattern. In HP associated with mutations in the cationic trypsinogen gene, studies have demonstrated that an additional presence of SPINK1 mutations affects neither the penetrance nor the disease severity nor the onset of a secondary diabetes mellitus[20]. While this does not rule out that SPINK1 is a 'weak' risk factor for the onset of pancreatitis in general, it makes a role for the onset of HP associated with 'strong' PRSS1 mutations very unlikely.

In studies that analysed the association of PSTI with tropical pancreatitis, an endemic variety of pancreatitis in Africa and Asia, several groups reported a strong association of N34S in populations in India and Bangladesh. Tropical pancreatitis is a type of idiopathic CP of so-far-unknown aetiology that can be categorized by its clinical manifestations into either tropical calcific pancreatitis (TCP) or fibrocalculous pancreatic diabetes (FCPD). While frequencies of the N34S mutation in the normal control population are comparable to previous reports from Europe and North America (1.3%), the mutation was found in 55% and 29% of FCDP patients and in 20% and 36% of TCP patients in Bangladesh and South India respectively[21,22]. Mutations in the PSTI gene may define a genetic predisposition for pancreatitis and apparently lower the threshold for pancreatitis caused by other factors.

CFTR

Two groups[23,24] reported in 1998 a strong association of cystic fibrosis transmembrane conductance regulator gene (CFTR) mutations with idiopathic chronic pancreatitis (ICP). While CFTR mutations are well known to cause cystic fibrosis (CF), the most frequent autosomal recessive inherited disease in Caucasians, typical features of CF include progressive obstructive pulmonary disease, pancreatic insufficiency, abnormal sweat secretion, and male infertility. Children with CFTR mutations are often born with a severely damaged, fibrotic pancreas and pancreatic insufficiency. CFTR, an adenosine 3',5'-cyclic monophosphare (cAMP) and phosphorylation-regulated chloride channel performs a critical role in the regulation of epithelial ion transport. The reduction in CFTR protein function by (to date) more than 1000 registered gene variations (www.genet.sickkids.on.ca/cftr/) appears to affect type and severity of epithelial disease phenotypes.

In the pancreas, CFTR is expressed in centroacinar and proximal intralobular duct cells and also in apical cell membranes[25] of acinar cells. In a recent study[26] insight into the pathomechanisms of CF-related pancreatic disease, expanding the theory of inspisated pancreatic secretions as a main factor for pancreatic injury, is provided. The study revealed that a proinflammatory, anti-apoptotic pathway is responsible for the susceptibility to acute pancreatitis.

To date more than 1000 CFTR mutations are known; however, commercial tests generally detect only a few severe mutations that are known to cause classical CF. While individuals with two identifiable deleterious CFTR mutations have at least mild CF, the risk of pancreatitis in humans with atypical CF so far is believed to apply to compound heterozygotes rather than simple heterozygotes. In a recent publication it was shown that CF carrier status for different types of CFTR mutations, including uncommon/mild mutations, also significantly increases the risk of developing pancreatitis[27]. These data also indicate that a co-occurrence of SPINK1 mutations in ICP is not required for CFTR mutations to confer their risk for developing pancreatitis. The degree of CFTR functional impairment obviously is important for an increased susceptibility to pancreatitis, but even uncommon/mild mutations must be considered as potential risk factors for the disease.

GENETIC PREDISPOSITION IN CHRONIC ALCOHOLIC PANCREATITIS

Alcohol remains one of the most important risk factors that are associated with chronic pancreatitis. In industrialized countries, long-term alcohol abuse accounts for approximately 70% of chronic pancreatitis, whereas in 25% the cause remains generally unknown. While acute pancreatitis is caused in approximately 50% by events unrelated to alcohol, alcohol-related pancreatitis presents in most cases as a chronic disease state. Recurrent episodes of acute inflammatory conditions may lead over a period of time to chronic inflammation and fibrosis. The correlation between alcohol abuse and chronic pancreatitis is not strict, as it appears that less than 5% of alcoholics develop pancreatitis as a consequence of excessive ethanol consumption. Why the pancreas of one individual is more susceptible to alcohol than that of others, and why the development of alcoholic pancreatitis appears to follow such different routes in individual alcoholics, has prompted many investigators to study genetic predisposition. The discovery of specific gene mutations in HP was therefore an opportunity to search for a potential role of these mutations on the association between alcohol intake and chronic pancreatitis.

A number of studies screened for HP-associated cationic trypsinogen mutations in alcoholic pancreatitis patients[28,29] but the results indicate that neither R122 nor N29I mutations represent a major risk factor in alcoholic pancreatitis. The frequency of the SPINK N34S mutation in alcoholics was also analysed by several groups and found to be slightly elevated compared to the control population[17,18].

This low but statistically significant frequency also rules out a major role of N34S mutations, but suggests some possible relevance for the intrapancreatic protease inhibitor function of SPINK1 in certain individuals with alcoholic pancreatitis. So far, however, detailed reports about the clinical characteristics of patients with SPINK1 N34S mutations and alcoholic pancreatitis are few, and it remains unclear whether SPINK1 mutations have an impact on the clinical course of alcoholic chronic pancreatitis.

Further studies have analysed mutations in some other genes such as the cystic fibrosis transmembrane conductance regulator (CFTR) gene or the gene for alcohol dehydrogenase[30–32], but they revealed no conclusive evidence for the existence of an association with alcoholic chronic pancreatitis. While the SPINK1 N34S mutation may represent a minor genetic risk factor for the development of alcoholic pancreatitis, it does not appear to be the initiating cause.

INBORN ERRORS OF METABOLISM

A number of metabolic disorders have been reported in families to be associated with chronic pancreatitis. While, in most of these diseases, pancreatitis is not the most serious clinical manifestation of the underlying metabolic defect, some disorders are known to cause dramatically increased plasma concentrations of chylomicrons and triglycerides. Hyperlipidaemia, as a consequence of familial disorders of lipid metabolism, is generally considered to put patients at a significant risk of developing pancreatitis[33–35]. An extensive plasma accumulation of chylomicrons and triglycerides is found in patients with lipoprotein lipase deficiency or apolipoprotein C-II deficiency. Both proteins confer an important metabolic function in the hydrolysis of triglycerides and the production of free fatty acids. Therefore, genetic disorders in either of these genes can lead to a genetic predisposition for pancreatitis. Carriers of currently more than 30 disease-relevant lipoprotein lipase gene mutations can be identified by reduced catalytic activity in post-heparin plasma or by genetic testing. The mode of inheritance is autosomal recessive and the disease has a low incidence of 1 in 1 000 000. The first symptoms arise in early childhood and nearly 30% of patients with lipoprotein lipase deficiency develop recurrent episodes of pancreatitis. Apolipoprotein C-II deficiency is usually diagnosed at a later age during adolescence or in young adults, often with a similar clinical presentation of recurrent episodes of pancreatitis. More than 10 disease-relevant mutations have so far been identified in the apolipoprotein C-II gene which apparently interfere with the biological function of apolipoprotein C-II as an activator of lipoprotein lipase. Up to 60% of affected patients develop pancreatitis as a frequent and severe complication which can result in chronic exocrine and endocrine pancreatic insufficiency[36,37].

Several other disorders of lipid metabolism have been reported which can lead to chylomicronaemia or hypertriglyceridaemia and which are independent of the lipoprotein lipase system. They represent a significant risk factor for the development of pancreatitis when plasma triglyceride levels rise above 2000 mg/dl. The most common familial disorders associated with chylomicronaemia are type I and type V hyperlipoproteinaemias (according to Levy and Fredrickson) that comprise a diverse family of disorders with moderate to severe hypertriglyceridaemia[38].

POLYMORPHISMS IN GENES OF THE INFLAMMATORY RESPONSE SYSTEM

Proinflammatory and regulatory cytokines such as tumour necrosis factor-alpha (TNF-α) and interleukin 10 (IL-10) play an important role in the initial stages of the disease and in the development of severe pancreatitis. In addition to mutations that act with environmental risk factors in affecting disease susceptibility, some genetic polymorphisms have been shown to influence the severity of diseases by their control of the inflammatory response. Even though polymorphic alleles sometimes have a high frequency in the population, and may be considered 'physiologically normal', they may have a moderate effect on the function of a gene product. Their disease-relevant mechanism may involve the transcription efficiency, the stability of mRNA or protein products or impaired protein–protein interactions that lead to a modulation in biological function. A recent study[39] investigated cytokine genotypes in 190 pancreatitis patients and found no differences in polymorphism frequencies of TNF-α, IL-10 and IL-1 receptor antagonist gene loci between pancreatitis patients and control individuals. In a similar report[40] it was concluded that TNF-α and IL-10 play no role in the determination of disease severity or susceptibility to acute pancreatitis. The same group, however, found that allele 1 of the IL-1RN polymorphism was significantly increased in patients with acute pancreatitis and appears to determine the disease phenotype[41].

Polymorphisms in α_1-antitrypsin and α_2-macroglobulin have been suggested to play a moderating but not a dominant role in the course of alcoholic pancreatitis[42]. Sequence variations in the TNF-α promoter region have also been analysed, and the variant TNF-238A has been reported to be a relevant risk factor for disease manifestation in families with HP[43].

PANCREATIC CARCINOMA

Pancreatic cancer is a disorder from which most affected patients die. It has the worst survival rate of any major cancer. In the US, and according to the latest estimates, 30 700 patients were diagnosed with this condition and 30 000 Americans died from it in the year 2004.

Survival rates are somewhat stage-dependent with a 5-year survival rate of only 17% for local disease, whereas only a minority of patients presents with local disease. This is a result of the clinical inability to diagnose pancreatic cancer early by symptoms alone, and the current lack of blood or imaging tests which can accurately detect cancer prior to symptom onset in the general population. The low incidence of pancreatic cancer in the general population does not make it practical to screen for this disease at this time; however, high-risk groups can be identified which may benefit by detecting a tumour at an earlier, more curable, stage. The most promising of those are subjects or patients from families in which a definitive gene has been identified, that conveys an increased risk of developing pancreatic cancer and can be genetically tested for. In addition to HP, which increases the pancreatic cancer risk 40–70-fold, and due to extensive research in recent years, many tumour syndromes such as HBOC (hereditary breast and ovarian cancer), PJS (Peutz–Jeghers syndrome), HNPCC (hereditary non-polyposis colorectal cancer) and FAMM (familial atypical multiple mole melanoma) are known to have an increased risk of developing pancreatic carcinoma.

Additionally a high number of other gene mutations than those in the PRSS1 gene has also been identified to be associated with pancreatic carcinoma.

HEREDITARY BREAST AND OVARIAN CANCER SYNDROME (HBOC)

Patients diagnosed with HBOC syndrome show a hereditary predisposition to develop early-onset breast and ovarian cancer, whereas other malignant tumours are also associated with this syndrome such as prostate, colon and pancreatic carcinoma[44]. Women diagnosed with HBOC have an approximate 80% lifetime risk of developing breast cancer and an approximate 40% lifetime risk of developing ovarian cancer. The disease is caused by germline mutations in the genes coding for BRCA1 on chromosome 17q21 and BRCA2 on chromosome 13q12–q13[45–47]. Two recently reported studies demonstrated that the relative risk for developing pancreatic cancer in BRCA1 carriers was found to be 2.26[48], whereas patients who carry a BRCA2 mutation have a 2.2 relative risk of developing pancreatic carcinoma[49]. Although the accumulated data suggest that the overall lifetime risk for pancreatic carcinoma in BRCA1 and BRCA2 carriers is likely to be low, genetic counselling to identify a potential genetic predisposition to pancreatic cancer should be referred if two or more family members (first-degree relatives of each other) with pancreatic cancer with or without breast or ovarian cancer exists, if one pancreatic cancer case exists with at least two relatives with early age onset (< 50 years) and onset of breast cancer or ovarian cancer at any age, if one pancreatic cancer case with at least three cases of breast cancer or one case of ovarian cancer and one or more cases of breast cancer exists. In Ashkenazi Jewish ancestries with one pancreatic cancer case and a single case (or more) of breast or ovarian cancer at any age in a first- or second-degree relative (testing for the three Ashkenazi Jewish founder mutations may be sufficient) should also be referred.

PEUTZ–JEGHERS SYNDROME (PJS)

PJS is an autosomal dominant inherited disease. It is characterized by the development of multiple gastrointestinal hamartomatous polyps and mucocutaneous pigmentation. Affected individuals with this disease show an increased risk for developing pancreas, colon, breast, endometrial, ovarian, lung or testes cancer with an estimated incidence of 1:25 000. Pancreatic carcinoma plays a prominent role with an estimated lifetime risk of 36%[50]. The syndrome is caused by germline mutations in the STK11/LKB1 gene, located on chromosome 19p13.3, which codes for a serine–threonine protein kinase which seems to have a tumour-suppressor function[51,52].

Individuals should be referred for genetic counselling to identify a potential genetic predisposition to pancreatic cancer if the individual can be clinically diagnosed with PJS based on an individual who has two or more histologically verified Peutz–Jeghers polyps, small bowel polyposis and mucocutaneous hyperpigmentation, or if an individual has small bowel polyposis, mucocutaneous hyperpigmentation and a family history of PJS.

HEREDITARY NON-POLYPOSIS COLORECTAL CANCER SYNDROME (HNPCC)

HNPCC is a condition that is characterized by an increased risk of colon cancer and other cancers that include malignant tumours of endometrium, ovary, stomach, small intestines, hepatobiliary tract, upper urinary tract, brain and skin.

The disease is caused by a germline mutation in mismatch repair genes, including MLH1 and MSH2[53]. Individuals diagnosed with HNPCC have an approximate 80% chance of developing colon cancer in their lifetime. The average age of onset for colorectal cancer in these individuals is 44 years. Women diagnosed with HNPCC have a 20–60% chance of developing endometrial cancer in their lifetime with an average of diagnosis of 46 years. In several HNPCC kindreds the development of pancreatic carcinoma was reported[54]. The relative risk of developing pancreatic cancer is increased 1.5-fold.

A clinical diagnosis of HNPCC can be based on one of the following two criteria:

1. The Amsterdam criteria states that an individual can be diagnosed with HNPCC if:

   (a) At least three individuals in the family are diagnosed with colorectal cancer.

   (b) The affected individuals represent two generations in the family.

(c) One of the affected individuals must be a first-degree relative (parent, sibling, or child) of the other two.

(d) At least one individual must be diagnosed with a colorectal cancer before the age of 50.

2. The Amsterdam II criteria states that an individual can be diagnosed with HNPCC if:

(a) At least three individuals in the family are diagnosed with an HNPCC-related cancer.

(b) The affected individuals represent two generations in the family.

(c) One of the affected individuals must be a first-degree relative (parent, sibling, or child) of the other two.

(d) At least one individual must be diagnosed with an HNPCC-related cancer before the age of 50.

FAMILIAL ATYPICAL MULTIPLE MOLE MELANOMA (FAMMM)

Individuals with FAMMM have a familial predisposition to developing atypical moles that can develop into melanoma. Melanoma can also develop *de novo* in these individuals. The average age of initial melanoma diagnosis is 34. Those diagnosed with FAMMM may have an increased risk of developing pancreatic cancer and astrocytomas[55]. The disease is associated with germline mutations in the P16INK4 (CDKN2A) gene on chromosome 9p21[56].

Whelan et al. described the occurrence of a p16 mutation in a pancreatic cancer-prone family that showed an excess of malignant melanomas. Genetic testing of asymptomatic members of these families has identified several healthy individuals who carry this mutation and thus are at high risk for the development of pancreatic cancer[57]. Goldstein et al. found a 13–22-fold prospective risk of pancreatic cancer in FAMMM kindreds with the p16 mutation[58]. Vasen et al. estimated the cumulative risk of developing pancreatic cancer of 17% by the age of 75 in putative p16 mutation carriers from 19 FAMMM families[59].

The Melanoma Genetics Consortium has recommended that clinical testing be confined to confirming research results and not routinely offered. With that in mind individuals diagnosed with FAMMM have the option of enrolling in research protocols if an individual has a personal history of melanoma and a first-degree relative with melanoma, if an individual has three or more primary melanomas or if an individual has two or more first-degree relatives with melanoma.

HEREDITARY PANCREATITIS (HP)

As mentioned above, HP is an autosomal dominant inherited disorder with an incomplete phenotypic penetrance of 80%. It is characterized by an onset of recurrent attacks of acute pancreatitis in childhood or young adulthood and frequent progression to chronic pancreatitis. Patients with HP have an approximately 60–70-fold increased risk of developing pancreatic cancer[60]. Tobacco smoking seems to further increase this risk[61,62].

Existing methods for diagnosing pancreatic cancer, such as tumour markers, endoscopy and radiological imaging, barely reach the sensitivity and specificity needed for an early diagnosis of tumours when they are still safely resectable. To date no prospective study has addressed the clinical utility of any of these diagnostic tools in screening patients with HP for early cancer, but some conclusions can be drawn from other clinical trials or personal experience with HP patients.

References

1. Lerch MM, Saluja AK, Dawra R, Ramarao P, Saluja M, Steer ML. Acute necrotizing pancreatitis in the opossum: earliest morphological changes involve acinar cells. Gastroenterology. 1992;103:205–13.
2. Comfort MW, Steinberg AG. Pedigree of a family with hereditary chronic relapsing pancreatitis. Gastroenterology. 1952;21:54–63.
3. Whitcomb DC, Gorry MC, Preston RA et al. Hereditary pancreatitis is caused by a mutation in the cationic trypsinogen gene. Nat Genet. 1996;14:141–5.
4. Gaboriaud C, Serre L, Guy-Crotte O, Forrest E, Fontecilla-Camps JC. Crystal structure of human trypsin 1: unexpected phosphorylation of Tyr151. J Mol Biol. 1996;259:995–1010.
5. Sahin-Toth M. Human cationic trypsinogen. Role of Asn-21 in zymogen activation and implications in hereditary pancreatitis. J Biol Chem. 2000;275:22750–5.
6. Le Marechal C, Chen JM, Quere I, Raguenes O, Ferec C, Auroux J. Discrimination of three mutational events that result in a disruption of the R122 primary autolysis site of the human cationic trypsinogen (PRSS1) by denaturing high performance liquid chromatography. BMC Genet. 2001;2:19.
7. Simon P, Weiss FU, Sahin-Toth M et al. Hereditary pancreatitis caused by a novel PRSS1 mutation (Arg-122 → Cys) that alters autoactivation and autodegradation of cationic trypsinogen. J Biol Chem. 2002;277:5404–10.
8. Pfutzer R, Myers E, Applebaum-Shapiro S et al. Novel cationic trypsinogen (PRSS1) N29T and R122C mutations cause autosomal dominant hereditary pancreatitis. Gut. 2002;50: 271–2.
9. Simon P, Weiss FU, Zimmer KP et al. Spontaneous and sporadic trypsinogen mutations in idiopathic pancreatitis. J Am Med Assoc. 2002;288:2122.
10. Sahin-Toth M. Hereditary pancreatitis-associated mutation asn(21) → ile stabilizes rat trypsinogen *in vitro*. J Biol Chem. 1999;274:29699–704.
11. Keim V, Bauer N, Teich N, Simon P, Lerch MM, Mossner J. Clinical characterization of patients with hereditary pancreatitis and mutations in the cationic trypsinogen gene. Am J Med. 2001;111:622–6.
12. Witt H, Luck W, Becker M. A signal peptide cleavage site mutation in the cationic trypsinogen gene is strongly associated with chronic pancreatitis. Gastroenterology. 1999;117:7–10.
13. Teich N, Ockenga J, Hoffmeister A, Manns M, Mossner J, Keim V. Chronic pancreatitis associated with an activation-peptide mutation that facilitates trypsin activation. Gastroenterology. 2000;119:461–5.
14. Ferec C, Raguenes O, Salomon R et al. Mutations in the cationic trypsinogen gene and evidence for genetic heterogeneity in hereditary pancreatitis. J Med Genet. 1999;36:228–32.
15. Witt H, Luck W, Hennies HC et al. Mutations in the gene encoding the serine protease inhibitor, Kazal type 1 are associated with chronic pancreatitis. Nat Genet. 2000;25: 213–6.
16. Pfutzer RH, Barmada MM, Brunskill AP et al. SPINK1/PSTI polymorphisms act as disease modifiers in familial and idiopathic chronic pancreatitis. Gastroenterology. 2000;119:615–23.

17. Threadgold J, Greenhalf W, Ellis I et al. The N34S mutation of SPINK1 (PSTI) is associated with a familial pattern of idiopathic chronic pancreatitis but does not cause the disease. Gut. 2002;50:675–81.
18. Drenth JP, te Morsche R, Jansen JB. Mutations in serine protease inhibitor Kazal type 1 are strongly associated with chronic pancreatitis. Gut. 2002;50:687–92.
19. Truninger K, Witt H, Kock J et al. Mutations of the serine protease inhibitor, Kazal type 1 gene, in patients with idiopathic chronic pancreatitis. Am J Gastroenterol. 2002;97:1133–7.
20. Weiss FU, Simon P, Witt H et al. SPINK1 mutations and phenotypic expression in patients with pancreatitis associated with trypsinogen mutations. J Med Genet. 2003;40:e40.
21. Schneider A, Suman A, Rossi L et al. SPINK1/PSTI mutations are associated with tropical pancreatitis and type II diabetes mellitus in Bangladesh. Gastroenterology. 2002;123:1026–30.
22. Chandak GR, Idris MM, Reddy DN, Bhaskar S, Sriram PV, Singh L. Mutations in the pancreatic secretory trypsin inhibitor gene (PSTI/SPINK1) rather than the cationic trypsinogen gene (PRSS1) are significantly associated with tropical calcific pancreatitis. J Med Genet. 2002;39:347–51.
23. Cohn JA, Friedman KJ, Noone PG, Knowles MR, Silverman LM, Jowell PS. Relation between mutations of the cystic fibrosis gene and idiopathic pancreatitis. N Engl J Med. 1998;339:653–8.
24. Sharer N, Schwarz M, Malone G et al. Mutations of the cystic fibrosis gene in patients with chronic pancreatitis. N Engl J Med. 1998;339:645–52.
25. Zeng W, Lee MG, Muallem S. Membrane-specific regulation of Cl- channels by purinergic receptors in rat submandibular gland acinar and duct cells. J Biol Chem. 1997;272:32956–65.
26. DiMagno MJ, Lee SH, Hao Y, Zhou SY, McKenna BJ, Owyang C. A proinflammatory, antiapoptotic phenotype underlies the susceptibility to acute pancreatitis in cystic fibrosis transmembrane regulator (–/–) mice. Gastroenterology. 2005;129:665–81.
27. Weiss FU, Simon P, Bogdanova N et al. Complete cystic fibrosis transmembrane conductance regulator gene sequencing in patients with idiopathic chronic pancreatitis and controls. Gut. 2005;54: 1456–60.
28. Creighton J, Lyall R, Wilson DI, Curtis A, Charnley R. Mutations of the cationic trypsinogen gene in patients with chronic pancreatitis. Lancet. 1999;354:42–3.
29. Monaghan KG, Jackson CE, KuKuruga DL, Feldman GL. Mutation analysis of the cystic fibrosis and cationic trypsinogen genes in patients with alcohol-related pancreatitis. Am J Med Genet. 2000;94:120–4.
30. Norton ID, Apte MV, Dixson H et al. Cystic fibrosis genotypes and alcoholic pancreatitis. J Gastroenterol Hepatol. 1998;13:496–9.
31. Haber PS, Norris MD, Apte MV et al. Alcoholic pancreatitis and polymorphisms of the variable length polythymidine tract in the cystic fibrosis gene. Alcohol Clin Exp Res. 1999;23:509–12.
32. Haber PS, Apte MV, Applegate TL et al. Metabolism of ethanol by rat pancreatic acinar cells. J Lab Clin Med. 1998; 132:294–302.
33. Hata A, Ridinger DN, Sutherland S et al. Binding of lipoprotein lipase to heparin. Identification of five critical residues in two distinct segments of the amino-terminal domain. J Biol Chem. 1993;268:8447–57.
34. Brunzell JD, Schrott HG. The interaction of familial and secondary causes of hypertriglyceridemia: role in pancreatitis. Trans Assoc Am Physicians. 1973;86:245–54.
35. Siafakas CG, Brown MR, Miller TL. Neonatal pancreatitis associated with familial lipoprotein lipase deficiency. J Pediatr Gastroenterol Nutr. 1999;29:95–8.
36. Breckenridge WC, Little JA, Steiner G, Chow A, Poapst M. Hypertriglyceridemia associated with deficiency of apolipoprotein C-II. N Engl J Med. 1978; 298:1265–73.
37. Cox DW, Breckenridge WC, Little JA. Inheritance of apolipoprotein C-II deficiency with hypertriglyceridemia and pancreatitis. N Engl J Med. 1978;299:1421–4.
38. Levy RI, Fredrickson DS. Familial hyperlipoproteinemia. In: Stanbury JB, Wyngaarden JB, Fredrickson DS, editors. The Metabolic Basis of Inherited Disease, 3rd edn. New York: MacGraw-Hill, 1972:545.
39. Powell JJ, Fearon KC, Siriwardena AK, Ross JA. Evidence against a role for polymorphisms at tumor necrosis factor, interleukin-1 and interleukin-1 receptor

antagonist gene loci in the regulation of disease severity in acute pancreatitis. Surgery. 2001;129:633–40.

40. Sargen K, Demaine AG, Kingsnorth AN. Cytokine gene polymorphisms in acute pancreatitis. J Pancreas. 2000;1:24–35.

41. Smithies AM, Sargen K, Demaine AG, Kingsnorth AN. Investigation of the interleukin 1 gene cluster and its association with acute pancreatitis. Pancreas. 2000;20:234–40.

42. Teich N, Mossner J, Keim V. Screening for mutations of the cationic trypsinogen gene: are they of relevance in chronic alcoholic pancreatitis? Gut. 1999;44:413–16.

43. Beranek H, Teich N, Witt H, Schulz GU, Mossner J, Keim V. Analysis of tumour necrosis factor alpha and interleukin 10 promotor variants in patients with chronic pancreatitis. Eur J Gastroenterol Hepatol. 2003;15:1223–7.

44. Tulinius H, Olafsdottir GH, Sigvaldason H, Tryggvadottir L, Bjarnadottir K. Neoplastic diseases in families of breast cancer patients. J Med Genet. 1994;31:618–21.

45. Phelan CM, Lancaster JM, Tonin P et al. Mutation analysis of the BRCA2 gene in 49 site-specific breast cancer families. Nat Genet. 1996;13:120–2.

46. Tonin P, Ghadirian P, Phelan C et al. A large multisite cancer family is linked to BRCA2. J Med Genet. 1995;32: 982–4.

47. Simard J, Tonin P, Durocher F et al. Common origins of BRCA1 mutations in Canadian breast and ovarian cancer families. Nat Genet. 1994;8:392–8.

48. Thompson D, Easton DF, Breast Cancer Linkage Consortium. Cancer incidence in BRCA1 mutation carriers. J Natl Cancer Inst. 2002;94:1358–65.

49. Risch HA, McLaughlin JR, Cole DE et al. Prevalence and penetrance of germline BRCA1 and MRCA2 mutations in a population series of 649 women with ovarian cancer. Am J Hum Genet. 2001;68:700–10.

50. Giardiello FM, Brensinger JD, Tersmette AC et al. Very high risk of cancer in familial Peutz–Jeghers syndrome. Gastroenterology. 2000;119:1447–53.

51. Hemminki A, Avizienyte E, Roth S et al. A serine/threonine kinase gene defective in Peutz–Jeghers syndrome. Nature. 1998;391:184–7.

52. Martin SG, St Johnston D. A role for *Drosophila* LKB1 in anterior-posterior axis formation and epithelial polarity. Nature. 2003;421:379–84.

53. Peltomaki P, Vasen HF. Mutations predisposing to hereditary nonpolyposis colorectal cancer: database and results of a collaborative study. International Collaborative Group on Hereditary Nonpolyposis Colorectal Cancer. Gastroenterology. 1997;113:1146–58.

54. Lynch HT, Voorhees GJ, Lanspa SJ, McGreevy PS, Lynch JF. Pancreatic carcinoma and hereditary nonpolyposis colorectal cancer: a family study. Br J Cancer. 1985;52:271–3.

55. Lynch HT, Fusaro RM, Kimberling WJ, Lynch JF, Danes BS. Familial atypical multiple mole-melanoma (FAMMM) syndrome: segregation analysis. J Med Genet. 1983;20:342–4.

56. Borg A, Sandberg T, Nilsson K et al. High frequency of multiple melanomas and breast and pancreas carcinomas in CDKN2A mutation-positive melanoma families. J Natl Cancer Inst. 2000;92:1260–6.

57. Whelan AJ, Bartsch D, Goodfellow PJ. Brief report: a familial syndrome of pancreatic cancer and melanoma with a with a mutation in the CDKN2 tumor-suppressor gene. N Engl J Med. 1995;333:975–7.

58. Goldstein AM, Struewing JP, Chidambaram A, Fraser MC, Tucker MA. Genotype–phenotype relationships in U.S. melanoma prone families with CDKN2A and CDK4 mutations. J Natl Cancer Inst. 2000;92:1006–12.

59. Vasen HF, Gruis NA, Frants RR, van der Velden PA, Hille ET, Bergman W. Risk of developing pancreatic cancer in families with familial atypical multiple melanoma associated with a specific 19 deletion of p16 (p16-Leiden). Int J Cancer. 2000;87:809–11.

60. Perrault J. Hereditary pancreatitis: historical perspectives. Med Clin N Am. 2000;84: 519–29.

61. Lowenfels AB, Maisonneuve P, DiMagno EP et al. Hereditary pancreatiis and the risk of pancreatic cancer: International Herediatry Pancreatitis Study Group. J Natl Cancer Inst. 1997;89:442–6.

62. Lowenfels AB, Maisonneuve P, Whitcomb DC, Lerch MM, DiMagno EP. Cigarette smoking as a risk factor for pancreatic cancer in patients with hereditary pancreatitis. J Am Med Assoc. 2001;286:169–70.

9
Surveillance and diagnostics of chronic pancreatitis

J. MÖSSNER

INTRODUCTION

One has to know the risk factors for the development of chronic pancreatitis: genes, alcohol, smoking, pancreas divisum[1-3]. If one does not find a known risk factor the term sporadic chronic pancreatitis is preferred. In so-called idiopathic chronic pancreatitis risk factors such SPINK mutations (serine protease inhibitor type Kasal) or mutations of CFTR (cystic fibrosis transmembrane conductance regulator) may be found[4-8]. Hereditary chronic pancreatitis is a rather rare autosomal dominant disease. In about 70% mutations of the cationic trypsinogen are found[9-16]. However, 80% of all cases of chronic pancreatitis are preceded by long-term alcohol abuse. In some of these alcoholic patients mutations of CFTR or SPINK may be found, but not of the cationic trypsinogen[17,18]. Tropical pancreatitis is associated with SPINK mutations in more than 30%[19].

Decades of existing chronic inflammation of the pancreas may impose a risk to develop pancreatic cancer[20,21]. The prognosis of patients with alcohol-induced chronic pancreatitis is not good. After 10 years of the disease up to 50% of all patients may have already died[22]. Death is often due not to complications of chronic pancreatitis such as severe relapses or complications of diabetes but due to the general 'life style', such as consequences of alcohol and smoking (lung cancer, cancers in the head, neck and throat region, oesophageal cancers, heart infarction, infectious complications such as pneumonia, accidents). Age at diagnosis, smoking, and drinking are major predictors of mortality in patients with chronic pancreatitis. The risk to develop pancreatic cancer is especially high in patients at ages above 40–50 with hereditary pancreatitis with early onset of chronic pancreatitis[21].

DIAGNOSIS

History, physical examination, symptoms

In about 80% of all cases in industrialized nations long-term alcohol consumption will be reported. However, there seems to be no real threshold regarding the amount of alcohol consumed. Nevertheless, most patients are heavy drinkers. Interestingly alcohol *per se* does not considerably increase the risk of developing pancreatitis since most heavy drinkers do not have chronic pancreatitis[23]. Heavy alcohol consumption usually precedes the first onset of symptoms by about 10–20 years. According to a recent study the diagnosis of chronic pancreatitis was made, on average, 4.7 years earlier in smokers than in non-smokers. In this study tobacco smoking was associated with earlier diagnosis of chronic alcoholic pancreatitis and with earlier appearance of calcifications and diabetes, independent of alcohol consumption[24].

The patient with chronic pancreatitis reports acute and relapsing upper abdominal pain. About 10% have continuous pain. Pain may radiate into the back. Meteorism, vomiting and both constipation and diarrhoea may be additional symptoms. Physical examination reveals deep pain by pressure without signs of peritonitis. Only a few patients present without any abdominal pain syndrome. In cases of severe exocrine dysfunction steatorrhoea and further symptoms of severe maldigestion may be present. Further diseases as a consequence of the lack of fat-soluble vitamins such as skin disorders (vitamin E deficiency), night-blindness (vitamin A deficiency), coagulopathy (vitamin K deficiency), or osteomalacia (vitamin D deficiency) are rather rare. Insulin-dependent diabetes mellitus is mostly a rather late symptom. Exocrine insufficiency is characterized by voluminous yellow, bad-smelling stools with a stool weight above 200 g per day and a fat excretion of more than 7 g per day. Lipase secretion must be decreased by more than 90% for the manifestation of steathorroea[25]. Carbohydrate and protein maldigestion can sometimes be compensated by enzymes of saliva (amylase), stomach (pepsin and HCl) and the gut mucosa (peptidases, saccharidases). However, lipase of gastric fundus is not able to compensate for the lack of pancreatic lipase.

Very often patients are already underweight and signs of heavy smoking (yellow fingers) and alcohol abuse may be seen (neglected body care). Symptoms may be widened by diseases related to nicotine and alcohol abuse such as symptoms due to arteriosclerosis, chronic bronchitis, lung cancer, fatty liver, liver cirrhosis with or without portal hypertension.

Disease progression and prognosis

Before clinical onset of the disease an oligosymptomatic latency phase may exist, followed by acute relapses of pancreatitis. The point of no return after alcohol-induced acute pancreatitis is not known. Some cases of alcohol-induced acute pancreatitis may be acute indeed with 'restitutio ad integrum'. However, in most cases chronic subclinical inflammation of the pancreas precedes the first attack of pancreatitis. The various signs of chronic pancreatitis, such as exocrine and endocrine insufficiency, calcifications and duct dilations, increase with the duration of the disease. Progression of the disease is faster in alcohol-related pancreatitis as compared to idiopathic and hereditary forms[26,27]. In alcohol-related chronic pancreatitis one may expect diabetes after 10 years of the disease in about 45%, whereas in hereditary pancreatitis having an autosomal-dominant mutation of cationic trypsinogen we have observed diabetes in less than 5% after 10 years. According to a retrospective study by the Mayo group the gender distribution was nearly equal in idiopathic chronic pancreatitis, but 72% of patients with alcoholic pancreatitis were men. In early-onset idiopathic pancreatitis, calcification and exocrine and endocrine insufficiency developed more slowly than in late-onset idiopathic and alcoholic pancreatitis. However, in early idiopathic chronic pancreatitis, pain frequently occurred initially and was more severe. In late-onset idiopathic pancreatitis, pain was absent in nearly 50% of patients. Patients with early-onset pancreatitis have initially and thereafter a long course of severe pain, but slowly develop morphological and functional pancreatic damage, whereas patients with late-onset pancreatitis have a mild and often painless course. Both forms differ from alcoholic pancreatitis in their equal gender distribution and a much slower rate of calcification[27].

As to the clinical picture, both alcoholic and hereditary (PRSS1 mutation-associated) chronic pancreatitis exhibit essentially identical clinical laboratory results, histopathology or morphological changes in imaging studies. However, there are marked differences in the clinical course, such as 30 years earlier age of onset, but less frequent pancreatic calcification and diabetes in PRSS1-associated pancreatitis[28]. In the first large investigation of clinical criteria in hereditary pancreatitis, the mean age of onset was 12.9 years[29,30]. Our own investigations revealed no difference in the age of onset between carriers of the N29I or R122H PRSS1 mutations. The median was 13 years in each group. Only 4% of our patients had severe chronic pancreatitis with exocrine and endocrine insufficiency, pancreatic calcifications and duct dilations as well as hospitalizations due to pancreatitis. In general, half of the mutation carriers had few or no complaints or complications[26].

According to the spontaneous course of chronic alcohol-related pancreatitis one can separate four stages:

Stage I, a preclinical stage with no or only minor clinical symptoms.

Stage II, typical signs of acute relapsing pancreatitis and secondary complications. However, definitive signs of chronic pancreatitis are still missing.

Stage III, continuous relapses of pancreatitis and appearance of definitive signs of chronic pancreatitis such as dilations and scars of pancreatic ducts, calcifications, and increasing loss of exocrine and endocrine functional tissue.

Stage IV, undoubted chronic pancreatitis with exocrine and endocrine insufficiency and calcifications. In this stage the severity and frequency of acute relapses may decrease.

In many patients pain decreases with time. According to a study by the Zürich group the average duration of chronic pancreatitis was 17 years. In early stages, episodes of recurrent pancreatitis predominated. Chronic pain was typically associated with local complications such as pseudocysts. All patients achieved complete pain relief in advanced stages[31]. According to another long-term study, alcoholic chronic pancreatitis seems to evolve from severe acute pancreatitis[32]. However, a subgroup of alcoholic acute pancreatitis does not seem to progress to advanced chronic pancreatitis[33]. Interestingly the same group reported that approximately one-third of patients with chronic pancreatitis showed a marked decrease of calcifications in late phases of their disease[34].

A cure for the disease is not possible. Lowenfels et al. undertook a multicentre historical cohort study of 2015 subjects with chronic pancreatitis who were recruited from clinical centres in six countries. A total of 56 cancers were identified among these patients during a mean follow-up of 7.4 years. The cumulative risk of pancreatic cancer in subjects who were followed for at least 2 years increased steadily, and 10 and 20 years after the diagnosis of pancreatitis it was 1.8% and 4.0%, respectively. Thus, the risk of pancreatic cancer is significantly elevated in subjects with chronic pancreatitis and appears to be independent of sex, country, and type of pancreatitis[20]. Another study reported on pancreatic cancers appearing 16–26 times more often in chronic pancreatitis as compared to controls[35]. Besides the chronic inflammation smoking may be a relevant further cause for the increased risk of pancreatic cancer or immune deficiency due to malnutrition and alcohol abuse. However, the importance of the inflammatory process is underlined by the significantly elevated risk of pancreatic cancer in autosomal-dominant inherited chronic pancreatitis[21].

Complications of chronic pancreatitis

There are numerous possible potential complications during the course of the disease, such as jaundice due to scarring of the distal bile duct or compression by a pseudocyst or an inflammatory mass of the pancreatic head. The most common complication is the development of pseudocysts; they cause various symptoms according to their speed of development, their size and location. Pseudocysts may be responsible for pain, jaundice, pancreatic ascites in cases of rupture, severe bleeding in cases of vessel erosions. Fistulas between necrotic pancreatic areas and the chest may lead to pleural effusions.

Diagnosis

Progressive organ destruction is usually preceded by numerous acute relapses of pancreatitis. Thus, diagnosis of chronic pancreatitis is often made on the occasion of such an acute relapse. Definitive signs of chronic pancreatitis such as ductal dilations or calcifications may not be present at an early stage. At this stage one cannot differentiate between acute or already chronic pancreatitis.

There are almost no studies evaluating which diagnostic procedure should be primarily used at a certain stage of the disease. Due to the lack of a 'gold standard' comparisons between various diagnostic procedures regarding sensitivity and specificity must be taken with care. Furthermore those comparisons are usually not performed at clearly defined stages of the disease. There are several reasons for the necessity of diagnosis:

1. Verification of the diagnosis of truly chronic pancreatitis.

2. Evaluation of the residual organ function.

3. Detection of complications that need therapeutic interventions such as either surgery or interventional endoscopy.

4. Clarification of the various causes of pain.

5. Early detection of pancreatic cancer.

Morphological changes do not parallel deteriorations in exocrine and endocrine function. However, a prospective study confirmed that both normal endoscopic retrograde pancreatographic findings and Cambridge III ductal changes on endoscopic retrograde pancreatography correlate well with normal pancreatic function and advanced functional insufficiency, respectively. As diagnostic tools, ultrasound and computed tomography are as sensitive as pancreatography only in chronic pancreatitis with considerable morphological changes[36]. Advanced stages are easily to diagnose both by various imaging procedures and by function tests.

Serum laboratory parameters

An elevation of serum lipase and amylase is usually seen in acute relapses. However, serum enzymes cannot differentiate between acute and chronic pancreatitis. Serum enzymes decrease in cases of severe organ destruction. However, the sensitivity is too low to correlate remaining exocrine function with the level of serum lipase or immunoreactive trypsinogen.

Cholestasis indicating parameters such as alkaline phosphatase and γ-glutamyltransferase are elevated in cases of biliary outlet obstruction. In severe cholestasis, bilirubin may also be elevated.

In diagnosis of a rather rare form of chronic pancreatitis, i.e. autoimmune pancreatitis, immunological parameters such as antibodies against carboanhydrase (CA-II) and pancreatic tissue are employed. It has been reported that the percentage of patients with increased serum CA-II antibodies was higher in idiopathic chronic pancreatitis (28%) than in controls (1.9%) and in patients with alcoholic chronic pancreatitis (CP) (10.5%), but lower than in patients with Sjögren syndrome (64%). The proportion with elevated IgG4 levels was higher in the idiopathic pancreatitis group (15%) compared with controls (1.9%) and Sjögren syndrome (0%) but not significantly different from alcoholic CP (8%). Most autoimmune pancreatitis patients with high IgG4 levels exhibited increased CA-II antibodies. Thus, determination of CA-II Ab and IgG4 may be recommended in suspicion of autoimmune pancreatitis[37].

Pancreatic function tests

Despite its numerous methodological variations, the direct pancreatic function test remains the gold standard in diagnosing a deterioration of exocrine pancreatic function. Pancreatic secretions are collected via a duodenal tube after stimulation of the pancreas by intravenous application of secretin and the synthetic cholecystokinin analogue caerulein. However, this test is cumbersome, expensive and not liked by patients. A recent meta-analysis discusses the sensitivity of non-invasive (tubeless) pancreatic function tests which have been compared with the gold standard, i.e. secretin-CCK direct pancreatic function test. For faecal chymotrypsin a sensitivity of 54% was found in slight, 53% in mild and 89% in severe pancreatic insufficiency. The values for the NBT-PABA test were 49%, 72%, 83%; for the pancreolauryl test 63%, 76%, 85%; for faecal elastase-1 54%, 75%, 79% respectively. Thus, none of the non-invasive pancreatic function tests is sensitive enough to diagnose reliably a slight to moderate exocrine pancreatic insufficiency[38].

IMAGING PROCEDURES

Plain X-ray of the abdomen

Calcifications of the pancreas are usually seen only in advanced stages of chronic pancreatitis. Thus, the specificity of this simple diagnostic tool is high but the sensitivity rather low.

Sonography

Transabdominal sonography is certainly the first diagnostic imaging procedure in the diagnostic algorithm of chronic pancreatitis. It enables an evaluation of an organ enlargement or decrease of organ size, changes in the echo structure, detection of pseudocysts, calcifications, dilation of the main pancreatic duct, and prestenotic dilation of the common bile duct. However, the diagnostic yield is highly dependent on the experience of the investigator and the quality of the instrument. Furthermore, the diagnostic sensitivity is dependent on the stage of the disease and ranges from 60% to 80%.

One recent study reports on sonographic evaluation before and after intravenous secretin application. In healthy pancreas the main pancreatic duct dilated immediately after a bolus injection of secretin and recovered gradually. For the maximal to basal duct diameter ratio, statistically significant differences were found between the control and chronic pancreatitis. Thus, the authors claim that exocrine pancreatic function and the morphological changes of the main pancreatic duct are significantly related. Dynamic ultrasonographic findings may reflect pancreatic function[39].

Oesophagogastro duodenoscopy

Endoscopy has to be performed to exclude other causes of pain such as peptic ulcers, or to detect portal hypertension. Fundic varices may be seen when the splenic vein is thrombotic due to chronic pancreatitis, an impression of the stomach or duodenum by pseudocysts or a stenosis of the duodenum by an inflammatory mass.

Endoscopic ultrasound (EUS)

Endosonography is regarded as the most sensitive imaging procedure to detect chronic pancreatitis, especially early forms. One may see echogenic foci within the gland, focal regions of either reduced or increased echogenicity of the main pancreatic duct wall, accentuation of the gland's lobular pattern, pseudocysts, an irregular contour or dilation of the main pancreatic duct and side branch dilation[40,41]. The usefulness and accuracy rate of EUS in the diagnosis of chronic pancreatitis were prospectively evaluated in 81 patients with suspected pancreatic disease. EUS, abdominal ultrasonography (AUS), computed tomography (CT), and endoscopic retrograde cholangiopancreatography (ERCP) were compared. According to this study the sensitivity of EUS for diagnosis of chronic pancreatitis was 88% versus AUS 58%, ERCP 74%, CT scan 75%. The specificity was 100% for ERCP and EUS, 95% for CT scan, and 75% for AUS[42]. In a recent study 80 consecutive patients with recurrent pancreatitis underwent ERCP, EUS, and secretin test. The secretin test had 100% agreement with normal and severe chronic pancreatitis by EUS criteria, but agreement was poor for mild (13%) and moderate (50%) disease. The agreement between ERCP- and EUS-specific criteria was excellent for normal (100%), moderate (92%), and severe (100%) chronic pancreatitis and poor for mild (17%) disease. Thus, EUS may assist in the diagnosis of early chronic pancreatitis not established by ERCP or secretin test[43]. The specificity of EUS was evaluated in a prospective follow-up study. Patients with normal endoscopic retrograde pancreatography but signs of chronic pancreatitis on EUS were included in a follow-up programme. All patients with chronic pancreatitis confirmed by retrograde pancreatography had ductal or parenchymal changes detectable with EUS. Among 38 patients with normal retrograde pancreatography, 32 presented with morphological features consistent with chronic pancreatitis by EUS. During follow-up of 6–25 months chronic pancreatitis was confirmed by repeat endoscopic retrograde pancreatography in 22 of these 32 patients. Thus, EUS detects chronic pancreatitis in all cases if endoscopic retrograde pancreatography was suggestive for chronic pancreatitis and EUS is more sensitive than endoscopic retrograde pancreatography in the detection of early morphological changes of chronic pancreatitis[44]. EUS seems to be the method of choice to exclude pancreatic dieases in patients with unexplained abdominal pain[45].

Diagnosis of autoimmune pancreatitis may be cumbersome. The EUS features may be mistaken for malignancy. However, a diffusely hypoechoic, enlarged pancreas, together with chronic inflammatory cells in aspirated cytologic specimens, is supportive of the diagnosis of autoimmune pancreatitis. When combined with clinical data, EUS and EUS-guided FNA may support the diagnosis of autoimmune pancreatitis[46].

EUS is the method of choice to measure the distance between the wall of a pseudocyst and either the gastric or duodenal wall. Furthermore, combination with Doppler sonography enables one to detect vessels in the pseudocyst wall. This information is important prior to endoscopic drainage procedures.

Endoscopic retrograde cholangiopancreatography (ERCP)

ERCP has been claimed to be the gold standard in diagnosing chronic pancreatitis. However, as mentioned above, EUS has a higher sensitivity, especially in early stages. A graduation of ductal changes is still made according to the Cambridge classification[47]. However, due to potential procedure-related complications, a merely diagnostic ERCP is seldom perfomed.

Computer tomotraphy

Computer tomography (CT) reveals similar abnormalities in chronic pancreatitis comparable to ultrasound. However, sensitivity and specificity seem to be somehow higher. Bowel gas disturbs the image quality in ultrasound but not in CT. Sensitivity is reported to be between 60% and 95% according to the stage of the disease[48].

Magnetic resonance cholangiopancreatography (MRCP)

ERCP has been the reference technique in the diagnosis of pancreatic duct pathology. MRCP, a non-invasive diagnostic method, could potentially be substituted for ERCP[49]. In a prospective 15-month study in 78 patients with suspected biliopancreatic pathology MRCP was compared with ERCP. Both techniques found the pancreatic tract to be normal and non-dilated in 60 patients. The specificity and sensitivity of MRCP in evaluating the normal pancreatic duct were 98% and 94%, respectively[50]. The sensitivity of MRCP in diagnosing chronic pancreatitis can be increased with dynamic secretin-enhanced magnetic resonance cholangiopancreatography[51-53]. Furthermore, MRCP can assist the diagnosis and management of patients in whom ERCP is not possible, e.g. when the papilla of Vater cannot be accessed in patients after Billroth II gastric resections[54].

Positron emission tomography (PET)

Early diagnosis of pancreatic cancer in chronic pancreatitis remains a major unsolved problem. One study claims that PET may be a solution. FDG-PET was negative in the large majority of chronic pancreatitis patients, which suggests that a positive PET scan in chronic pancreatitis patients must lead to efforts to exclude a malignancy [55].

DIFFERENTIAL DIAGNOSIS AND CONCOMITANT ALCOHOL-RELATED DISEASES

The prevalence of chronic pancreatitis in patients with alcohol-related liver cirrhosis is uncertain. In 72 patients with alcoholic cirrhosis additional chronic pancreatitis was diagnosed in 19% by both EUS and ERCP and an additional 25% had isolated pancreatic parenchymal changes at EUS[56]. The most important differential diagnosis is certainly pancreatic cancer. In some cases this differential diagnosis may be rather cumbersome[57]. According to a study by the Ludwigsburg group MRCP is as sensitive as ERCP in detecting pancreatic carcinomas. The use of MRCP may prevent inappropriate explorations of the pancreatic and common bile ducts in cases of suspected pancreatic carcinomas, where interventional endoscopic therapy is unlikely[58]. A very important study included 510 patients who had a final diagnosis available and who had undergone ultrasound-guided fine-needle biopsy of the pancreas. Sensitivity and specificity, and overall diagnostic accuracy, were evaluated by three different bioptic procedures, i.e. cytology, histology, and cytology plus histology. The reliability of ultrasound-guided fine-needle biopsy to allow a correct diagnosis in the different pancreatic pathologies was calculated. For cytology, histology, and cytology plus histology sensitivity was 87%, 94%, and 94%, specificity 100%; and diagnostic accuracy 91%, 90%, and 95%, respectively[59]. Further studies have to clarify whether EUS-guided fine-needle biopsy may help to solve the problem of diagnosing pancreatic cancer in chronic pancreatitis. An early diagnosis would be especially mandatory in patients with hereditary pancreatitis.

References

1. Bourliere M, Barthet M, Berthezene P, Durbec JP, Sarles H. Is tobacco a risk factor for chronic pancreatitis and alcoholic cirrhosis? Gut. 1991;32:1392–5.
2. DiMagno MJ, DiMagno EP. Chronic pancreatitis. Curr Opin Gastroenterol. 2005;21:544–54.
3. Durbec JP, Sarles H. Multicenter survey of the etiology of pancreatic diseases. Relationship between the relative risk of developing chronic pancreaitis and alcohol, protein and lipid consumption. Digestion. 1978;18:337–50.
4. Audrezet M P, Chen JM, Le Marechal C et al. Determination of the relative contribution of three genes – the cystic fibrosis transmembrane conductance regulator gene, the cationic trypsinogen gene, and the pancreatic secretory trypsin inhibitor gene – to the etiology of idiopathic chronic pancreatitis. Eur J Hum Genet. 2002;10:100–6.
5. Chen JM, Mercier B, Audrezet MP, Ferec J. Mutational analysis of the human pancreatic secretory trypsin inhibitor (PSTI) gene in hereditary and sporadic chronic pancreatitis. J Med Genet. 2000;37:67–9.
6. Cohn JA, Friedman KJ, Noone PG, Knowles MR, Silverman LM, Jowell PS. Relation between mutations of the cystic fibrosis gene and idiopathic pancreatitis. N Engl J Med. 1998;339:653–8.
7. Sharer N, Schwarz M, Malone G et al. Mutations of the cystic fibrosis gene in patients with chronic pancreatitis. N Engl J Med. 1998;339:645–52.
8. Witt H, Luck W, Hennies HC et al. Mutations in the gene encoding the serine protease inhibitor, Kazal type 1 are associated with chronic pancreatitis. Nat Genet. 2000;25:213–16.
9. Gorry MC, Gabbaizedeh D, Furey W et al. Mutations in the cationic trypsinogen gene are associated with recurrent acute and chronic pancreatitis. Gastroenterology. 1997;113:1063–8.

10. Howes N, Lerch MM, Greenhalf W et al. European Registry of Hereditary Pancreatitis and Pancreatic Cancer (EUROPAC). Clinical and genetic characteristics of hereditary pancreatitis in Europe. Clin Gastroenterol Hepatol. 2004;2:252–61.
11. Pfützer RH, Whitcomb DC. Trypsinogen mutations in chronic pancreatitis. Gastroenterology. 1999;117:1507–8.
12. Teich N, Mossner J, Keim V. Mutations of the cationic trypsinogen in hereditary pancreatitis. Hum Mutat. 1998;12:39–43.
13. Teich N, Ockenga J, Hoffmeister A, Manns M, Mössner J, Keim V. Chronic pancreatitis associated with an activation peptide mutation that facilitates trypsin activation. Gastroenterology. 2000;19:461–5.
14. Teich N, Bauer N, Mössner J, Keim V. Mutational screening of patients with nonalcoholic chronic pancreatitis: identification of further trypsinogen variants. Am J Gastroenterol. 2002;97:341–6.
15. Whitcomb DC, Preston RA, Aston CE et al. A gene for hereditary pancreatitis maps to chromosome 7q35. Gastroenterology. 1996;110:1975–80.
16. Whitcomb DC, Gorry MC, Preston RA et al. Hereditary pancreatitis is caused by a mutation in the cationic trypsinogen gene. Nat Genet. 1996;14:141–45.
17. Monaghan KG, Jackson CE, KuKuruga DL, Feldman GL. Mutation analysis of the cystic fibrosis and cationic trypsinogen genes in patients with alcohol-related pancreatitis. Am J Med Genet. 2000;94:120–4.
18. Teich N, Mössner J, Keim V: Screening for mutations of the cationic trypsinogen gene: are they of relevance in chronic alcoholic pancreatitis? Gut. 1999;44:413–16.
19. Hassan Z, Mohan V, Ali L et al. SPINK1 is a susceptibility gene for fibrocalculous pancreatic diabetes in subjects from the Indian subcontinent. Am J Hum Genet. 2002;71: 964–8.
20. Lowenfels AB, Maisonneuve P, Cavallini G et al. Pancreatitis and the risk of pancreatic cancer. International Pancreatitis Study Group. N Engl J Med. 1993;328:1433–7.
21. Lowenfels AB, Maisonneuve P, Whitcomb DC. Risk factors for cancer in hereditary pancreatitis. International Hereditary Pancreatitis Study Group. Med Clin N Am. 2000; 84:565–73.
22. Lowenfels AB, Maisonneuve P, Cavallini G et al. Prognosis of chronic pancreatitis: an international multicenter study. International Pancreatitis Study Group. Am J Gastroenterol. 1994;89:1467–71.
23. Lankisch PG, Lowenfels AB, Maisonneuve P. What is the risk of alcoholic pancreatitis in heavy drinkers? Pancreas. 2002;25:411–12.
24. Maisonneuve P, Lowenfels AB, Mullhaupt B et al. Cigarette smoking accelerates progression of alcoholic chronic pancreatitis. Gut. 2005;54:510–14.
25. DiMagno EP, Go VL, Summerskill WH. Relations between pancreatic enzyme ouputs and malabsorption in severe pancreatic insufficiency. N Engl J Med. 1973;288:813–15.
26. Keim V, Bauer N, Teich N, Simon P, Lerch MM, Mössner J. Clinical characterization of patients with hereditary pancreatitis and mutations in the cationic trypsinogen gene. Am J Med. 2001;111:622–6.
27. Layer P, Yamamoto H, Kalthoff L, Clain JE, Bakken LJ, DiMagno EP. The different courses of early- and late-onset idiopathic and alcoholic chronic pancreatitis. Gastroenterology. 1994;107:1481–7.
28. Keim V, Witt H, Bauer N et al.The course of genetically determined chronic pancreatitis. JOP. 2003;4:146–54.
29. Lowenfels AB, Maisonneuve P, DiMagno EP et al. Hereditary pancreatitis and the risk of pancreatic cancer. International Hereditary Pancreatitis Study Group. J Natl Cancer Inst. 1997;89:442–6.
30. Sossenheimer MJ, Aston CE, Preston RA et al. Clinical characteristics of hereditary pancreatitis in a large family, based on high-risk haplotype. The Midwest Multicenter Pancreatic Study Group (MMPSG). Am J Gastroenterol. 1997;92:1113–16.
31. Ammann RW, Muellhaupt B. The natural history of pain in alcoholic chronic pancreatitis. Gastroenterology. 1999;116:1132–40.
32. Ammann RW, Heitz PU, Klöppel G. Course of alcoholic chronic pancreatitis: a prospective clinicomorphological long-term study. Gastroenterology. 1996;111:224–31.

33. Ammann RW, Muellhaupt B, Meyenberger C, Heitz PU. Alcoholic nonprogressive chronic pancreatitis: prospective long-term study of a large cohort with alcoholic acute pancreatitis (1976–1992). Pancreas. 1994;9:365–73.
34. Ammann RW, Muench R, Otto R, Buehler H, Freiburghaus AU, Siegenthaler W. Evolution and regression of pancreatic calcification in chronic pancreatitis. A prospective long-term study of 107 patients. Gastroenterology. 1988;95:1018–28.
35. Malka D, Hammel P, Maire F et al. Risk of pancreatic adenocarcinoma in chronic pancreatitis. Gut. 2002;51:849–52.
36. Bozkurt T, Braun U, Leferink S, Gilly G, Lux G. Comparison of pancreatic morphology and exocrine functional impairment in patients with chronic pancreatitis. Gut. 1994;35: 1132–6.
37. Aparisi L, Farre A, Gomez-Cambronero L et al. Antibodies to carbonic anhydrase and IgG4 levels in idiopathic chronic pancreatitis: relevance for diagnosis of autoimmune pancreatitis. Gut. 2005;54:703–9.
38. Siegmund E, Löhr JM, Schuff-Werner P. The diagnostic validity of non-invasive pancreatic function tests – a meta-analysis. Z Gastroenterol. 2004;42:1117–28.
39. Osawa S, Kataoka K, Sakagami J et al. Relation between morphologic changes in the main pancreatic duct and exocrine pancreatic function after a secretin test. Pancreas. 2002;25: 12–19.
40. Wallace MB, Hawes RH, Durkalski V et al. The reliability of EUS for the diagnosis of chronic pancreatitis: interobserver agreement among experienced endosonographers. Gastrointest Endosc. 2001;53:294–9.
41. Wiersema MJ, Hawes RH, Lehman GA, Kochman ML, Sherman S, Kopecky KK. Prospective evaluation of endoscopic ultrasonography and endoscopic retrograde cholangiopancreatography in patients with chronic abdominal pain of suspected pancreatic origin. Endoscopy. 1993;25:555–64.
42. Buscail L, Escourrou J, Moreau J et al. Endoscopic ultrasonography in chronic pancreatitis: a comparative prospective study with conventional ultrasonography, computed tomography, and ERCP. Pancreas. 1995;10:251–7.
43. Catalano MF, Lahoti S, Geenen JE, Hogan WJ. Prospective evaluation of endoscopic ultrasonography, endoscopic retrograde pancreatography, and secretin test in the diagnosis of chronic pancreatitis. Gastrointest Endosc. 1998;48:11–17.
44. Leodolter A, Pross M, Schulz HU, Malfertheiner P. EUS in the diagnosis of early chronic pancreatitis: a prospective follow-up study. Gastrointest Endosc. 2002;55:507–11.
45. Sahai AV, Mishra G, Penman ID et al. EUS to detect evidence of pancreatic disease in patients with persistent or nonspecific dyspepsia. Gastrointest Endosc. 2000;52:153–9.
46. Farrell JJ, Garber J, Sahani D, Brugge WR. EUS findings in patients with autoimmune pancreatitis. Gastrointest Endosc. 2004;60:927–36.
47. Sarner M, Cotton PB. Classification of pancreatitis. Gut. 1984;25:756–9.
48. Luetmer PH, Stephens DH, Ward EM. Chronic pancreatitis: reassessment with current CT. Radiology. 1989;171:353–7.
49. Sica GT, Braver J, Cooney MJ, Miller FH, Chai JL, Adams DF. Comparison of endoscopic retrograde cholangiopancreatography with MR cholangiopancreatography in patients with pancreatitis. Radiology. 1999;210:605–10,
50. Calvo MM, Bujanda L, Calderon A et al. Comparison between magnetic resonance. Am J Gastroenterol. 2002;97:347–53.
51. Bali MA, Sztantics A, Metens T et al. Quantification of pancreatic exocrine function with secretin-enhanced magnetic resonance cholangiopancreatography: normal values and short-term effects of pancreatic duct drainage procedures in chronic pancreatitis. Initial results. Eur Radiol. 2005;15:2110–21.
52. Hellerhoff KJ, Helmberger H 3rd, Rosch T, Settles MR, Link TM, Rummeny EJ. Dynamic MR pancreatography after secretin administration: image quality and diagnostic accuracy. Am J Roentgenol. 2002;179:121–9.
53. Manfredi R, Costamagna G, Brizi MG et al. Severe chronic pancreatitis versus suspected pancreatic disease: dynamic MR cholangiopancreatography after secretin stimulation. Radiology. 2000;214:849–55.
54. Czako L, Takacs T, Morvay Z, Csernay L, Lonovics J. Diagnostic role of secretin-enhanced MRCP in patients with unsuccessful ERCP. World J Gastroenterol. 2004;10:3034–8.

55. van Kouwen MC, Jansen JB, van Goor H, de Castro S, Oyen WJ, Drenth JP. FDG-PET is able to detect pancreatic carcinoma in chronic pancreatitis. Eur J Nucl Med Mol Imaging. 2005;32:399–404.
56. Hastier P, Buckley MJ, Francois E et al. A prospective study of pancreatic disease in patients with alcoholic cirrhosis: comparative diagnostic value of ERCP and EUS and long-term significance of isolated parenchymal abnormalities. Gastrointest Endosc. 1999; 49:705–9.
57. Böhmig M, Rosewicz S. Pankreaskarzinom. Z Gastroenterol. 2004;42:261–8.
58. Adamek HE, Albert J, Breer H, Weitz M, Schilling D, Riemann JF. Pancreatic cancer detection with magnetic resonance cholangiopancreatography and endoscopic retrograde cholangiopancreatography: a prospective controlled study. Lancet. 2000;356:1607–8.
59. Di Stasi M, Lencioni R, Solmi L et al. Ultrasound-guided fine needle biopsy of pancreatic masses: results of a multicenter study. Am J Gastroenterol. 1998;93:1329–33.

10
Medical management of pancreatic cancer

J.-M. LÖHR, M. GEISSLER and M. P. LUTZ

INTRODUCTION

Pancreatic ductal carcinoma (PDAC) is a disastrous disease with a dismal prognosis[1]; the only cure is surgery[2]. The vast majority of patients is inoperable at the time of diagnosis and will require palliative treatment[3]. With a median survival time oscillating around 6 months, any treatment has to subscribe to the oncological paradigm that the treatment must not be worse than the disease itself. The quality of life is the utmost important feature for these patients. Beside the standard in best supportive care (BSC), some issues specific for pancreatic cancer need attention that will be covered in this chapter. Most importantly, all aspects of palliative anti-tumour treatment will be presented in detail and discussed. This will include preliminary communications such as presentations at ASCO[4]. Finally, some outlooks are given into the future of pancreatic cancer treatment.

BEST SUPPORTIVE CARE

The basics of palliative therapy in patients with pancreatic carcinoma are made up by symptom-oriented BSC. Besides the obvious symptoms, reduced appetite, anorexia, weight loss and pain, some special problems arise in pancreatic cancer: obstructive jaundice, gastric outlet obstruction/duodenal stenosis and psychic alterations.

Almost every patient with PDAC has lost weight at the time of diagnosis[5]. Several factors contribute to the loss of appetite and food intake: pain, anxiety and sorrow[6], gastrointestinal problems related to anatomical pathology and metabolic factors such as islet amyloid polypeptide (IAPP)[7]. Patients with PDAC have a special wasting with increased caloric demand at rest but reduced in total[5]. The serum CRP correlates with weight (loss), reduced food intake and survival[8]; therefore, patients need nutritional counselling by a specialized expert, trained nutritionalist or nurse (in Germany Ökotrophologe/ErnährungsberaterIn). Enteral feeding is preferable for many reasons and should be aimed for. If needed, surgical or endoscopic measures to restore the duodenal passage should be considered (see below). There is no clinical or scientific evidence for drugs stimulating appetite such as synthetic anabolics (megesteronacetate, Farlutal[®]). Even though they increase appetite, this does not result in weight gain or improvement of performance status[9] – besides being rather expensive. Synthetic androgens such as flutamide (Fugarel[®]) have demonstrated in a single though well-designed study an increase of weight and a small positive effect on the survival of patients with PDAC[10]. Larger subsequent studies are missing.

Weight loss in pancreatic cancer patients is mostly due to tumour cachexia. However, tumours in the pancreatic head, the most frequent site, will also obstruct the main pancreatic duct and cause exocrine pancreatic insufficiency. This is prevalent in most if not all patients with PDAC in the pancreatic head[11]. It is mandatory to treat these patients to prevent further wasting[12]. Patients therefore must receive enzyme substitution with pancreatin (such as Creon[®]) in a sufficient dose to ensure complete digestion of high molecular weight sugars and fat. If administered early on, weight loss can be ameliorated[13]. Besides exocrine pancreatic insufficiency, many patients also suffer from endocrine pancreatic insufficiency. Diabetes mellitus may even precede the diagnosis of PDAC[14] and must also be treated, preferably with insulin. However, a tight glycaemic control is certainly not the most pressing treatment goal.

The weight loss in cancer patients is not only a simple concern of supportive care. Underweight, malnourished cancer patients such as those with PDAC will also receive less chemotherapy due to more/more severe side-effects[15] and thus have a worse outcome.

The treatment of pain[16] follows established guidelines according to the WHO Step-by-step scheme[17]. Because of the anatomical site close to the solaric plexus and the preference of pancreatic carcinoma cells for neural invasion along nerve sheets, patients with PDAC will early require opioids that should be administered without hesitation. Due to the specific problems with food intake/appetite, transcutaneous applications have proven favourable[18], e.g. fentanyl plasters (Durogesic[®]) or buprenorphin plasters (Transtec[®]). Patients and physicians should be aware of the constipation following opioids, and mild laxatives such as lactulose or macrogol (Laxofalk[®]) should be prescribed as a concomitant medication.

Psychic alterations are known in cancer patients with a variety of tumours; however, they seem to be more prominent in patients with PDAC, with anxiety, depression and panic being the most prominent symptoms. Understandably, this is triggered by the inescapable poor prognosis of the disease. Pancreatic cancer patients seem to have specific depressive symptoms[19]. There is some evidence that these symptoms, similar to diabetes, may precede the diagnosis of pancreatic carcinoma[20]. As a consequence, patients with PDAC presenting with such symptoms will profit from antidepressant therapy.

There is one substance that may potentially ameliorate several of the above-mentioned symptoms (weight loss, appetite, pain, anxiety) in patients with PDAC: cannabis[21]. This natural substance is known for increasing appetite, being anxiolytic and relieving pain[22]. Synthetic formulations of the active ingredient, tetrahydrocannabiol (THC) are available in capsules and liquid

(Dronabiol, Marinol®)[23]. They should be administered with care since many older patients with PDAC may come down with adverse reactions such as so-called bad trips.

ENDOSCOPIC THERAPY

Due to the anatomical location of the pancreas, and the preferred localization of the adenocarcinoma in the head of the pancreas, local growth of the tumour will result in obstructive jaundice and/or duodenal obstruction. If this is expected, a definite surgical procedure can treat both obstructions with a biliary bypass (hepaticojejunostomy) and a gastric bypass (gastroenterostomy) should be preferred. For biliary obstruction alone, endoscopic stenting is superior to surgery. Biliary obstruction may precede duodenal obstruction, which can also be treated by endoscopic measures. Therefore, patients may require both endoscopic procedures. While biliary obstruction may be treated with plastic stents in those patients with a rather short life expectancy[24], duodenal obstruction can be treated only with self-expandable metals stents[25]. Current stent systems fit through the instrumentation channel of the endoscope (TTS = through the scope)[26]. For obvious reasons this has dramatically improved the technical success rate to place such stents into the pylorus/duodenum (Figure 1).

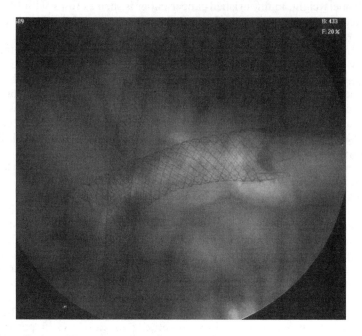

Figure 1 Palliative endoscopic treatment in a patient with pancreatic head carcinoma. Self-expandable metal stents in the distal bile duct and the pylorus/duodenum. Radiograph of both stents

PALLIATIVE CHEMOTHERAPY

Due to the nature and biology of pancreatic cancer, chemotherapy will only be palliative[27]. Placed on Sigmund Freud's famous couch for psychoanalysis, and being honest to oneself, few anticancer drugs work convincingly and demonstrate significant, i.e. 30%, improvement of survival time over BSC or standard therapy[28]. Patients with a metastasized disease and treated with BSC have a median survival of 2–4 months. The quasi-standard still is gemcitabine, based on a study which demonstrated a relevant increase in survival at 12 months (18%) when compared to an underdosed 5-fluorouracyl (5-FU) regimen (2%)[29]. Nevertheless, the response rate with gemcitabine is only about 15%, and time to progression 2.2–3.8 months[30]. Gemcitabine improves quality of life as measured by a clinical benefit questionnaire (pain, performance status, weight) significantly compared to 5-FU (23.8% vs 4.5%). Preclinical evidence indicated that the converting enzyme is dose-limiting. As a consequence a fixed-dose regimen with prolonged infusion time has been developed that showed increased response and survival[31].

In the meantime, several studies have been conducted with combinations of gemcitabine of which the results are now available (Table 1). So far all combinations of gemcitabine with oxaliplatin, cisplatin, pemetrexed, exatecan or capecitabine have resulted in no significant increase in survival. Nevertheless, even in this dismal situation, second-line therapies have been offered to those patients who had some benefit during the initial treatment, usually gemcitabine. Apparently second-line therapy is feasible, e.g. treatment with an oxaliplatin/5-FU-based regimen after failure of gemcitabine (Table 1).

TARGETED THERAPY

Based on the profound knowledge in tumour biology gathered during recent years, several targets for therapy on different levels in a tumour cell have been identified (Figure 2). Therefore, the concept of targeted therapy has come to pancreatic cancer rather early on. On the level of a single tumour cell the target may be a surface receptor, its ligand, the receptor tyrosine kinaseses and finally the subsequent signal transduction pathway involving a multitude of transcription factors and enzymes. Beyond the tumour cell there are also some additional targets, e.g. metalloproteinases. For all levels and targets, compounds of various natures (antibodies, small molecule inhibitors) have been developed[32]. Although some of the substances are already registered for other tumour entities, studies in pancreatic carcinoma are still ongoing or just completed (Table 2).

Cetuximab (Erbitux®), an antibody against the EGF receptor, has shown efficacy during an uncontrolled phase II study with 32% 1-year survival, 12% partial response and 63% stable disease[33], and is currently being tested in phase III trials. Blocking another EGF receptor, her2/neu with trastuzumab (Herceptin®), resulted in a response rate of 24% and 1-year survival of 24%. A phase II study is ongoing in Germany (AIO).

Table 1 Recent randomized controlled trials for chemotherapy in patients with inoperable/advanced pancreatic ductal adenocarcinoma

Regimen	Study	Phase	No. of patients	Survival		Reference
				Median survival	One year survival	
GEM+5-FU/FA vs GEM	CONKO-002	III	473	5.85 6.2 (n.s.)		Riess et al., ASCO 2005 #4009
GEM+CAP vs GEM+OX vs CAP+OX		II	190	7.9 6.9 8.2	n.s.	Heinemann et al., ASCO 2005 #4030
GEM+CAP vs GEM	SAKK	III	319	8.4 7.3	7.9 6.9 8.2	Hermann et al., ASCO 2005 #4010
GEM+DOC vs CISP+DOC	EORTC-GI 40984	II	96	7.4 7.1	30% 16%	47
5-FU/FA+OX vs BSC	OFF	III	46	21 weeks 10 weeks (p = 0.007)		Oettle et al., ASCO 2005 #4031

GEM = gemcitabine; 5-FU/FA = 5-fluorouracil/folinic acid; CAP = capecitabine; OX = oxaliplatin; CISP = cisplatin; BSC = best supportive care; n.s. = not significant

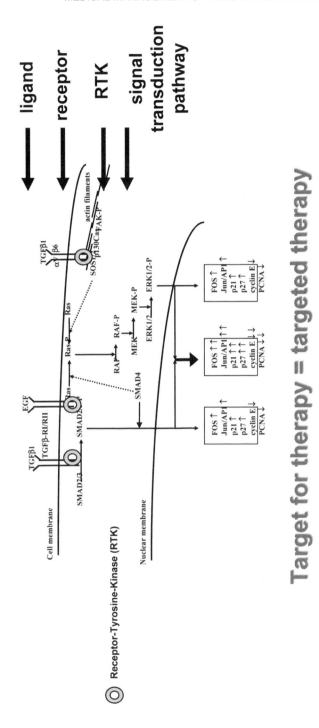

Figure 2 Levels of action for targeted therapy. RTK = receptor tyrosine kinases

Table 2 Randomized controlled trials for targeted therapy in patients with inoperable/advanced pancreatic ductal adenocarcinoma

Target	Substance	Class	Chemo	Phase	No. of patients	Survival — Median survival	Survival — 1-year survival	Reference
EGF-R	Cetuximab	Moab		II	41	7.1 months	32%	33
Her2/neu	Trastuzumab	Moab	GEM	II	32	7.5 months	24%	Safran et al., ASCO 2001 #517
EGF-R RTK	Erlotinib	Small molecule	GEM	III	569	6.37 months vs 5.91 months	24% vs 17%	Moore et al., ASCO 2005 #1
Ras oncogene/farnesyl transferase	R115777	Small molecule	Ø	II	20	19.7 weeks		39
Ras oncogene/farnesyl transferase	R115777	Small molecule	GEM	III	688	193 days vs 182 days		36
Multi-folate dependent enzyme	Permetrexed	Small molecule	GEM	III	565	6.2 vs 6.3	21.4 vs 20.1	Richards et al., ASCO 2004 #4007
Thymidilate synthetase	Raltitrexed	Small molecule	GEM	II	25	199 days		34
Matrix metallo-proteinase	Marimastat	Small molecule	GEM	III	Xxx	5.0 vs 6.9 months	15% vs 19%	37
Matrix metallo-proteinase	Tanomastat	Small molecule	GEM	III	227	3.74 months vs 6.59 months	10% vs 20%	38
VEGF	Bevacizumab	Moab	GEM	II	52	8.7 months	29%	Kindler et al., ASCO 2004 #4009

Erlotinib (Tarceva®), targeting the EGF-R on the level of its RTK, showed marginally increased 1-year (24%) and median survival (6.37 months) compared to gemcitabine (17% and 5.91 months, respectively) (Moore et al., ASCO 2005 #1). To date most experts argue that these data do not translate in a new standard as a first-line chemotherapy. An inhibitor of thymidilate synthetase, raltitrexed (Tomudex®), could not demonstrate any benefit in a phase II study with gemcitabine[34].

Most pancreatic ductal adenocarcinomas show mutations in the k-ras oncogene. This led to a permant activity of small G proteins. These have a so-called CAAX box at the carboxyterminal end of the protein, which represents the recognition site for an enzyme called farnesyl transferase, leading to the first post-translational modification, a thio-alkylation of the CAAX box. This in turn results in the anchorage of ras in the cell membrane facilitating the (permanent) activity. It was therefore a very rational approach to develop inhibitors of the farnesyl transferase (FTI) which was accomplished by several pharmaceutical companies. A phase II study with one of these compounds (R115777, Zarnestra®) demonstrated reduction of farnesyl transferase activity by 50%; however, it showed no response and no improvement in median survival (5 months)[35]. A subsequent phase III study with this FTI did not produce any better results than gemcitabine alone[36] (Table 2).

Inhibitors covering several target molecules are attractive from our understanding of tumour biology. Pemetrexed (Alimta), an inhibitor of multiple folate-dependent enzymes, is such a candidate. While a phase II study was promising, a large phase III study ($\pm$ gemcitabine) did not show any benefit either for TTP or mOS (Richards et al., ASCO 2004 #4007). Another multiplex inhibitor, BAY92037, inhibiting ras/raf kinases, is currently under investigation.

Targeting matrix metalloproteinases (MMP) as one of the tumour-promoting factors in PDAC again was a well-thought-out idea in antitumoral treatment. Those enzymase help the tumour cells to remodel the stroma (extracellular matrix). MMP are overexpressed not only by the tumour cells themselves but also in high amounts by the stromal cells in the immediate vicinity to the tumour cells. Several MMP inhibitors (against MMP-1, -2, -3, -9, 11), marimastat and tanomastat, have been tested in patients with PDAC, leading to a worse outcome than gemcitabine alone[37,38]. This is as disappointing as the failure of the farnesyl transferase inhibitors, since both approaches had an extremely good scientifc reasoning based on our understanding of pancreatic carcinoma tumour biology.

The tumour environment/stroma offers other targets for therapy. Among those the tumour vasculature and the capability of the growing tumour to promote tumour neoangiogenesis appears to be most rewarding. Pancreatic carcinomas, as other solid tumours, secrete a multitude of proangiogenic factors such as VEGF and FGF2[39]; indeed, an antibody against VEGF, Bevacizumab, has demonstrated a significant response in advanced colorectal carcinoma[40]. A phase II study in pancreatic carcinoma has demonstrated efficacy, particularly in those with high VEGF serum levels (Kindler et al., ASCO 2004 #4009). A phase III study (CALGB 80303) is ongoing.

Table 3 Clinical trials using gene therapy in patients with pancreatic ductal adenocarcinoma

Indication	Type of gene therapy	Vector	Therapeutic construct	Additional therapy	Outcome	Remarks	Reference
Palliative	Direct/virus	Adenovirus	Onyx 015	Ø	No effect	Oncolytic virus	48
Adjuvant	Ex-vivo/immunstimuli	Conventional/CMV	GM-CSF	5-FU/LV+Mito	mOS >25 months	Immune vaccination plus adjuvant radio-chemotherapy (Johns–Hopkins protocol)	43
Palliative	Ex vivo/fibroblasts	Retrovirus	IL-2 LXSN-tIL2	Ø	No effect	Subcutaneous injection of transfected autologous fibro-blasts with tumour cells (irradiated)	49
Palliative	Indirect/intravenous	Retrovirus	Cyclin D	Ø	Claimed SD in 3/3	Original data not published	50
Palliative	Indirect/GDEPT	Conventional/CMV	CYP2B1		Doubling of mOS (44 weeks); 1 year 32%	Ex-vivo, micro encapsulation	44

Ø, no additional therapy

110

GENE THERAPY

Since pancreatic cancer has such a dismal prognosis this tumour has already been subject to gene therapy studies in patients. Nevertheless, following the first swell of enthusiasm after its inauguration in 1992, this concept stalled with the patient who died due to reckless investigators[41]. There is no other area in medicine where the reviews outnumber the original work by such a magnitude. Several concepts have been applied to pancreatic cancer: direct oncolytic viruses, gene-directed enzyme prodrug therapy (GDEPT) and genetic vaccination[42], both in advanced disease and as adjuvant treatment (Table 3). The two concepts which demonstrated tumour response were genetic vaccination with GM-CSF in allogenic, irradiated tumour cells in the adjuvant setting (plus radiochemotherapy) resulting in a median survival in excess of 24 months[43], and the application of microencapsulated cells, genetically modified to express cytochrome 2B1 (plus low-dose ifosfamide) in the palliative setting resulting in a doubling of the median survival from 22 to 44 weeks and 32% 1-year survival[44]. Due to the prospects of targeted therapy, very few if any gene therapy protocols are out and clinical studies running.

OUTLOOK

Under stringent oncological criteria, as mentioned[28], conventional cytotoxic chemotherapy in pancreatic carcinoma is close to ineffective apart from individual patients. The advent of targeted therapy has changed the scenario significantly. Although the median survival times do not change that impressively, a subset of patients who respond seem to profit from this kind of treatment, with 1-year survival times now being in the range of 25%. To date, very few of the available targeted therapies have been applied to pancreatic carcinoma[32]. The current global gene expression approaches employing transcriptomics and proteomics will provide us with even more therapeutic targets[45,46]. Further, no combination of several of such targeted therapies, e.g. antibody plus small molecule targeting the vessels and tyrosine kinases has been tested so far. The clever selection for such a combined approach could be a concept that may significantly improve survival – as does second-line therapy. Gene therapy, due to several conceptual problems, still remains experimental.

References

1. Jemal A, Murray T, Ward E et al. Cancer statistics, 2005. CA Cancer J Clin. 2005;55:10–30.
2. Büchler MW, Wagner M, Schmied BM, Uhl W, Friess H, Z'Graggen K. Changes in morbidity after pancreatic resection: toward the end of completion pancreatectomy. Arch Surg. 2003;138):1310–4; discussion 1315.
3. Rosewicz S, Wiedenmann B. Pancreatic carcinoma. Lancet. 1997;349:485–9.
4. Hohler T, Heike M, Lutz MP, Graeven U, Seufferlein T. [ASCO-Update 2005 – Highlights of the 41st Meeting of the American Society of Clinical Oncology/ASCO 2005.]. Z Gastroenterol. 2005;43:1253–9.
5. Wigmore SJ, Plester CE, Richardson RA, Fearon KCH. Changes in nutritional status associated with unresectable pancreatic cancer. Br J Cancer. 1997;75:106–9.
6. Holland JC. Anorexia and cancer: psychological aspects. CA Cancer J Clin. 1977;27:363–7.

7. Permert J, Larsson J, Westermark GT et al. Islet amyloid polypeptide in patients with pancreatic cancer and diabetes. N Engl J Med. 1994;330:313–18.
8. Wigmore SJ, Fearon KC, Maingay JP, Ross JA. Down-regulation of the acute-phase response in patients with pancreatic cancer cachexia receiving oral eicosapentaenoic acid is mediated via suppression of interleukin-6. Clin Sci (Lond). 1997;92:215–21.
9. Downer S, Joel S, Albright A et al. A double blind placebo controlled trial of medroxyprogesterone acetate (MPA) in cancer. Br J Cancer. 1993;67:1102–5.
10. Greenway BA. Effect of flutamide on survival in patients with pancreatic cancer: results of a prospective, randomized, double blind, placebo controlled trial. Br Med J. 1998;316: 1935–8.
11. Braganza JM, Howat HT. Cancer of the pancreas. In: Howat HT, editor. The Exocrine Pancreas. London: WB Saunders, 1972:219–37.
12. Friess H, Bohm J, Ebert M, Büchler M. Enzyme treatment after gastrointestinal surgery. Digestion. 1993;54(Suppl. 2):48–53.
13. Bruno MJ, Haverkort EB, Tijssen GP, Tytgat GN, van Leeuwen DJ. Placebo controlled trial of enteric coated pancreatin microsphere treatment in patients with. Gut. 1998;42:92–6.
14. Gullo L, Pezzilli R, Morselli-Labate AM. Diabetes and the risk of pancreatic cancer. Italian pancreatic cancer study group. N Engl J Med. 1994;331:81–4.
15. Andreyev HJ, Norman AR, Oates J, Cunningham D. Why do patients with weight loss have a worse outcome when undergoing chemotherapy for gastrointestinal malignancies? Eur J Cancer. 1998;34:503–9.
16. Caraceni AG, Portenoy RK. Pain management in patients with pancreatic carcinoma. Cancer. 1996;78(Suppl. 3):639–53.
17. (WHO) WHO. Cancer Pain Relief and Palliative Care, 2 edn. New York: WHO, 1990.
18. Grond S, Zech D, Lehmann KA, Radbruch L, Breitenbach H, Hertel D. Transdermal fentanyl in the long-term treatment of cancer pain: a prospective study of 50. Pain. 1997;69: 191–8.
19. Passik SD, Breitbart WS. Depression in patients with pancreatic carcinoma. Cancer. 1996; 78(Suppl. 3):615–26.
20. Passik SD, Roth AJ. Anxiety sympoms and panic attacks preceding pancreatic cancer diagnosis. Psychooncology. 1999;8:268–72.
21. Gorter RW. Cancer cachexia and cannabinoids. Forsch Komplementarmed 1999;6(Suppl. S3):21–2.
22. Hall W, Christie M, Currow D. Cannabinoids and cancer: causation, remediation, and palliation. Lancet Oncol. 2005;6:35–42.
23. Radbruch L, Elsner F. [Palliative pain therapy, cannabinoids.]. Internist (Berl). 2005;46: 1105–14.
24. Binmoeller KF, Seitz U, Seifert H, Thonke F, Sikka S, Soehendra N. The Tannenbaum stent: a new plastic biliary stent without side holes. Am J Gastroenterol. 1995;90:1764–8.
25. Löhr M, Ell C. Interventionelle endoskopische Therapie des inoperablen Pankreaskarzinoms. In: Hopt UT, Brinkmann W, editors. Pankreaskarzinom. Neckargemünd: Weller Verlag, 2000.
26. Kim GH, Kang DH, Lee DH et al. Which types of stent, uncovered or covered, should be used in gastric outlet obstructions? Scand J Gastroenterol. 2004;39:1010–14.
27. Lutz MP. [Chemotherapy of pancreatic carcinoma]. Schweiz Rundsch Med Prax. 2005;94:933–5.
28. Atkins JH, Gershell LJ. Selective anticancer drugs. Nat Rev Drug Discov. 2002;1:491–2.
29. Burris HA, Moore MJ, Andersen J et al. Improvements in survival and clinical benefit with gemcitabine as first-line therapy for patients with advanced pancreatic cancer: a randomized trial. J Clin Oncol. 1997;15:2403–13.
30. Storniolo AM, Enas NH, Brown CA, Voi M, Rothenberg ML, Schilsky R. An investigational new drug treatment program for patients with gemcitabine. Cancer. 1999; 85:1261–8.
31. Tempero M, Plunkett W, Ruiz Van Haperen V et al. Randomized phase II comparison of dose-intense gemcitabine: thirty-minute infusion and fixed dose rate infusion in patients with pancreatic adenocarcinoma. J Clin Oncol. 2003;21:3402–8.
32. Wiedmann MW, Caca K. Molecularly targeted therapy for gastrointestinal cancer. Curr Cancer Drug Targets. 2005;5:171–93.

33. Xiong HQ, Rosenberg A, LoBuglio A et al. Cetuximab, a monoclonal antibody targeting the epidermal growth factor receptor, in combination with gemcitabine for advanced pancreatic cancer: a multicenter phase II Trial. J Clin Oncol. 2004;22:2610–16.
34. Kralidis E, Aebi S, Friess H, Buchler MW, Borner MM. Activity of raltitrexed and gemcitabine in advanced pancreatic cancer. Ann Oncol. 2003;14:574–9.
35. Cohen SJ, Ho L, Ranganathan S et al. Phase II and pharmacodynamic study of the farnesyltransferase inhibitor R115777 as initial therapy in patients with metastatic pancreatic adenocarcinoma. J Clin Oncol. 2003;21:1301–6.
36. Van Cutsem E, van de Velde H, Karasek P et al. Phase III trial of gemcitabine plus tipifarnib compared with gemcitabine plus placebo in advanced pancreatic cancer. J Clin Oncol. 2004;22:1430–8.
37. Bramhall SR, Rosemurgy A, Brown PD, Bowry C, Buckels JA. Marimastat as first-line therapy for patients with unresectable pancreatic cancer: a randomized trial. J Clin Oncol. 2001;19:3447–55.
38. Moore MJ, Hamm J, Dancey J et al. Comparison of gemcitabine versus the matrix metalloproteinase inhibitor BAY 12-9566 in patients with advanced or metastatic adenocarcinoma of the pancreas: a phase III trial of the National Cancer Institute of Canada Clinical Trials Group. J Clin Oncol. 2003;21:3296–302.
39. Korc M. Pathways for aberrant angiogenesis in pancreatic cancer. Mol Cancer. 2003;2:8.
40. Hurwitz H, Fehrenbacher L, Novotny W et al. Bevacizumab plus irinotecan, fluorouracil, and leucovorin for metastatic colorectal cancer. N Engl J Med. 2004;350:2335–42.
41. Raper SE, Chirmule N, Lee FS et al. Fatal systemic inflammatory response syndrome in a ornithine transcarbamylase deficient patient following adenoviral gene transfer. Mol Genet Metab. 2003;80:148–58.
42. Löhr M. Gentherapeutische Ansätze bei gastrointestinalen Tumoren. Z Gastroenterol. 2006 (In press).
43. Jaffee EM, Hruban RH, Biedrzycki B et al. Novel allogeneic granulocyte–macrophage colony-stimulating factor-secreting tumor vaccine for pancreatic cancer: a phase I trial of safety and immune activation. J Clin Oncol. 2001;19:145–56.
44. Löhr M, Hoffmeyer A, Kroger J et al. Microencapsulated cell-mediated treatment of inoperable pancreatic carcinoma. Lancet. 2001;357:1591–2.
45. Brandt R, Grutzmann R, Bauer A et al. DNA microarray analysis of pancreatic malignancies. Pancreatology. 2004;4:587–97.
46. Chen R, Yi EC, Donohoe S et al. Pancreatic cancer proteome: the proteins that underlie invasion, metastasis, and immunologic escape. Gastroenterology. 2005;129:1187–97.
47. Lutz MP, Van Cutsem E, Wagener T et al. Docetaxel-gemcitabine or docetaxel-cisplatin in advanced pancreatic carcinoma. Randomized phase II study #40984 of the EORTC-GI group. J Clin Oncol. 2005;23:9250–6.
48. Mulvihill S, Warren R, Venook A et al. Safety and feasibility of injection with an E1B-55 kDa gene-deleted, replication-selective adenovirus (ONYX-015) into primary carcinomas of the pancreas: a phase I trial. Gene Ther. 2001;8:308–15.
49. Sobol RE, Shawler DL, Carson C et al. Interleukin 2 gene therapy of colorectal carcinoma with autologous irradiated tumour cells and genetically engineered fibroblasts: a Phase I study. Clin Cancer Res. 1999;5:2359–65.
50. Gordon EM, Cornelio GH, Lorenzo CC 3rd et al. First clinical experience using a 'pathotropic' injectable retroviral vector (Rexin-G) as intervention for stage IV pancreatic cancer. Int J Oncol. 2004;24:177–85.

11
Pancreatic carcinoma: surgery, palliative resection and value of lymph node resection

C. MICHALSKI, J. KLEEFF, M. W. BÜCHLER and H. FRIESS

INTRODUCTION

Pancreatic ductal adenocarcinoma (PDAC) is the most common malignancy of the pancreas, most likely arising from the ductal epithelium of the pancreas. With its incidence (10–11 per 100 000 people) almost equalling its prevalence in Western countries, it is one of the most aggressive human tumours[1]. In the United States alone, 420 000 life-years are lost due to pancreatic cancer every year[2].

The 5-year survival rate for all stages of PDAC combined has risen from less than 1% in the 1950s to approximately 4% today[2]. Yet even these dismal numbers are controversial[3,4], since it has been suggested recently that a high percentage of the long-term survivors were wrongly classified as PDAC and were actually affected by other benign or malignant pancreatic diseases[5]. Its aggressive growth with retroperitoneal and perineural infiltration, angioinvasion, formation of metastases, and resistance to most of the available treatment regimens, makes patient management a complex and challenging task.

Although the concept of cure following 'curative' resection has been challenged[4], surgical resection is the only therapy that gives a patient a significantly increased survival (and a chance for cure). The median survival following resection is 14–20 months and 20–25% will be true 5-year survivors[6,7]. In contrast, patients in whom resection is not possible due to advanced disease have a median survival of only 4–6 months.

The standard operation is a pancreaticoduodenectomy (PD) for tumours of the pancreatic head, and a left pancreatectomy or distal pancreatectomy for tumours of the body/tail. Ductal adenocarcinoma is by far the most frequent tumour of the pancreas, with a predominant localization within the pancreatic head (78%)[8]. Furthermore, adenocarcinoma of the body or tail is seldom resectable on presentation due to the often late diagnosis in an advanced stage. It is thus not surprising that PD is the most commonly performed surgical procedure for pancreatic tumours. The Kausch–Whipple operation in its early years (named in honor of Walter Kausch and Allen Whipple)[9,10] was associated with high rates of morbidity and mortality with poor long-term outcome. However, in the 1980s the surgical mortality rates dropped significantly due to a combination of better perioperative and postoperative supportive care and surgical techniques. In centres with high case-load, pancreatic resections can be performed nowadays with mortality rates below 5%[11]. Randomized controlled trials are increasingly carried out to define the best palliative and adjuvant therapy for this disease. Translational research combined with clinical trials will hopefully lead to improved survival and better quality of life for pancreatic cancer patients in the future.

SURGERY OF PANCREATIC CANCER

In 1995 Gudjonsson[4] stated that 'pancreatic resections have had minimal impact on survival rates in patients with carcinoma and are wasteful of resources'. He based this statement on the fact that overall survival rates remained low despite 20–25% 5-year survival rates following potentially curative resection. This statement has led to some controversial discussion, but a number of studies have clearly shown that curative resection offers a chance for cure or at least a substantial survival benefit.

CURATIVE AND PALLIATIVE RESECTION

Yeo et al.[12] showed in 1995 that curatively resected patients had a 5-year survival rate of 26% (median survival 18 months), while R1/R2 resected patients (palliative resections) fared significantly worse, with a 5-year survival rate of 8% (median survival 10 months). Richter et al.[13] and Wagner et al.[14] have reported similar results with 5-year survival rates in the R0 groups of 25% and 24%, respectively. Besides these reports from high-volume centres there is also evidence from controlled studies. A randomized multicentre trial by Imamura et al.[15], for example, compared surgical resection with radiochemotherapy and revealed a clear survival benefit for the surgically treated patients, with 1-year survival rates of 62% in the resection group versus 32% in the chemoradiation group (mean survival 17 months versus 11 months, respectively).

TECHNICAL ASPECTS OF THE PANCREATICODUODENECTOMY

The most demanding step in resectional surgery for pancreatic cancer is the pancreaticojejunal anastomosis. A small main pancreatic duct and soft texture of the pancreatic tissue render this part of the operation particularly difficult. Thus, pancreatic fistula rates of greater than 10% are common and are responsible for considerable mortality. Fistulas are less frequent in chronic pancreatitis because of the harder texture of the chronically inflamed pancreatic tissue in this disease[16]. In large series from single institutions it has been shown that pancreatic fistula rates vary between 2.1% and 14%, a difference that can – at least in part – be attributed to different fistula definitions[17–19].

The pancreatico-enteric anastomosis has been an ongoing challenge for surgeons. Many techniques have been described to lower the risk of pancreatic leak (and thus subsequent morbidity/mortality), but successful management probably depends primarily on the surgeon's meticulous execution of a familiar technique[7].

SURGEONS AS PROGNOSTIC FACTORS

As resection-related mortality and morbidity have decreased in recent decades, survival after surgery has also improved[20]. Importantly, Birkmeyer and co-workers[21] have shown that mortality rates strikingly correlate with the number of resections per year and institution. This effect, with high case-load correlating with safer surgery, is especially true for pancreatic cancer, and has been shown in a number of single-centre studies and in a recent well-designed meta-analysis.[22–24]. In addition, long-term survival after pancreatic cancer resection is also superior in high-volume centres[25].

FACTORS INFLUENCING THE PROGNOSIS AFTER PANCREATICODUODENECTOMY

Wagner et al.[14] have shown that curative resection is the single most important factor determining outcome in patients with PDAC. However, other factors also significantly influence postoperative survival. These are the presence or absence of blood vessel infiltration, of nerve invasion, and of lymph node metastasis. An analysis of 650 consecutive PD also revealed curative resection as an important factor influencing survival[19]. Among others, lymph node status and poor tumour differentiation were also important factors in patient survival. Interestingly, Lim et al.[26] identified surgery in a teaching hospital and adjuvant therapy as further important prognostic factors in addition to tumour size and the nodal status. These results were confirmed by another study demonstrating the prognostic value of the resection and nodal status[13]. Thus it can be concluded that potentially curative resection is the most important prognostic factor, and lymph node status, vascular infiltration and perineural invasion are also important factors influencing long-term outcome after surgery for PDAC.

EXTENDED LYMPHADENECTOMY

In order to improve the long-term survival of surgically treated patients, extended lymphadenectomy after partial duodenopancreatectomy has been suggested. A large number of retrospective studies from the late 1980s showed improved 5-year survival for patients in whom PD was performed together with extended lymphadenectomy. However, consecutive randomized controlled studies did not confirm these results[27–30]. A recent large multicentre trial from Japan has also demonstrated that there is no survival benefit from extended lymphadenectomy, although the procedure itself was not associated with increased morbidity or mortality[31]. A feasibility analysis revealed that adequately powered randomized trials addressing the potential benefit of extended lymphadenectomy would require an enormously large sample size and are thus not feasible[32]. In conclusion, there are now four well-designed randomized controlled trials from three continents including over 500 patients, reporting essentially the same outcome – i.e. that extended lymphadenectomy does not offer a survival benefit but potentially compromises safety and quality of life. Extended lymphadenectomy with retroperitoneal clearance should therefore no longer be routinely performed.

ADJUVANT THERAPY

Few studies have investigated the effects of adjuvant therapies on survival of PDAC patients. Among those, the largest is the ESPAC-1 study, which demonstrated a significant survival benefit from adjuvant chemotherapy with 5-FU/FA versus no chemotherapy[33]. A similar benefit of adjuvant chemotherapy has been observed with gemcitabine, although longer follow-up is necessary to analyse the overall survival benefit[34]. The ESPAC-3 study is currently comparing 5-FU/FA with gemcitabine (the observation arm has been closed due to the results of the ESPAC-1 study), with more than 1000 patients having been recruited so far. Further ESPAC trials addressing different questions are currently under development. Interestingly, a study by Picozzi et al.[35] in which PD was followed by interferon-based chemoradiation demonstrated encouraging results, with 1-, 2- and 5-year survival rates of 95%, 64% and 55%, respectively. As these results are promising, the CapRI study has been initiated to compare interferon-alpha, cisplatin, radiation and 5-fluorouracil with leucovorin and 5-fluorouracil alone in a randomized, controlled fashion[36]. Together, these studies strengthen the hope that surgery, together with multimodal therapy consisting of chemotherapy, radiotherapy, immunotherapy and/or targeted therapy, will significantly improve overall patient survival.

CONCLUSION

Curative resection and favourable tumour biology are the most important prognostic factors for prolonged survival in (resectable) pancreatic cancer patients. Pancreatic operations today are safe procedures with acceptable morbidity and low mortality in specialized centres. Current evidence does not support extended lymphadenectomy as a standard procedure. Adjuvant chemotherapy significantly improves outcome after surgical resection, while chemoradiation in the adjuvant setting is still controversially discussed.

Gemcitabine remains the standard for palliative therapy despite proven low effectiveness, but combination therapies are increasingly being evaluated. Greater understanding of the pathophysiological basis of PDAC, and the molecular-targeted therapies that result, promise to be extraordinarily helpful in prolonging patient survival after surgical resection, as well as in the palliative setting.

References

1. Jemal A, Murray T, Ward E et al. Cancer statistics. CA Cancer J Clin. 2005;55:10–30.
2. Ries L, Eisner M, Kosary C et al., editors. SEER Cancer Statistics Review. Bethesda, MD: NC Institute, 1975–2001.
3. Gudjonsson B. Cancer of the pancreas. 50 years of surgery. Cancer. 1987;60:2284–303.
4. Gudjonsson B. Carcinoma of the pancreas: critical analysis of costs, results of resections, and the need for standardized reporting. J Am Coll Surg. 1995;181:483–503.
5. Carpelan-Holmstrom M, Nordling S, Pukkala E et al. Does anyone survive pancreatic ductal adenocarcinoma? A nationwide study re-evaluating the data of the Finnish Cancer Registry. Gut. 2005;54:385–7.
6. Conlon KC, Klimstra DS, Brennan MF. Long-term survival after curative resection for pancreatic ductal adenocarcinoma. Clinicopathologic analysis of 5-year survivors. Ann Surg. 1996;223:273–9.
7. Trede M, Richter A, Wendl K. Personal observations, opinions, and approaches to cancer of the pancreas and the periampullary area. Surg Clin N Am. 2001;81:595–610.
8. Schafer M, Mullhaupt B, Clavien PA. Evidence-based pancreatic head resection for pancreatic cancer and chronic pancreatitis. Ann Surg. 2002;236:137–48.
9. Kausch W. Das Carcinom der Papilla duodeni und seine radikale Entfernung. Beitr Klin Chir. 1912;78:439–86.
10. Whipple AO, Parsons WB, Mullins CR. Treatment of carcinoma of the ampulla of Vater. Ann Surg. 1935;102:763–79.
11. Beger HG, Rau B, Gansauge F, Poch B, Link KH. Treatment of pancreatic cancer: challenge of the facts. World J Surg. 2003;27:1075–84.
12. Yeo CJ, Cameron JL, Lillemoe KD et al. Pancreaticoduodenectomy for cancer of the head of the pancreas. 201 patients. Ann Surg. 1995;221:721–31; discussion 731–3.
13. Richter A, Niedergethmann M, Sturm JW, Lorenz D, Post S, Trede M. Long-term results of partial pancreaticoduodenectomy for ductal adenocarcinoma of the pancreatic head: 25-year experience. World J Surg. 2003;27:324–9.
14. Wagner M, Redaelli C, Lietz M, Seiler CA, Friess H, Buchler MW. Curative resection is the single most important factor determining outcome in patients with pancreatic adenocarcinoma. Br J Surg. 2004;91:586–94.
15. Imamura M, Doi R, Imaizumi T et al. A randomized multicenter trial comparing resection and radiochemotherapy for resectable locally invasive pancreatic cancer. Surgery. 2004; 136:1003–11.
16. Bartoli FG, Arnone GB, Ravera G, Bachi V. Pancreatic fistula and relative mortality in malignant disease after pancreaticoduodenectomy. Review and statistical meta-analysis regarding 15 years of literature. Anticancer Res. 1991;11:1831–48.
17. Bassi C, Dervenis C, Butturini G et al. Postoperative pancreatic fistula: an international study group (ISGPF) definition. Surgery. 2005;138:8–13.
18. Buchler MW, Friess H, Wagner M, Kulli C, Wagener V, Z'Graggen K. Pancreatic fistula after pancreatic head resection. Br J Surg. 2000;87:883–9.
19. Yeo CJ, Cameron JL, Sohn TA et al. Six hundred fifty consecutive pancreatico-duodenectomies in the 1990s: pathology, complications, and outcomes. Ann Surg. 1997;226:248–57; discussion 257–60.
20. Bramhall SR, Allum WH, Jones AG, Allwood A, Cummins C, Neoptolemos JP. Treatment and survival in 13,560 patients with pancreatic cancer, and incidence of the disease, in the West Midlands: an epidemiological study. Br J Surg. 1995;82:111–15.
21. Birkmeyer JD, Siewers AE, Finlayson EV et al. Hospital volume and surgical mortality in the United States. N Engl J Med. 2002;346:1128–37.

22. Cameron JL, Pitt HA, Yeo CJ, Lillemoe KD, Kaufman HS, Coleman J. One hundred and forty-five consecutive pancreaticoduodenectomies without mortality. Ann Surg. 1993;217: 430–5; discussion 435–8.

23. Trede M, Schwall G, Saeger HD. Survival after pancreatoduodenectomy. 118 consecutive resections without an operative mortality. Ann Surg. 1990;211:447–58.

24. van Heek NT, Kuhlmann KF, Scholten RJ et al. Hospital volume and mortality after pancreatic resection: a systematic review and an evaluation of intervention in the Netherlands. Ann Surg. 2005;242:781–8, discussion 788–90.

25. Fong Y, Gonen M, Rubin D, Radzyner M, Brennan MF. Long-term survival is superior after resection for cancer in high-volume centers. Ann Surg. 2005;242:540–4; discussion 544–7.

26. Lim JE, Chien MW, Earle CC. Prognostic factors following curative resection for pancreatic adenocarcinoma: a population-based, linked database analysis of 396 patients. Ann Surg. 2003;237:74–85.

27. Farnell MB, Pearson RK, Sarr MG et al. A prospective randomized trial comparing standard pancreatoduodenectomy with pancreatoduodenectomy with extended lymphadenectomy in resectable pancreatic head adenocarcinoma. Surgery. 2005;138:618–28; discussion 628–30.

28. Henne-Bruns D, Vogel I, Luttges J, Kloppel G, Kremer B. Ductal adenocarcinoma of the pancreas head: survival after regional versus extended lymphadenectomy. Hepato-gastroenterology. 1998;45:855–66.

29. Pedrazzoli S, DiCarlo V, Dionigi R et al. Standard versus extended lymphadenectomy associated with pancreatoduodenectomy in the surgical treatment of adenocarcinoma of the head of the pancreas: a multicenter, prospective, randomized study. Lymphadenectomy Study Group. Ann Surg. 1998;228:508–17.

30. Yeo CJ, Cameron JL, Lillemoe KD et al. Pancreaticoduodenectomy with or without distal gastrectomy and extended retroperitoneal lymphadenectomy for periampullary adenocarcinoma, part 2: randomized controlled trial evaluating survival, morbidity, and mortality. Ann Surg. 2002;236:355–66; discussion 366–58.

31. Nimura Y, Nagino M, Kato H et al. Standard versus extended lymphadenectomy for pancreatic cancer: a multicenter, randomized controlled trial. Pancreatology. 2004;4:274 (Abstract).

32. Pawlik TM, Abdalla EK, Barnett CC et al. Feasibility of a randomized trial of extended lymphadenectomy for pancreatic cancer. Arch Surg. 2005;140:584–89; discussion 589–91.

33. Neoptolemos JP, Stocken DD, Friess H et al. A randomized trial of chemoradiotherapy and chemotherapy after resection of pancreatic cancer. N Engl J Med. 2004;350:1200–10.

34. Neuhaus P, Oettle H, Post S. A randomised, prospective, multicenter, phase III trial of adjuvant chemotherapy with gemcitabine vs. observation in patients with resected pancreatic cancer. ASCO Annual Meeting. 2005: Abstract 4013.

35. Picozzi VJ, Kozarek RA, Traverso LW. Interferon-based adjuvant chemoradiation therapy after pancreaticoduodenectomy for pancreatic adenocarcinoma. Am J Surg. 2003;185:476–80.

36. Knaebel HP, Marten A, Schmidt J et al. Phase III trial of postoperative cisplatin, interferon alpha-2b, and 5-FU combined with external radiation treatment versus 5-FU alone for patients with resected pancreatic adenocarcinoma – CapRI: study protocol [ISRCTN62866759]. BMC Cancer. 2005;5:37.

12
Special Lecture: Development compounds with different modes of action for the treatment of pancreatic and hepatocellular carcinomas: ZK 304709 and L19-IL-2

G. SIEMEISTER, A. MENRAD, C. WAGNER, K. DETJEN, D. NERI, L. ZARDI, C. McCOY, H. D. MENSSEN and K. BOSSLET

INTRODUCTION

Adenocarcinoma of the pancreas and hepatocellular carcinoma both belong to the most devastating cancers. These cancers can neither be cured nor can survival be prolonged in a clinically really meaningful way. It seems that both diseases are largely resistant to conventional chemotherapeutic drugs, asking for the application of novel and innovative compounds working by modes of action clearly different from standard non-targeted antiproliferative drugs.

Here we present two novel development compounds (ZK 304709 and L19-IL-2) having modes of action different from standard chemotherapy and showing strong anti-tumour efficacy in a variety of standard human xenotransplantation models as well as orthotopic models for pancreatic and hepatocellular carcinomas.

ZK 304709

ZK 304709 is a first-in-class, oral Multi-target Tumor Growth Inhibitor® (MTGI®) that blocks tumour cell proliferation and induces apoptosis by inhibiting a unique combination of disease progression driving pathways. This is accomplished by potent inhibition of (a) serine/threonine kinases CDK 1, 2 and 4, leading to inhibition of cell cycle progression; (b) serine/threonine kinases CDK 7 and 9 leading to apoptosis in resting tumour cells; (c) receptor tyrosine kinases VEGF-R1, R2 and R3, and PDGF-Rβ inhibiting tumour angiogenesis.

Table 1   Selectivity: kinase IC50 (nM)

CDK2/CycE	4
CDK1/CycB	50
CDK4/CycD1	61
CDK7/CycH	85
CDK9/CycT1	5
CHK1	500
GSK3ß	9000
Akt2/PDK1	1300
PKC	6000
PKA	1000
MK2	> 10 000
Plk1	> 10 000
T-Fyn	10 000
EGF-R	> 10 000
Insulin-R	> 10 000
VEGF-R1 (Flt1)	10
VEGF-R2 (KDR)	34
VEGF-R3 (Flt4)	1
PDGF-Rß	27
Ckit	1000

The compound concentration which inhibits kinase activity in a biochemical kinase assay is given in Table 1.

These data show that ZK 304709 inhibits cell cycle kinases cdk 2, 1 and 4 with IC50 of 4, 50 and 61 nM, respectively. Additionally, the compound inhibits the kinases associated with angiogenesis such as VEGF-R 1, 2, 3 and PDGF-R with IC50 values of 10, 34, 1 and 27 nM respectively. Kinases such as the EGF-R and insulin receptor are not inhibited at pharmacologically relevant concentrations.

After having determined the biochemical specificity of ZK 304709 the compound was tested for its antiproliferative potential on six human tumour cell lines. Concentrations of 100–300 nM were found to be sufficient to block the growth of human tumour cell lines under standard assay conditions *in vitro*.

Thereafter the *in-vivo* efficacy of ZK 304709 was evaluated using human tumour xenografts transplanted subcutaneously in nude mice and compared to clinically approved as well as to experimental competitive compounds (see Table 2).

As is shown, ZK 304709 was the most efficacious compound as judged by T/C ratio describing the ratio between the tumour weight of the compound-treated group divided by the tumour weight of the vehicle-treated group. This observation confirms our assumption that blocking cell cycle and angiogenesis at the same time with a single compound will result in very strong anti-tumoral effects.

These impressive data were confirmed using orthotopic pancreatic carcinoma models. Superior therapeutic effects of ZK 304709 compared to gemcitabine, not only on primary tumours but also on their metastases, were shown for the human Capan pancreatic carcinoma model (see Figure 1).

Table 2 ZK 304709: summary of efficacy in human tumour xenograft models (T/C, based on tumour weight)

	ZK 304709	Doxorubicin	Paclitaxel	Flavopiridol	CYC 202	Gemcitabine
Breast						
MaTu	0.01	0.43	0.02	0.19	0.62	n.d.
MX-1	0.01	0.19	n.d.	0.38	n.d.	n.d.
MCF-7	0.01	n.d.	n.d.	n.d.	n.d.	n.d.
MaTu/ADR-Res	0.08	0.53	>1	0.17	n.d.	n.d.
NCI/ADR-RES	0.03	0.37	0.75	0.54	n.d.	n.d.
Prostate						
DU145	0.19	0.57	0.80	0.49	n.d.	n.d.
CWR-22	0.16	0.35	0.46	0.55	n.d.	n.d.
Pancreas						
MIA PaCa-2 (s.c.)	0.04	0.26	n.d.	0.63	n.d.	0.48
MIA PaCa-2 (orthotop.)	0.11	n.d.	n.d.	n.d.	n.d.	n.d.
Capan-1 (s.c.)	0.18	0.26	0.26	0.37	n.d.	0.58
Capan-1 (orthotop.)	0.2	n.d.	n.d.	n.d.	n.d.	0.8
BON (orthotop.)	0.2	n.d.	n.d.	n.d.	n.d.	n.d.
Kidney						
Caki-1	0.17	0.41	0.77	0.65	n.d.	n.d.
Caki-2	0.23	0.34	0.26	>1	n.d.	n.d.
786-O	0.43	0.43	1	>1	n.d.	n.d.
NSC lung						
A549	0.35	0.39	n.d.	n.d.	n.d.	n.d.
NCI-H460	0.49	0.38	0.91	n.d.	n.d.	n.d.
SC lung						
NCI-H69	0.05	n.d.	0.86	n.d.	n.d.	n.d.
Colon						
HCT-116	0.16	0.58	0.39	0.4	n.d.	n.d.
HCT-15	0.41	0.45	0.58	0.39	n.d.	n.d.
Glioblastoma						
U-87 MG	0.04	0.04	0.55	0.39	n.d.	n.d.
Melanoma						
A375	0.19	0.36	>1	0.36	n.d.	n.d.
Haematological tumours						
RL (non-Hodgkin)	0.31	n.d.	n.d.	0.34	n.d.	n.d.
RAMOS (Burkitt's)	0.03	n.d.	n.d.	0.01	n.d.	n.d.
KG-1 (AML)	0.03	0.19	n.d.	0.22	n.d.	n.d.
MOLM-13 (AML)	0.03	0.37	n.d.	n.d.	n.d.	n.d.

Summing up, combined inhibition of cell cycle and angiogenesis by ZK 304709 resulted in superior efficacy compared to standard chemotherapeutic compounds both in subcutaneous human tumour xenografts and in orthotopic human pancreatic carcinoma models.

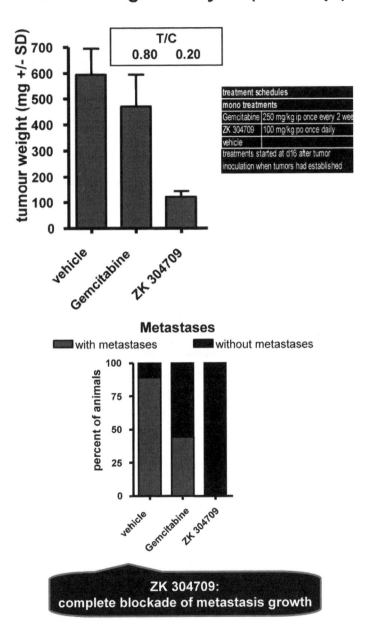

Figure 1   Capan-1 human pancreatic tumour model

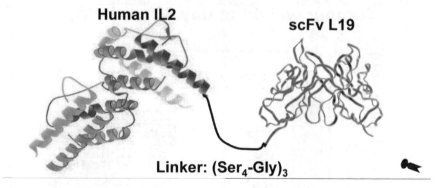

Human IL2

scFv L19

Linker: (Ser₄-Gly)₃

Figure 2 L19-IL-2: a recombinant fusion protein for the treatment of solid tumours

Tumour implantation:
Day -48 => fully established orthotopic tumour

Treatment schedule:

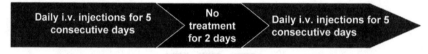

Daily i.v. injections for 5 consecutive days | No treatment for 2 days | Daily i.v. injections for 5 consecutive days

Figure 3 Treatment regimen of established tumour mass

L19-IL-2

L19-IL-2 is a recombinant fusion protein consisting of a scFv targeting moiety selective for the ED-B domain of fibronectin and IL-2 as an effector moiety able to attract and stimulate NK and T cells (see Figure 2).

Hepatocellular and pancreatic cancers show perivascular and stromal ED-B fibronectin expression within the tumour tissue, whereas corresponding normal tissues and liver biopsies from patients with pancreatitis or liver cirrhosis do not.

In previous studies it was shown that cyanine dye-labelled fusion protein is able to localize ED-B expressing human tumours and to retain within human tumour xenografts. Based on these earlier findings we anticipated that targeting and retention of IL-2 to human tumour xenografts might induce therapeutic effects superior to those achievable with systemically applied IL-2 alone.

To test this hypothesis human MPS pancreatic carcinoma cells or human HU17 hepatocellular carcinoma cells were implanted orthotopically in the pancreas or the liver, respectively. Animals were treated as shown in Figure 3.

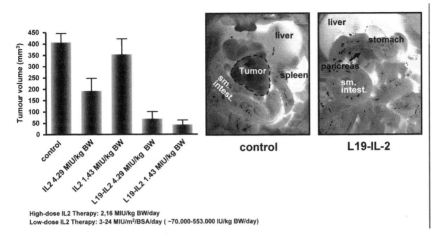

High-dose IL2 Therapy: 2,16 MIU/kg BW/day
Low-dose IL2 Therapy: 3-24 MIU/m²/BSA/day (~70.000-553.000 IU/kg BW/day)

Figure 4 Therapeutic effects after two treatment cycles with L19-IL-2 in orthotopic MPS pancreatic cancer model in nu/nu

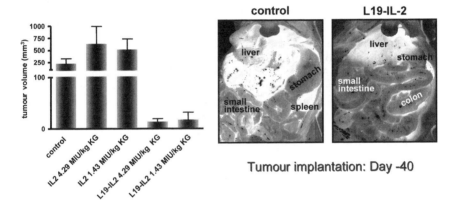

Tumour implantation: Day -40

Figure 5 Therapeutic effect after two treatment cycles using L19-IL-2 in the orthotopic HuH7-model for HCC

Very strong anti-tumour effects were observed in the fusion protein-treated animals, resulting in nearly complete eradication of pancreatic carcinomas or hepatocelllular carcinomas at targeted IL-2 doses which did not result in significant efficacy of systemically applied IL-2 (see Figures 4 and 5).

Interestingly, these therapeutic effects were achieved at fusion protein doses which did not result in any increase of liver or pancreas enzymes or any body weight loss. In summary it can be concluded that fusion protein-targeted IL-2 induces strong therapeutic effects in orthotopic models for human pancreatic carcinoma and hepatocellular carcinoma without any detectable side effects.

Both experimental cancer compounds, ZK 304709 and L19-IL-2 are in Phase I clinical studies.

13
Special Lecture: Anti-apoptotic intervention as a novel treatment option in liver diseases

A. CANBAY and G. J. GORES

INTRODUCTION

Hepatocyte death by apoptosis is a prominent feature in human liver diseases. For example, liver damage by apoptosis has been well documented in alcoholic hepatitis, non-alcoholic fatty liver disease, viral hepatitis, and ischaemia–reperfusions injury. Apoptosis and fibrosis are both ubiquitous features of chronic liver injury[1,2]. Apoptosis has been linked to fibrosis by two opposing processes. Hepatocyte apoptosis by death receptors appears to be pro-fibrogenic. For example, genetic or siRNA ablation of Fas expression, a death receptor richly expressed in the liver, attenuates fibrosis in murine models of liver injury[3,4]. In contrast, hepatic stellate cell (HSC) apoptosis is thought to be essential for the resolution phase of fibrosis[5]. Activated HSC appear to undergo an activation associated cell death terminating their life span and limiting hepatic fibrogenesis. Inhibition of HSC apoptosis would be expected to be pro-fibrogenic by permitting the accumulation of these activated cells within the liver. Therefore, the net effect of broadly inhibiting liver cell apoptosis is unclear; it may be anti-fibrogenic by blocking hepatocyte apoptosis or pro-fibrogenic by inhibiting HSC apoptosis. Further, different drugs might have different cellular specificity; however, the net effect of the drug's administration on hepatic fibrosis is probably the most important.

Although inhibition of Fas death receptor-mediated apoptosis reduces hepatic fibrosis, studies cannot be equated with broad inhibition of apoptosis. Death receptors signal through several intracellular cascades, many of which are proinflammatory rather than death-producing. For example, activation of NF-κB by death receptors is proinflammatory[6]. Consistent with this concept, Fas-activation in the liver is proinflammatory and triggers the production of several inflammatory chemokines[7]. The resulting inflammation from Fas activation may result in HSC activation and fibrosis[8]. In this context, blocking Fas stimulation may prevent hepatic fibrosis by blocking inflammation, not apoptosis. Therefore the elegant studies examining the relationship between

126

Fas expression and hepatic fibrosis do not directly address the question as to whether broad-based anti-apoptotic therapy would be pro- or anti-fibrogenic. Given the complexity of the relationships between apoptosis, inflammation and fibrosis, it is important that the *in-toto* effects are evaluated experimentally, and then clinically.

The use of a pan-caspase pharmacological inhibitor which is very effective in blocking cell death[9,10] can help to ascertain if blocking liver cell apoptosis is pro- or anti-fibrogenic. Thus, the overall objectives of this study were to examine the potential role of pharmacological inhibition of hepatocyte apoptosis in liver inflammation and fibrogenesis in the bile duct ligated (BDL) mouse. We sought to answer the following questions: Does the pan-caspase inhibitor, IDN-6556, attenuate hepatocyte apoptosis and liver injury in the BDL mouse? Does the pan-caspase inhibition reduce liver inflammation? Is liver fibrogenesis and HSC activation reduced following treatment with IDN-6556?

METHODS

Bile duct ligation, drug, alanine aminotransferase values (ALT), terminal deoxynucleotidyl transferase-mediated deoxyuridine triphosphate nick-end labelling (TUNEL) assay

The common bile duct ligation (BDL) was performed as previously described by us in detail[11]. After 3 days of BDL the animal was re-anaesthetized and blood samples and liver tissue procured. In selected experiments the mice were treated with the pan-caspase inhibitor, IDN-6556, which binds irreversibly to activated caspases with a K_i in the low to subnanomolar concentrations. The binding is selective, as it does not bind to other cysteine or serine enzymes at nanomolar or even low micromolar concentrations (> 10 μM). IDN-6556 (10 mg/kg) was given intraperitoneally 3 h after the BDL, and twice a day thereafter. The dosing was based on preliminary data demonstrating that IDN-6556 at doses of 10 mg/kg were required to prevent liver injury in this model. The agent was obtained from Idun Pharmaceuticals, Inc. (San Diego, CA).

Serum samples were used for the measurements of ALT levels using a commercially available assay kit following the manufacturer's instructions (Sigma Diagnostics Kit no. 505; Sigma Chemical Co., St Louis, MO). The liver tissues were used for TUNEL assay following the manufacturer's instructions (In Situ Cell Death Detection Kit; Roche Diagnostics, Indianapolis, IN).

Liver fibrosis

Liver fibrosis was quantified using Sirius red as previously described[3]. Direct red 80 and Fast green FCF (colour index 42053) were obtained from Sigma–Aldrich Diagnostics St Louis, MO). Red-stained collagen fibres were quantitated by using digital image analysis as described (Slide Scanner, BLISS

System, Bacus Laboratories, Lombard, IL). The red area was mathematically divided by the RGB area and multiplied by 100%. This determined the percentage area staining positively for collagen fibres providing a quantitative value on a continuous scale.

Statistical analysis

All data represent at least three independent experiments and are expressed as the mean $\pm$ SD unless otherwise indicated. Differences between groups were compared using ANOVA for repeated measures and a post-hoc Bonferroni test to correct for multiple comparisons.

RESULTS AND DISCUSSION

We used the BDL model of murine extrahepatic cholestasis for these studies because it is well characterized with regard to the nature of the hepatic injury. Liver injury in this model occurs by the death receptors Fas and death receptor 5/tumour necrosis factor related apoptosis inducing ligand (TRAIL)-receptor 2[12]. Apoptosis by death receptors is caspase-dependent[13]; therefore our current observations demonstrating that IDN-6556 inhibits hepatocyte apoptosis and fibrogenesis in cholestasis is relevant to death receptor-mediated liver injury. Each of these observations is discussed in greater detail below.

The observations demonstrate that, in the BDL animal, pharmacological inhibition of caspases reduces: (a) hepatocyte apoptosis, serum ALT values and histological evidence of liver injury (Figure 1); (b) hepatic inflammation (data not shown); (c) mRNA expression for markers of HSC activation (data not shown); and (d) collagen expression and deposition (Figure 1). Taken together, these observations suggest a critical role for hepatocyte apoptosis in the initiation of stellate cell activation and hepatic fibrogenesis during cholestatic liver injury.

Also as observed in this study, prior publications have linked hepatocyte apoptosis with liver injury and elevated ALT values, and a reduction in these parameters by inhibiting apoptosis (Figure 1).

Our study suggests that apoptosis not only is associated with liver injury but is also proinflammatory in the liver during cholestasis. In this study the inhibition of apoptosis with the pan-caspase inhibitor reduced hepatic expression of chemokines. Apoptosis may induce inflammation by several mechanisms. First, dysregulated apoptosis in pathological conditions can disrupt hepatocyte integrity. For example, after experimental induction of apoptosis with Fas agonists mice develop fulminant hepatic failure, with massive necrosis and inflammation[14]. Second, death receptor-mediated apoptosis may contribute to liver inflammation, possibly by initiating proinflammatory signalling cascades[15]. For example, Fas agonists induce chemokine expression[7], and hepatocyte apoptosis is a potent stimulus for neutrophil extravasation[16]. The disposition of apoptotic bodies may also link apoptosis to inflammation in the liver. For example, engulfment of neutrophil

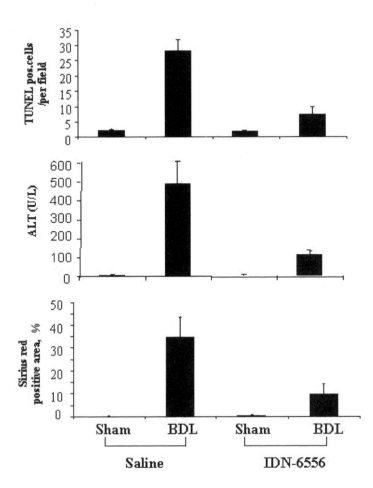

Figure 1 Hepatocyte apoptosis, liver injury and liver fibrosis are attenuated in IDN-6556-treated BDL mice. TUNEL-positive cells/field were significantly reduced in IDN-6556-treated mice compared to saline-treated BDL mice ($p < 0.001$, $n = 4$ for each group). Serum ALT values are significantly greater in saline-treated than in IDN-6556-treated BDL mice ($p < 0.005$, $n = 4$ for each experimental group). Sirius red staining was quantitatively greater in BDL than in and IDN-6556-treated BDL mice ($p < 0.001$, $n = 4$ for each group)

apoptotic bodies by macrophages and/or Kupffer cells can induce expression of death ligands, especially Fas ligand[17–19], thereby accelerating apoptosis. Finally, caspases may directly contribute to liver inflammation[15]. A pan-caspase inhibitor such as IDN-6556 may also block liver inflammation by inhibiting these caspases, in addition to reducing cellular apoptosis. Thus, probably by a combination of mechanisms, broad-spectrum caspase inhibition is salutary against liver inflammation during cholestasis.

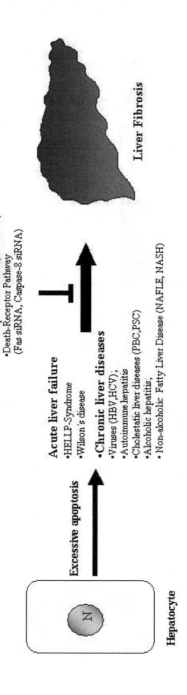

Figure 2 Anti-apoptotic therapy in liver diseases

Rather than promoting accumulation of activated HSC, the caspase inhibitor actually blocked their activation. The results suggest apoptosis plays an instrumental if not a pivotal role in HSC activation and hepatic fibrogenesis. Without significant HSC activation, the fear that a caspase inhibitor would block apoptosis of activated HSC, thereby promoting fibrosis, is not a concern. The mechanism by which hepatocyte apoptosis results in HSC activation may be direct or indirect. A direct pathway linking hepatocyte apoptosis to HSC activation is HSC engulfment of hepatocyte apoptotic bodies as has been documented *in vitro*[20]. Phagocytosis of apoptotic bodies by HSC results in their activation and promotes collagen expression. An indirect mechanism coupling hepatocyte apoptosis to HSC activation is via a secondary inflammatory response. As described above, hepatocyte apoptosis elicits an inflammatory response associated with chemokine expression and neutrophil infiltration[16,21]. This inflammatory response has been well established to cause HSC activation[8]. In either model, hepatocyte apoptosis is an apical event resulting in liver injury, HSC activation and liver scarring.

In summary, our findings suggest that, during extrahepatic cholestasis in the mouse, liver injury, inflammation, markers of stellate cell activation, and elevation of indices of hepatic fibrogenesis are, in part, hepatocyte apoptosis-dependent. Inhibition of hepatocyte apoptosis with a selective caspase inhibitor appears to be a viable therapeutic option for cholestatic liver injury, inflammation and fibrosis. These data also implicate a mechanistic link between hepatocyte apoptosis and HSC activation, and suggest inhibition of apoptosis would diminish liver fibrosis in chronic cholestatic liver diseases.

CONCLUSION

Taken together, it appears that increased hepatocyte apoptosis plays a dominant role in the development and progression of liver diseases. Although still preliminary, one may make a convincing case for the potentially high therapeutic benefit of inhibiting hepatocyte apoptosis in patients with liver injury. Such a strategy obviously might prevent liver inflammation, fibrosis, and their sequelae. To this end, caspase inhibitors are currently being developed for clinical use. Treatment of HCV-positive patients with this inhibitor significantly reduces ALT values and, therefore, liver injury[22]. In line with this observation, Bantel et al. have demonstrated the correlation of hepatocyte apoptosis with fibrosis in HCV patients[23]. More recently, Eichhorst et al. have demonstrated that the FDA-approved drug, suramin, inhibits apoptosis in a mouse model of liver damage[24,25]. Their results appear highly encouraging but caution is needed, because the therapeutic long-term employment of anti-apoptotic drugs, by tipping the balance to the opposite side of the spectrum, might potentially promote excessive cell growth. Although much work still has to be done, recent findings provide exciting new treatment options as therapeutic strategies for liver diseases (Figure 2).

References

1. Canbay A, Friedman S, Gores GJ. Apoptosis: the nexus of liver injury and fibrosis. Hepatology. 2004;39:273–8.
2. Yoon JH, Gores GJ. Death receptor-mediated apoptosis and the liver. J Hepatol. 2002;37: 400–10.
3. Canbay A, Higuchi H, Bronk SF, Taniai M, Sebo TJ, Gores GJ. Fas enhances fibrogenesis in the bile duct ligated mouse: a link between apoptosis and fibrosis. Gastroenterology. 2002;123:1323–30.
4. Song E, Lee SK, Wang J et al. RNA interference targeting Fas protects mice from fulminant hepatitis. Nat Med. 2003;9:347–51.
5. Iredale JP, Benyonn RC, Pickering J et al. Mechanism of spontaneous resolution of rat liver fibrosis. J Clin Invest. 1998;102:538–49.
6. Jaeschke H, Fisher MA, Lawson JA, Simmons CA, Farhood A, Jones DA. Activation of caspase 3 (CPP32)-like proteases is essential for TNF- alpha-induced hepatic parenchymal cell apoptosis and neutrophil- mediated necrosis in a murine endotoxin shock model. J Immunol. 1998;160:3480–6.
7. Faouzi S, Burckhardt BE, Hanson JC et al. Anti-Fas induces hepatic chemokines and promotes inflammation by an NF- kappa B-independent, caspase-3-dependent pathway. J Biol Chem. 2001;276:49077–82.
8. Maher JJ. Interactions between hepatic stellate cells and the immune system. Semin Liver Dis. 2001;21:417–26.
9. Valentino KL, Gutierrez M, Sanchez R, Winship MJ, Shapiro DA. First clinical trial of a novel caspase inhibitor: anti-apoptotic caspase inhibitor, IDN-6556, improves liver enzymes. Int J Clin Pharm Ther. 2003;41:441–9.
10. Natori S, Higuchi H, Contreras P, Gores GJ. The caspase inhibitor IDN-6556 prevents caspase activation and apoptosis in sinusoidal endothelial cells during liver preservation injury. Liver Transplant. 2003;9:278–84.
11. Miyoshi H, Rust C, Roberts PJ, Burgart LJ, Gores GJ. Hepatocyte apoptosis after bile duct ligation in the mouse involves Fas. Gastroenterology. 1999;117:669–77.
12. Higuchi H, Bronk SF, Taniai M, Canbay A, Gores GJ. Cholestasis increases tumor necrosis factor-related apoptotis-inducing ligand (TRAIL)-R2/DR5 expression and sensitizes the liver to TRAIL- mediated cytotoxicity. J Pharmacol Exp Ther. 2002;303:461–7.
13. Hengartner MO. The biochemistry of apoptosis. Nature. 2000;407:770–6.
14. Ogasawara J, Watanabe-Fukunaga R, Adachi M et al. Lethal effect of the anti-Fas antibody in mice. Nature. 1993;364:806–9.
15. Chen JJ, Sun Y, Nabel GJ. Regulation of the proinflammatory effects of Fas ligand (CD95L). Science. 1998;282:1714–17.
16. Lawson JA, Fisher MA, Simmons CA, Farhood A, Jaeschke H. Parenchymal cell apoptosis as a signal for sinusoidal sequestration and transendothelial migration of neutrophils in murine models of endotoxin and Fas-antibody-induced liver injury. Hepatology. 1998;28: 761–7.
17. Kurosaka K, Watanabe N, Kobayashi Y. Production of proinflammatory cytokines by resident tissue macrophages after phagocytosis of apoptotic cells. Cell Immunol. 2001;211: 1–7.
18. Geske FJ, Monks J, Lehman L, Fadok VA. The role of the macrophage in apoptosis: hunter, gatherer, and regulator. Int J Hematol. 2002;76:16–26.
19. Canbay A, Feldstein AE, Higuchi H et al. Kupffer cell engulfment of apoptotic bodies stimulates death ligand and cytokine expression. Hepatology. 2003;38:1188–98.
20. Canbay A, Taimr P, Torok N, Higuchi H, Friedman S, Gores GJ. Apoptotic body engulfment by a human stellate cell line is profibrogenic. Lab Invest. 2003;83:655–63.
21. Canbay A, Guicciardi ME, Higuchi H et al. Cathepsin B inactivation attenuates hepatic injury and fibrosis during cholestasis. J Clin Invest. 2003;112:152–9.
22. Valentino KL, Gutierrez M, Sanchez R, Winship MJ, Shapiro DA. First clinical trial of a novel caspase inhibitor: anti-apoptotic caspase inhibitor, IDN-6556, improves liver enzymes. Int J Clin Pharmacol Ther. 2003;41:441–9.

23. Bantel H, Lugering A, Heidemann J et al. Detection of apoptotic caspase activation in sera from patients with chronic HCV infection is associated with fibrotic liver injury. Hepatology. 2004;40:1078–87.
24. Eichhorst ST, Krueger A, Muerkoster S et al. Suramin inhibits death receptor-induced apoptosis *in vitro* and fulminant apoptotic liver damage in mice. Nat Med. 2004;10:602–9.
25. Guicciardi ME, Gores GJ. Cheating death in the liver. Nat Med. 2004;10:587–8.

Section Liver I
Diagnosis and surveillance in liver disease

Chair: A. LOHSE and G. RAMADORI

14
Imaging modalities in hepatic tumours

L. CROCETTI and R. LENCIONI

INTRODUCTION

Hepatocellular carcinoma (HCC) is increasingly diagnosed at an early, asymptomatic stage owing to surveillance of high-risk patients[1,2]. However, it has been shown by pathological studies that many small nodules detected by ultrasound (US) in cirrhotic livers do not correspond to HCC[3]. Diagnostic confirmation of small nodules as true HCC may be challenging, as pathological changes inherent in cirrhosis – such as dysplastic nodules (DN) – mimic a small tumour[4]. Percutaneous US-guided biopsy could appear to be the most straightforward approach. Unfortunately, biopsy of small nodular lesions in cirrhosis is not entirely reliable. Needle placement may be difficult and a sampling error may occur. Moreover, it is very difficult to distinguish well-differentiated HCC from DN on small biopsy specimens, as there is no clear-cut dividing line between dysplasia and well-differentiated tumour. Therefore, a positive biopsy – as assessed by an expert pathologist – is helpful, but a negative biopsy can never be taken as a criterion to rule out malignancy[5,6]. In addition, biopsy is associated with a low but not negligible rate of complications, including tumour seeding along the needle track.

Both the European Association for the Study of the Liver (EASL) Monothematic Conference on HCC and the American Association for the Study of Liver Diseases (AASLD) practice guidelines have recommended further investigation of nodules detected during US surveillance with dynamic imaging techniques – including contrast-enhanced US, contrast-enhanced multidetector computed tomography (CT), and contrast-enhanced magnetic resonance imaging (MRI)[5,6]. One of the key pathological factors for differential diagnosis that is reflected in dynamic imaging studies is the vascular supply to the lesion. Through the progression from regenerative nodule, to low-grade DN, to high-grade DN, to frank HCC, one sees loss of visualization of portal tracts and development of new arterial vessels, termed non-triadal arteries, which become the dominant blood supply in overt HCC lesions[4]. Careful assessment of lesion vascularity – through the use of state-of-the-art dynamic imaging techniques – can provide a reliable non-invasive diagnosis in cirrhotic patients.

ULTRASOUND

US is the imaging technique most commonly used worldwide for early detection of HCC in surveillance programmes[5]. US enables rapid and non-invasive evaluation of liver parenchyma, although a comprehensive assessment may be impossible because of the patient's body habitus or colonic interposition. When careful imaging–pathological correlation was performed, the sensitivity of US in the detection of small HCC lesions was shown to be much lower than previously estimated. In seven series that reported the correlation between pretransplantation US and pathological examination of explanted liver, lesion sensitivity ranged from 20% to 72% (Table 1)[7–13]. The ability to detect the emergence of a small HCC is highly dependent on the expertise of the operator performing the examination. Of interest, no improvement in sensitivity has been observed over the past decade, despite the advances in US technology (Table 1).

Table 1 Sensitivity of US in the detection of HCC in series with pathologic examination of the explanted liver as term of reference

Reference	No. of patients	No. of lesions	Lesion sensitivity
Dodd et al. (1992)[7]	200	80	36/80 (45%)
Shapiro et al. (1996)[8]	21	40	21/40 (51%)
Kim et al. (2001)[9]	52	18	6/18 (33%)
Rode et al. (2001)[10]	43	13	6/13 (46%)
Bennett et al. (2002)[11]	200	39	8/39 (20%)
Liu et al. (2003)[12]	118	51	14/51 (27%)
Teefey et al. (2003)[13]	25	18	13/18 (72%)

At US, small, nodular type HCC usually appears as a round or oval mass lesion with sharp and smooth boundaries, that may exhibit a hypoechoic, an isoechoic, or a hyperechoic appearance with respect to surrounding liver parenchyma. Nodular type HCC with extranodular growth and contiguous multinodular type HCC show a nodular configuration with irregular or blurred margins. The hyperechoic pattern of small HCC usually indicates fatty change or, less frequently, pseudoglandular arrangement of the cancer cells or peliotic changes of tumour vascular spaces. Small, nodular type HCC is usually indistinguishable from large regenerative nodule and DN. In addition, small hyperechoic HCC may be indistinguishable from haemangioma[14].

Doppler US techniques have long been used in attempts to evaluate the tumour vascularity of HCC. With colour or power Doppler US, HCC is usually displayed as a vascular-rich lesion containing intratumoral flow signals with an arterial Doppler spectrum. A basket pattern, which is a fine blood-flow network surrounding the nodule, and tumour vessels flowing into the lesion and branching within it, are typically observed in large HCC. Doppler interrogation shows a pulsatile Doppler waveform with high-frequency shifts and abnormally elevated resistive and pulsatility indexes. Since large regenerative nodule and DN usually do not show intratumoral arterial vessels, detection of neovascularity with Doppler US imaging supports the diagnosis of HCC[15]. In small HCC lesions, however, the sensitivity of Doppler techniques in showing arterial hypervascularity is low, and a pulsatile flow with arterial waveform can be demonstrated in less than 50% of the lesions[15].

Recently the introduction of microbubble contrast agents and the development of contrast-specific scanning techniques have opened new prospects in liver US[16]. Contrast-specific techniques produce images based on non-linear acoustic effects of microbubbles and display enhancement in grey scale, with high contrast and spatial resolution. Over the past few years several reports have shown that contrast-enhanced studies substantially increase the ability of US to characterize focal liver lesions[17–20]. The advent of second-generation agents and low mechanical index real-time scanning techniques has been instrumental in improving the ease and reproducibility of the examination, and has prompted the European Federation of Societies for Ultrasound in Medicine and Biology (EFSUMB) to define the indications and recommendations for the use of contrast agents in clinical practice[21].

According to EFSUMB guidelines, performing a contrast-enhanced US study is recommended to characterize any lesion or suspect lesion detected at baseline US in the setting of liver cirrhosis[21]. HCC typically shows strong intratumoral enhancement in the arterial phase (i.e. within 25–35 s after the start of contrast injection) followed by rapid washout with isoechoic or hypoechoic appearance in the portal venous and delayed phases. In contrast, large regenerative nodule and DN usually do not show any early contrast uptake, and resemble the enhancement pattern of liver parenchyma. In two recent series, selective arterial enhancement at contrast US was observed in 91–96% of HCC lesions, confirming that contrast US may be a tool to show arterial neoangiogenesis of HCC[22,23]. Assuming findings at spiral CT as the gold standard, the sensitivity of contrast US in the detection of arterial hypervascularity was 97% in lesions larger than 3 cm, 92% in lesions of 2–3 cm, 87% in lesions of 1–2 cm, and 67% in lesions smaller than 1 cm[23].

SPIRAL COMPUTED TOMOGRAPHY

With the introduction of spiral scanners the role of CT in liver imaging has dramatically changed. Owing to the possibility to scan the whole liver during a single breath-hold, a comprehensive evaluation of the hepatic parenchyma during the different phases of contrast enhancement has become feasible. The standard spiral CT examination protocol for detection and characterization of HCC should include unenhanced and contrast-enhanced images obtained in the arterial phase (scanning initiated at about 25–30 s after the start of contrast injection), the portal venous phase (scanning initiated at about 70–80 s after the start of contrast injection), and the delayed phase (scanning initiated at about 180–210 s after the start of contrast injection). Proper timing of arterial phase imaging is crucial to identify hypervascular nodules, and requires the use of a test dose injection or a bolus track system to initiate the scanning at an optimal phase of opacification[24].

The recent coupling of multidetector-row scan technology with spiral image acquisition has further enhanced the performance of CT in liver imaging. Multidetector spiral CT offers a marked reduction in the time required for thin-section imaging of the entire liver relative to standard single-detector spiral CT. The resulting substantial improvement in spatial resolution was shown to increase CT sensitivity in the detection of hypervascular HCC[25]. In addition, the increased temporal resolution permits hepatic imaging during two distinct arterial phases: the early arterial phase and the late arterial phase, acquired during the same breath-hold[26]. Doubling the classic arterial phase of single-detector spiral CT may offer advantages. The early arterial phase is a true CT arteriography, and can be used to assess vascular anatomy. However, in most studies acquiring a double arterial phase did not improve the detection rate of HCC with respect to late arterial phase imaging alone[27–30]. A further evolution of the scanning protocol includes triple arterial phase scanning, with the middle arterial phase imaging claimed as the most sensitive for HCC detection[31].

Despite these substantial technological advances, CT remains relatively insensitive for the detection of tiny HCC lesions. In six series that reported careful lesion-by-lesion imaging–pathological correlation in explanted livers, the sensitivity of spiral CT in detection of HCC lesions was 52–79% (Table 2)[10,13,31–35]. In particular, only 10–43% of lesions smaller than 1 cm and 44–65% of lesions of 1–2 cm were identified (Table 2).

Another important issue is the specificity of CT findings. It is accepted that overt HCC lesions show a hypervascular CT pattern, with clear-cut enhancement in the arterial phase and rapid washout in the portal venous and delayed phases. In contrast, large regenerative nodule and DN usually fail to exhibit this feature and appear isoattenuating or hypoattenuating to surrounding liver parenchyma[36,37]. However, the positive predictive value of CT findings is 59–88%, as non-malignant lesions may show increased arterial blood supply and be indistinguishable from a small HCC. In one study only 17 (24%) of 71 hypervascular hepatic nodules detected during arterial phase CT scans were confirmed as HCC at histopathology of explanted livers[38]. Non-malignant hepatocellular lesions – histologically diagnosed as large regenerative nodule or DN – showed the following characteristics: 0.5–2 cm in diameter, distinct margins, internal homogeneity, and isoattenuation to surrounding liver on precontrast, portal venous, and delayed phase scanning[38].

False-positive interpretations can occasionally be caused by small (less than 1.5 cm) flash-filling haemangiomas, that may enhance homogeneously in the arterial phase[39]. However, these lesions usually do not exhibit contrast washout and show attenuation equivalent to that of the aorta during portal venous and delayed phase CT imaging[40]. Non-tumorous arterioportal shunts can also be a cause of pseudolesions, although in most cases they have the typical wedge-shaped and homogeneous appearance (with or without internal linear branching structures representing early opacification of portal veins during the arterial phase) and are isoattenuating or slightly hyperattenuating during the portal venous phase[41].

Table 2 Sensitivity and positive predictive value of spiral CT in the detection of HCC in series with pathological examination of the explanted liver as term of reference

Reference	No. of patients/ no. of lesions	Overall lesion sensitivity	Sensitivity for lesions <1 cm	Sensitivity for lesions 1–2 cm	Sensitivity for lesions >2 cm	Positive predictive value
Lim et al. (2000)[32]	41/21	15/21 (71%)	–	6/10 (60%)	9/11 (82%)	N/A
Rode et al. (2001)[10]	43/13	7/13 (54%)	3/7 (43%)	3/5 (60%)	1/1 (100%)	N/A
de Lédinghen et al. (2002)[33]	34/54	28/54 (52%)	2/8 (25%)	15/34 (44%)	11/12 (92%)	28/37 (76%)
Burrel et al. (2002)[34]	50/76	43/70 (61%)	2/20 (10%)	17/26 (65%)	24/24 (100%)	43/49 (87%)
Teefey et al. (2003)[13]	25/18	13/18 (72%)	N/A	N/A	N/A	13/22 (59%)
Valls et al. (2004)[35]	85/85	67/85 (79%)	–	23/38 (61%)	44/47 (94%)	67/76 (88%)

N/A, not available.

141

Identification of morphological features of HCC may support the diagnosis of HCC in questionable cases. Tumour capsule appears as a peripheral rim, that is hypoattenuating on unenhanced and arterial-phase images and hyperattenuating on delayed phase images. Unfortunately, the CT detection rate of the capsule is strongly dependent on lesion size, and is low in small tumours because the capsule itself is thin and poorly developed[42]. Internal mosaic architecture, with components showing various attenuation index on CT images, is another typical feature of HCC that, however, is usually detected in large nodular lesions. Invasion of portal vein branches, with partial or complete neoplastic thrombosis, is quite frequent in advanced tumours and is best shown on portal venous phase images. Neoplastic thrombi, however, may enhance in the arterial phase, like the main tumour. While invasion of main portal vein branches may be clearly detected by CT, identification of tumour spread into peripheral–segmental or subsegmental–branches, remains a substantial limitation of the technique[43].

MAGNETIC RESONANCE IMAGING

Over the past few years MR imaging of the liver has progressed significantly. Technical advances in hardware and software have allowed the acquisition of images with excellent anatomical detail, largely free of artifacts secondary to respiratory motion. Fast sequences have reduced image acquisition time, thereby improving patient acceptance and allowing more efficient utilization of machine time. New volumetric sequences have enabled three-dimensional serial dynamic imaging of the liver with a very high spatial and temporal resolution, reducing section misregistration and motion artifacts while improving multiplanar reformations[44]. A number of novel liver-specific contrast agents, including hepatocyte-targeted and reticuloendothelial system (RES)-targeted compounds, have been developed, permitting manipulation of the tissue signal in different ways, according to the relevant diagnostic issue[4,45].

The standard examination protocol for the detection and characterization of HCC includes T1-weighted fast spoiled gradient-echo sequences with fat suppression, respiratory-triggered or breath-hold T2-weighted fast spin-echo sequences with fat suppression, and serial dynamic T1-weighted fast spoiled gradient-echo sequences after bolus injection of a gadolinium chelate[45]. Additional sequences, such as out-of-phase spoiled gradient-echo T1-weighted sequences, may be performed to provide a comprehensive information or to solve specific diagnostic issues[46].

HCC shows a variety of MR imaging features, that reflect the variable characteristics of this malignancy in tumour architecture, grading, stromal component, as well as intracellular content of certain substances, such as fat, glycogen, or metal ions, that greatly affect the appearance of the lesion on baseline T1-weighted and T2-weighted MR images[45]. The signal intensity may range from hypointensity to isointensity to hyperintensity on T1-weighted images and from isointensity to hyperintensity on T2-weighted images. Hyperintensity on T1-weighted images and isointensity on T2-weighted images are typical features of well-differentiated tumours, while hypointensity on T1-weighted images and hyperintensity on T2-weighted images are usually associated with moderately or poorly differentiated tumours[47]. The signal intensity of HCC lesions may be inhomogeneous, reflecting the presence of areas with different degree of differentiation. Lesion signal intensity on baseline T1-weighted and T2-weighted images may help differentiate HCC from large regenerative nodule or DN, although considerable overlap exists[48].

Dynamic contrast-enhanced MR imaging allows selective imaging of the entire liver in the arterial, the portal venous, and the delayed phases[49–53]. The acquisition protocol should be optimized for proper timing of arterial phase imaging by using automated bolus-detection three-dimensional sequences and may include double or triple arterial phase imaging, as in multidetector CT[54,55]. Dynamic MR imaging well demonstrates the typical vascular features of overt HCC; that is, arterial phase enhancement with portal venous phase washout. This feature enables differentiation of frank HCC from large regenerative nodule or DN, that usually are not hypervascular[49]. Nevertheless, as discussed for CT imaging, non-malignant hepatocellular lesions – especially high-grade DN – may show increased arterial blood supply and be indistinguishable from a small HCC. In addition, non-tumorous arterioportal shunts may cause false-positive interpretations[56,57]. In one study, 54 (52%) of 104 small (less than 2 cm), round or oval, early-enhancing hepatic lesions at serial contrast-enhanced dynamic MR imaging were not confirmed as HCC at follow-up[56].

Despite technical improvements, MR imaging remains relatively insensitive for the detection of tiny HCC nodules and for the identification of tumour vascular invasion into peripheral portal vein branches. In series in which MR imaging findings were correlated with histopathological results after thin-section slicing of the explanted liver, lesion-by-lesion analysis revealed a sensitivity of 33–78%, with positive predictive values of 54–90% (Table 3)[10,13,33,34,58,59]. In particular, only 4–71% of lesions smaller than 1 cm and 52–92% of lesions of 1–2 cm were identified (Table 3). Nevertheless, state-of-the-art dynamic MR imaging outperforms single-detector spiral CT in the detection of small nodules: in one comparative study with explant correlation the sensitivity for the identification of additional HCC lesions was significantly higher for MR imaging than for spiral CT in the range 1–2 cm[34].

While the dynamic study performed by using gadolinium chelates is currently a key part of the MR examination, a variety of liver-specific contrast agents have been used in attempts to improve the information provided by MR imaging in HCC detection and characterization[45]. It has been shown that some well-differentiated HCC may show a positive enhancement after the administration of the hepatocyte-targeted agent Mn-DPDP because of their affinity with normal hepatocytes. In one study, owing to this peculiar feature, early-stage tumours that were missed by spiral CT because of their immature neovascularity were detected[60]. HCC conspicuousness after the administration of RES-specific contrast agents depends on differences in the number of Kupffer cells within the nodule and the surrounding cirrhotic liver[61]. While moderately or poorly differentiated HCC containing few or no Kupffer cells show high contrast-to-noise ratio, well-differentiated HCC have a Kupffer cell population that may not significantly differ from that of surrounding

Table 3 Sensitivity and positive predictive value of dynamic MR imaging in the detection of HCC in series with pathological examination of the explanted liver as term of reference

Reference	No. of patients / no. of lesions	Overall lesion sensitivity	Sensitivity for lesions <1 cm	Sensitivity for lesions 1–2 cm	Sensitivity for lesions >2 cm	Positive predictive value
Rode et al. (2001)[10]	43/13	10/13 (77%)	5/7 (71%)	4/5 (80%)	1/1 (100%)	N/A
de Lédinghen et al. (2002)[33]	34/54	33/54 (61%)	2/8 (25%)	19/34 (56%)	12/12 (100%)	33/37 (89%)
Burrel et al. (2002)[34]	50/76	58/76 (76%)	8/23 (34%)	25/28 (89%)	25/25 (100%)	58/64 (90%)
Krinsky et al. (2002)[58]	24/118	39/118 (33%)	3/72 (4%)	11/21 (52%)	25/25 (100%)	39/45 (87%)
Teefey et al. (2003)[13]	22/18	14/18 (77%)	N/A	N/A	N/A	14/19 (74%)
Bhartia et al.* (2003)[59]	31/32	25/32 (78%)	3/8 (38%)	12/13 (92%)	10/11 (91%)	25/46 (54%)

Note. N/A, not available.

*MR protocol included dynamic imaging plus liver-specific imaging after administration of a RES-targeted agent.

Table 4 Comparison of MR imaging with use of liver-specific contrast agents with dynamic MR imaging for the detection of HCC

Reference	No. of patients/ no. of lesions	Overall lesion sensitivity	Sensitivity for lesions < 1.5 cm	Positive predictive value
Pauleit et al. (2001)[63]	43/77	Fe-MRI 63/77 (82%) Dy-MRI 69/77 (90%) p = NS	Fe-MRI 19/31 (61%) Dy-MRI 26/31 (84%) p = 0.039	N/A
Youk et al. (2004)[64]	46/96	Mn-MRI 139/192 (72%)* Dy-MRI 168/192 (87%)* $p < 0.05$	N/A	N/A
Kwak et al. (2005)[65]	49/61	Fe-MRI 148/183 (81%)* Dy-MRI 165/183 (90%)* p = 0.03	Fe-MRI 75/108 (69%)* Dy-MRI 92/108 (85%)* $p < 0.05$	Fe-MRI 148/173 (85%)* Dy-MRI 165/188 (88%)* p = NS

Fe-MRI, MR imaging with use of the RES-targeted contrast agent ferumoxide; Dy-MRI, dynamic contrast-enhanced MR imaging; Mn-MRI, MR imaging with use of the hepatocyte-targeted contrast agent Mn-DPDP; N/A, not available.

*Sum of observers with mean sensitivity and positive predictive values.

parenchyma, which results in a signal-to-noise ratio close to zero and, thus, in low detectability rates[61]. Despite, in one series, MR imaging with use of a RES-targeted agent being superior to spiral CT for the detection of HCC nodules[62], in comparative studies the sensitivity of MR imaging with use of either hepatocyte-targeted or RES-targeted contrast agents was shown to be inferior to dynamic MR imaging (Table 4)[63–65]. It has to be considered, however, that recently introduced liver-specific agents can deliver dynamic imaging in addition to the liver-specific phase[4,45].

DIAGNOSTIC WORK-UP

A rational diagnostic protocol should be structured according to the actual risk of malignancy and the possibility of achieving a reliable diagnosis. Since the prevalence of HCC among US-detected nodules is strongly related to the size of the lesion, the diagnostic work-up depends on the size of the lesion[6].

Lesions less than 1 cm in diameter

Lesions smaller than 1 cm in diameter have a low likelihood of being HCC. However, minute hepatic nodules detected by US may become malignant over time. Therefore, these nodules need to be followed up in order to detect growth suggestive of malignant transformation. A reasonable protocol is to repeat US every 3 months, until the lesion grows to more than 1 cm, at which point additional diagnostic techniques are applied[5]. It has to be emphasized, however, that the absence of growth during the follow-up period does not rule out the malignant nature of the nodule, because even an early HCC may take more than 1 year to increase in size[5].

Lesions 1–2 cm in diameter

When the nodule exceeds 1 cm in size the lesion is more likely to be HCC, and diagnostic confirmation should be pursued. It is accepted that the diagnosis of HCC in cirrhosis can be made without biopsy in a nodule larger than 1 cm that shows characteristic vascular features of HCC – i.e. arterial hyper-vascularization with washout in the portal venous or delayed phase – even in patients with a normal alpha-fetoprotein value. Such lesions should be treated as HCC, since the positive predictive value of the clinical and radiological findings exceeds 95%, provided that examinations are conducted by using state-of-the-art equipment and interpreted by radiologists with extensive expertise in liver imaging[66]. For lesions of 1–2 cm the current guidelines require typical imaging findings to be confirmed by two coincident dynamic imaging modalities to allow a non-invasive diagnosis[6]. If the imaging findings are not characteristic, or the vascular profile is not coincidental among techniques, biopsy is recommended[6].

Lesions more than 2 cm in diameter

For nodules above 2 cm a single imaging technique – from contrast-enhanced US, contrast-enhanced multidetector CT, and contrast-enhanced MRI – showing the characteristic vascular profile of HCC mentioned above, may confidently establish the diagnosis[6]. It should be pointed out, however, that if the diagnosis is made by using contrast-enhanced US, additional investigation with multidetector CT or MRI is required to provide a comprehensive assessment of the liver parenchyma and rule out additional tumour foci. Moreover, it should be stressed that non-invasive criteria based on imaging findings can be applied only in patients with established cirrhosis[5]. For nodules detected in non-cirrhotic livers, as well as for those showing atypical vascular patterns, biopsy is recommended.

References

1. Llovet JM, Burroughs A, Bruix J. Hepatocellular carcinoma. Lancet. 2003;362:1907–17.
2. Sherman M. Hepatocellular carcinoma: epidemiology, risk factors, and screening. Semin Liver Dis. 2005;25:143-54.
3. Kojiro M, Roskams T. Early hepatocellular carcinoma and dysplastic nodules. Semin Liver Dis. 2005;25:133–42.
4. Lencioni R, Cioni D, Della Pina C et al. Imaging diagnosis. Semin Liver Dis. 2005;25:162–70.
5. Bruix J, Sherman M, Llovet JM et al. and EASL Panel of Experts on HCC. Clinical management of hepatocellular carcinoma. Conclusions of the Barcelona-2000 EASL conference. European Association for the Study of the Liver. J Hepatol. 2001;35:421–30.
6. Bruix J, Sherman M. Management of hepatocellular carcinoma. Hepatology. 2005;42:1208–36.
7. Dodd GD 3rd, Miller WJ, Baron RL et al. Detection of malignant tumors in end-stage cirrhotic livers: efficacy of sonography as a screening technique. Am J Roentgenol. 1992;159:727–33.
8. Shapiro RS, Katz R, Mendelson DS et al. Detection of hepatocellular carcinoma in cirrhotic patients: sensitivity of CT and ultrasonography. J Ultrasound Med. 1996;15:497–502.
9. Kim CK, Lim JH, Lee WJ. Detection of hepatocellular carcinomas and dysplastic nodules in cirrhotic liver: accuracy of ultrasonography in transplant patients. J Ultrasound Med. 2001;20:99–104.
10. Rode A, Bancel B, Douek P et al. Small nodule detection in cirrhotic livers: evaluation with US, spiral CT, and MRI and correlation with pathologic examination of explanted liver. J Comput Assist Tomogr. 2001;25:327–36.
11. Bennett GL, Krinsky GA, Abitbol RJ et al. Sonographic detection of hepatocellular carcinoma and dysplastic nodules in cirrhosis: correlation of pretransplantation sonography and liver explant pathology in 200 patients. Am J Roentgenol. 2002;179:75–80.
12. Liu WC, Lim JH, Park CK et al. Poor sensitivity of sonography in detection of hepatocellular carcinoma in advanced liver cirrhosis: accuracy of pretransplantation sonography in 118 patients. Eur Radiol. 2003;13:1693–8.
13. Teefey SA, Hildeboldt CC, Dehdashti F et al. Detection of primary hepatic malignancy in liver transplant candidates: prospective comparison of CT, MR imaging, US, and PET. Radiology. 2003;226:533–42.
14. Caturelli E, Pompili M, Bartolucci F et al. Hemangioma-like lesions in chronic liver disease: diagnostic evaluation in patients. Radiology. 2001;220:337–42.
15. Lencioni R, Pinto F, Armillotta N, Bartolozzi C. Assessment of tumor vascularity in hepatocellular carcinoma: comparison of power Doppler US and color Doppler US. Radiology. 1996;201:353–8.

16. Lencioni R, Cioni D, Bartolozzi C. Tissue harmonic and contrast-specific imaging: back to gray scale in ultrasound. Eur Radiol. 2002;12:151–65.
17. Fracanzani AL, Burdick L, Borzio M et al. Contrast-enhanced Doppler ultrasonography in the diagnosis of hepatocellular carcinoma and premalignant lesions in patients with cirrhosis. Hepatology. 2001;34:1109–12.
18. Lencioni R, Cioni D, Crocetti L et al. Ultrasound imaging of focal liver lesions with a second-generation contrast agent. Acad Radiol. 2002;9(Suppl. 2):S371–4.
19. Wen YL, Kudo M, Zheng RQ et al. Characterization of hepatic tumors: value of contrast-enhanced coded phase-inversion harmonic angio. Am J Roentgenol. 2004;182:1019–26.
20. Quaia E, Calliada F, Bertolotto M et al. Characterization of focal liver lesions with contrast-specific US modes and a sulfur hexafluoride-filled microbubble contrast agent: diagnostic performance and confidence. Radiology. 2004;232:420–30.
21. Albrecht T, Blomley M, Bolondi L et al. and EFSUMB Study Group. Guidelines for the use of contrast agents in ultrasound. January 2004. Ultraschall Med. 2004;25:249–56.
22. Nicolau C, Catala V, Vilana R et al. Evaluation of hepatocellular carcinoma using SonoVue, a second generation ultrasound contrast agent: correlation with cellular differentiation. Eur Radiol. 2004;14:1092–9.
23. Gaiani S, Celli N, Piscaglia F et al. Usefulness of contrast-enhanced perfusional sonography in the assessment of hepatocellular carcinoma hypervascular at spiral computed tomography. J Hepatol. 2004;41:421–6.
24. Kim T, Murakami T, Hori M et al. Small hypervascular hepatocellular carcinoma revealed by double arterial phase CT performed with single breath-hold scanning and automatic bolus tracking. Am J Roentgenol. 2002;178:899–904.
25. Kawata S, Murakami T, Kim T et al. Multidetector CT: diagnostic impact of slice thickness on detection of hypervascular hepatocellular carcinoma. Am J Roentgenol. 2002;179:61–6.
26. Murakami T, Kim T, Takamura M et al. Hypervascular hepatocellular carcinoma: detection with double arterial phase multi-detector row helical CT. Radiology. 2001;218: 763–7.
27. Ichikawa T, Kitamura T, Nakajima H et al. Hypervascular hepatocellular carcinoma: can double arterial phase imaging with multidetector CT improve tumor depiction in the cirrhotic liver? Am J Roentgenol. 2002;179:751–8.
28. Kim SK, Lim JH, Lee WJ et al. Detection of hepatocellular carcinoma: comparison of dynamic three-phase computed tomography images and four-phase computed tomography images using multidetector row helical computed tomography. J Comput Assist Tomogr. 2002;26:691–8.
29. Laghi A, Iannaccone R, Rossi P et al. Hepatocellular carcinoma: detection with triple-phase multi-detector row helical CT in patients with chronic hepatitis. Radiology. 2003; 226:543–9.
30. Francis IR, Cohan RH, McNulty NJ et al. Multidetector CT of the liver and hepatic neoplasms: effect of multiphasic imaging on tumor conspicuity and vascular enhancement. Am J Roentgenol. 2003;180:1217–24.
31. Murakami T, Kim T, Kawata S et al. Evaluation of optimal timing of arterial phase imaging for the detection of hypervascular hepatocellular carcinoma by using triple arterial phase imaging with multidetector-row helical computed tomography. Invest Radiol. 2003; 38:497–503.
32. Lim JH, Kim CK, Lee WJ et al. Detection of hepatocellular carcinomas and dysplastic nodules in cirrhotic livers: accuracy of helical CT in transplant patients. Am J Roentgenol. 2000;175:693–8.
33. de Lédinghen V, Laharie D, Lecesne R et al. Detection of nodules in liver cirrhosis: spiral computed tomography or magnetic resonance imaging? A prospective study of 88 nodules in 34 patients. Eur J Gastroenterol Hepatol. 2002;14:159–65.
34. Burrel M, Llovet JM, Ayuso C et al. and Barcelona Clinic Liver Cancer Group. MRI angiography is superior to helical CT for detection of HCC prior to liver transplantation: an explant correlation. Hepatology. 2003;38:1034–42.
35. Valls C, Cos M, Figueras J et al. Pretransplantation diagnosis and staging of hepatocellular carcinoma in patients with cirrhosis: value of dual-phase helical CT. Am J Roentgenol. 2004;182:1011–17.

36. Hayashi M, Matsui O, Ueda K et al. Progression to hypervascular hepatocellular carcinoma: correlation with intranodular blood supply evaluated with CT during intraarterial injection of contrast material. Radiology. 2002;225:143–9.
37. Baron RL, Brancatelli G. Computed tomographic imaging of hepatocellular carcinoma. Gastroenterology. 2004;127(5 Suppl. 1):S133–43.
38. Freeny PC, Grossholz M, Kaakaji K, Schmiedl UP. Significance of hyperattenuating and contrast-enhancing hepatic nodules detected in the cirrhotic liver during arterial phase helical CT in pre-liver transplant patients: radiologic–histopathologic correlation of explanted livers. Abdom Imaging. 2003;28:333–46
39. Brancatelli G, Baron RL, Peterson MS, Marsh W. Helical CT screening for hepatocellular carcinoma in patients with cirrhosis: frequency and causes of false-positive interpretation. Am J Roentgenol. 2003;180:1007–14.
40. Kim T, Federle MP, Baron RL et al. Discrimination of small hepatic hemangiomas from hypervascular malignant tumors smaller than 3 cm with three-phase helical CT. Radiology. 2001;219:699–706.
41. Colagrande S, Fargnoli R, Dal Pozzo F et al. Value of hepatic arterial phase CT versus lipiodol ultrafluid CT in the detection of hepatocellular carcinoma. J Comput Assist Tomogr. 2000;24:878–83.
42. Iannaccone R, Laghi A, Catalano C et al. Hepatocellular carcinoma: role of unenhanced and delayed phase multi-detector row helical CT in patients with cirrhosis. Radiology. 2005;234:460–7.
43. Tsai TJ, Chau GY, Lui WY et al. Clinical significance of microscopic tumor venous invasion in patients with resectable hepatocellular carcinoma. Surgery. 2000;127:603–8.
44. Keogan MT, Edelman RR. Technologic advances in abdominal MR imaging. Radiology. 2001;220:310–20.
45. Lencioni R, Cioni D, Crocetti L et al. Magnetic resonance imaging of liver tumors. J Hepatol. 2004;40:162-71.
46. Sugihara E, Murakami T, Kim T et al. Detection of hypervascular hepatocellular carcinoma with dynamic magnetic resonance imaging with simultaneously obtained in-phase and opposed-phase echo images. J Comput Assist Tomogr. 2003;27:110–16.
47. Bartolozzi C, Cioni D, Donati F, Lencioni R. Focal liver lesions: MR imaging–pathologic correlation. Eur Radiol. 2001;11:1374–88.
48. Hussain HK, Syed I, Nghiem HV et al. T2-weighted MR imaging in the assessment of cirrhotic liver. Radiology. 2004;230:637–44.
49. Lencioni R. Mascalchi M, Caramella D, Bartolozzi C. Small hepatocellular carcinoma: differentiation from adenomatous hyperplasia with color Doppler US and dynamic Gd-DTPA-enhanced MR imaging. Abdom Imaging. 1996;21:41–8.
50. Noguchi Y, Murakami T, Kim T et al. Detection of hypervascular hepatocellular carcinoma by dynamic magnetic resonance imaging with double-echo chemical shift in-phase and opposed-phase gradient echo technique: comparison with dynamic helical computed tomography imaging with double arterial phase. J Comput Assist Tomogr. 2002;26:981–7.
51. Eubank WB, Wherry KL, Maki JH et al. Preoperative evaluation of patients awaiting liver transplantation: comparison of multiphasic contrast-enhanced 3D magnetic resonance to helical computed tomography examinations. J Magn Reson Imaging. 2002;16:565–75.
52. Noguchi Y, Murakami T, Kim T et al. Detection of hepatocellular carcinoma: comparison of dynamic MR imaging with dynamic double arterial phase helical CT. Am J Roentgenol. 2003;180:455–60.
53. Taouli B, Losada M, Holland A, Krinsky G. Magnetic resonance imaging of hepatocellular carcinoma. Gastroenterology. 2004;127:S144–152.
54. Hussain HK, Londy FJ, Francis IR et al. Hepatic arterial phase MR imaging with automated bolus-detection three-dimensional fast gradient-recalled-echo sequence: comparison with test-bolus method. Radiology. 2003;226:558–66.
55. Mori K, Yoshioka H, Takahashi N et al. Triple arterial phase dynamic MRI with sensitivity encoding for hypervascular hepatocellular carcinoma: comparison of the diagnostic accuracy among the early, middle, late, and whole triple arterial phase imaging. Am J Roentgenol. 2005;184:63–9.
56. Shimizu A, Ito K, Koike S et al. Cirrhosis or chronic hepatitis: evaluation of small (< or = 2-cm) early-enhancing hepatic lesions with serial contrast-enhanced dynamic MR imaging. Radiology. 2003;226:550–5.

57. Ito K, Fujita T, Shimizu A et al. Multiarterial phase dynamic MRI of small early enhancing hepatic lesions in cirrhosis or chronic hepatitis: differentiating between hypervascular hepatocellular carcinomas and pseudolesions. Am J Roentgenol. 2004;183:699–705.
58. Krinsky GA, Lee VS, Theise ND et al. Transplantation for hepatocellular carcinoma and cirrhosis: sensitivity of magnetic resonance imaging. Liver Transplant. 2002;8:1156–64.
59. Bhartia B, Ward J, Guthrie JA, Robinson PJ. Hepatocellular carcinoma in cirrhotic livers: double-contrast thin-section MR imaging with pathologic correlation of explanted tissue. Am J Roentgenol. 2003;180:577–84.
60. Bartolozzi C, Donati F, Cioni D et al. MnDPDP-enhanced MRI vs dual-phase spiral CT in the detection of hepatocellular carcinoma in cirrhosis. Eur Radiol. 2000;10:1697–702.
61. Lim JH, Choi D, Cho SK et al. Conspicuity of hepatocellular nodular lesions in cirrhotic livers at ferumoxides-enhanced MR imaging: importance of Kupffer cell number. Radiology. 2001;220:669–76.
62. Kang BK, Lim JH, Kim SH et al. Preoperative depiction of hepatocellular carcinoma: ferumoxides-enhanced MR imaging versus triple-phase helical CT. Radiology. 2003;226: 79–85.
63. Pauleit D, Textor J, Bachmann R et al. Hepatocellular carcinoma: detection with gadolinium- and ferumoxides-enhanced MR imaging of the liver. Radiology. 2002;222: 73–80.
64. Youk JH, Lee JM, Kim CS. MRI for detection of hepatocellular carcinoma: comparison of mangafodipir trisodium and gadopentetate dimeglumine contrast agents. Am J Roentgenol. 2004;183:1049–54.
65. Kwak HS, Lee JM, Kim YK et al. Detection of hepatocellular carcinoma: comparison of ferumoxides-enhanced and gadolinium-enhanced dynamic three-dimensional volume interpolated breath-hold MR imaging. Eur Radiol. 2005;15:140–7.
66. Levy I, Greig PD, Gallinger S et al. Resection of hepatocellular carcinoma without preoperative tumor biopsy. Ann Surg. 2001;234:206–9.

15
Hepatocellular tumours and tumour-like conditions: role of liver biopsy

T. LONGERICH and P. SCHIRMACHER

INTRODUCTION

The histological assessment of focal hepatocellular liver lesions plays a central role in liver pathology. In 1995 the terminology of nodular liver lesions was improved by an International Working Party (IWP)[1]. Based on this first standardized classification, two additional widely used schemes have been established. The actual WHO classification was introduced in 2000 and the last AFIP series was published in 2001[2-5]. Principally, all three classifications use a comparable nomenclature and distinguish benign from premalignant as well as malignant hepatocellular lesions, but their respective grouping differs slightly. Whereas the IWP distinguishes regenerative from dysplastic and neoplastic lesions, the WHO classification separates benign epithelial tumours, epithelial abnormalities, malignant epithelial tumours and miscellaneous lesions, and the AFIP-classification divides benign hepatocellular proliferations from putative precancerous lesions and malignant tumours. The detailed classification schemes are shown in Table 1.

Many focal liver lesions show characteristic radiological imaging features, especially by contrast-enhanced techniques, which are based on different vascularization patterns (e.g. focal nodular hyperplasia). Even diagnosis of hepatocellular carcinoma (HCC) can usually be made non-invasively with imaging procedures if the lesion is more than 2 cm in diameter[6-10]. Despite rapid advances in imaging techniques, the radiological sensitivity for diagnosis of smaller lesions is comparably low[11,12]. The major role of liver biopsy in the assessment of hepatocellular lesions is to establish a definite diagnosis of malignancy, when it is of therapeutic consequence, or to resolve cases of uncertain or inconsistent imaging results. Additionally, lesions that appear benign but show unusual imaging features or unexpected clinical behaviour are candidates for a liver biopsy. In general, a liver biopsy is indicated when diagnostic benefit exceeds the risks of intervention (see below) and when therapeutic strategy may be influenced.

Nowadays, imaging-guided, percutaneous liver biopsy is the standard procedure for biopsy of focal liver lesions; its accuracy is high and the

Table 1 Classification of hepatocellular tumours

International Working Party (1995), modified	*WHO (2000), modified*	*AFIP (2001), modified*

1. Regenerative lesions
1.1 Monoacinar regenerative nodule
  1.1.1 Diffuse nodular hyperplasia without fibrous septa (nodular regenerative hyperplasia)
  1.1.2 Diffuse nodular hyperplasia with fibrous septa or in cirrhosis
1.2 Multiacinar regenerative nodule
1.3 Lobar or segmental hyperplasia
1.4 Cirrhotic nodule
  1.4.1 Monoacinar cirrhotic nodule
  1.4.2 Mulitacinar cirrhotic nodule
1.5 Focal nodular hyperplasia (FNH)
  1.5.1 Focal nodular hyperplasia, solid type
  1.5.2 Focal nodular hyperplasia, teleangiectatic type
 	
2 Dysplastic or neoplastic lesions
2.1 Hepatocellular adenoma (LCA)
2.2 Dysplastic focus
2.3 Dysplastic nodule (DN)
  2.3.1 Dysplastic nodule with low atypia (low-grade, LGDN)
  2.3.2 Dysplastic nodule with high atypia (high-grade, HGDN)
2.4 Hepatocellular carcinoma (HCC)
	1. Benign epithelial tumours
	1.1 Hepatocellular adenoma
	1.2 Focal nodular hyperplasia
	
	2. Epithelial abnormalities
	2.1 Liver cell dysplasia
	  2.1.1 Large cell change
	  2.1.2 Small cell change
	2.2 Dysplastic nodules (adenomatous hyperplasia)
	  2.2.1 Low-grade dysplastic nodule
	  2.2.2 High-grade dysplastic nodule
	
	3. Malignant epithelial tumours
	3.1 Hepatocellular carcinoma
	3.2 Combined hepatocellular and cholangiocarcinoma
	3.3. Hepatoblastoma
	
	4. Miscellaneous lesions
	Nodular transformation (nodular regenerative hyperplasia)
		1. Benign hepatocellular proliferations
		1.1.1 Hepatocellular adenoma
		1.1.2 Hepatocellular adenomatosis
		1.2.1 Nodular regenerative hyperplasia
		1.2.2 Nodular regenerative hyperplasia with adenoma-like nodules
		1.3 Partial nodular transformation
		1.4 Focal nodular hyperplasia
		1.5 Compensatory hypertrophy (associated with lobar atrophy)
		1.6 Postnecrotic regenerative nodule
		1.7 Multiacinar regenerative nodule
		
		2. Putative precancerous lesions
		2.1 Dysplastic focus
		2.2 Dysplastic nodule
		  2.2.1 Low-grade dysplastic nodule
		  2.2.2 High-grade dysplastic nodule
		
		3. Malignant hepatocellular tumours
		3.1 Hepatocellular carcinoma
		3.2 Fibrolamellar hepatocellular carcinoma
		3.3 Combined hepatocellular-cholangiocarcinoma
		3.4 Hepatoblastoma

procedure is considered safe. Complications are observed in about 1% of patients, but nearly all are minor (pain, vagal symptoms, minor haemoperitoneum). Death following diagnostic liver biopsy has been reported to occur in up to 0.08% of cases. A specific complication following biopsy of HCC is needle-tract seeding, which has reported frequencies of 0.003% to 4.8% with an increasing frequency concurrent with the number of needle passes. Furthermore, the risk is increased for lesions exceeding 2 cm in diameter[13–18]. Therefore, some authors recommend resection of the needle track during surgery[15,16,19].

The diagnosis of well-differentiated hepatocellular tumours (especially in biopsy specimens) represents a challenging diagnostic problem and has gained increasing impact, because imaging-guided biopsies of small lesions (0.5–2 cm) are now technically possible. However, hepatopathological assessment has also improved significantly and several groups have elaborated differential diagnostic criteria for these lesions[20–26]. Despite improvements in morphological assessment, the establishment of a diagnosis requires close interdisciplinary cooperation. The pathologist needs clinical information about the patient's history (underlying liver disease and duration/progression, medication) and the size of the lesion, which give valuable additional information. Assessment of the non-tumorous liver tissue improves the likelihood of a certain tumour type (matrix diagnosis). For example, coexisting liver cirrhosis dramatically increases the likelihood of HCC. Additionally, the diagnostic power of liver biopsies depends on the amount of (tumour) tissue included.

The following sections will focus on the histological characteristics and differential diagnoses of well-differentiated hepatocellular lesions in biopsy. Relevant entities in this context include the tumour-like conditions multiacinar regenerative nodule (cirrhotic nodule) and focal nodular hyperplasia (FNH), the neoplastic, but benign liver cell adenoma (LCA), the premalignant dysplastic nodule (DN) and well-differentiated HCC. The diagnostic evaluation of liver metastasis is not discussed, although it may play a role in the differential diagnosis of moderately and poorly differentiated HCC.

MULTIACINAR REGENERATIVE NODULE/NODULAR TRANSFORMATION

Multiacinar regenerative nodules (MRN, cirrhotic nodule (IWP, AFIP)) do not pose specific clinical problems, but they represent a relevant differential diagnosis for the other focal lesions; they generally occur in diseased livers and represent a focal, regenerative parenchymal process including more than one acinar structure. Generally, these nodules measure between 0.2 and 5 cm. They are mostly seen in cirrhotic livers and to a lesser extent in other diseases where hepatic blood flow is impaired (e.g. Budd–Chiari syndrome). MRN themselves contain portal tracts, which sometimes show ductular proliferations. Obliteration of portal vein branches may be observed in the nearby parenchyma. Thus, recognition of MRN or differential diagnosis with FNH may occasionally pose problems in biopsy specimens. In contrast to dysplastic nodules, MRN does not show an expansive, clonal growth pattern. Hepatocyte plates of MRN are one or two cells wide and the reticulin framework is well formed and complete. Differentiating MRN from liver cell adenoma usually poses no problem in biopsy specimens, since portal tracts are present (20, 27). The relevant criteria for differential diagnosis are summarized in Table 2.

FOCAL NODULAR HYPERPLASIA

FNH is nowadays regarded as a tumour-like condition, which occurs as a consequence of a focal intrahepatic vascular malformation[28]. Two types are distinguished: the more frequent, classical, solid type and the teleangiectatic form, which are both easily distinguishable by histology. Although the genesis of FNH depends on an altered blood supply, there are a few reports of clonal characteristics in FNH, which would imply a neoplastic rather than a regenerative process.

The incidence of FNH is higher in women than in men, and there is some evidence that oral contraceptives may promote growth but not development of FNH. Diagnosis is mainly established by imaging techniques due to the unique vascularization pattern[29]. Therefore, histological diagnosis is typically limited to cases with unclear imaging results or an unusual clinical course. In about one-fourth of cases the FNH is multifocal, in part as the so-called FNH syndrome, which shows angiomatous lesions or intracerebral tumours[30]. The natural growth course of FNH is frequently stable and sometimes even regressive, especially when oral contraceptives are discontinued[31]. Spontaneous, intra-abdominal bleeding is exceedingly rare in FNH and malignant transformation has not been described unambiguously, therefore 'watch and wait' is the recommended primary strategy[32]. Surgical resection of FNH is mainly performed in cases of uncertain diagnosis or persistent growth of the lesion.

Whereas in resection specimens the pathomorphological diagnosis is straightforward, and even macroscopy with its central scar and radiating septa, ochre cut surface, absence of capsule and normal peritumorous liver tissue is characteristic, the diagnosis can be difficult in liver biopsy specimens (Figure 1A and 1B), especially when diagnostic features are not present and clinical information is lacking. Careful histological analysis in the search for abnormal vessels and ductular proliferations is essential. The arterial vessels of FNH show variable malformations including eccentric, subintimal fibrosis, fibromuscular hyperplasia and distortion of the elastica, whereas the veins are more frequently inconspicuous. FNH consists of a hepatocellular as well as a ductular component. Typically, there are polycyclic proliferations of hepatocytes, which are not encircled by capsular structures and lack regular central veins. In most cases hepatocytes of FNH are slightly smaller compared to normal hepatocytes and are surrounded by a proper reticulin framework[3,33]. The ductular proliferates are localized at the junction between the fibrous septa and the hepatocytes. The fibrous septa of FNH are often infiltrated by a predominantly lymphocytic infiltrate of variable density.

Table 2 Morphological characteristics of well-differentiated hepatocellular nodules (modified according to ref. 24)

Multiacinar regenerative nodule	Focal nodular hyperplasia	Liver cell adenoma	Dysplastic nodule	HCC
Histology No clonal expansion Inclusion of portal tracts Plates ≤2 cells thick Peripheral capillarization of sinusoids	Central scar with radial septa Central malformed vessel with media hyperplasia Ductular proliferation Focal lymphocytic aggregates	Scar or septa absent Trabecular growth pattern No ductular proliferation Solitary thin-walled vessels	Clonal growth pattern Slight trabecular disarrangement, sometimes pseudogland formation (HGDN) Peripheral (LGDN) and sometimes diffuse (HGDN) capillarization of sinusoids Focal loss of reticulin framework (HGDN) Sometimes nuclear peripheral alignment Unpaired arteries (low-grade > high grade) No definite signs of malignancy	'Nuclear crowding' and nuclear peripheral alignment Trabecular disarrangement (plates >2 cell thick, 'floating' trabecular ending) Loss of reticulin framework Capillarization of sinusoids Unpaired arteries Interstitial/vascular invasion
Cytology Atypia absent	Atypia absent Small hepatocytes Normal nuclear–cytoplasmic ratio	Atypia normally absent Frequently glycogen inclusion Normal nuclear–cytoplasmic ratio Adenoma cells frequently larger than normal cells	Sometimes increased cytoplasmic basophilia (HGDN) Slightly increased nuclear-cytoplasmic ratio	Increased cytoplasmic baophilia Increased nuclear–cytoplasmic ratio
Matrix diagnosis Cirrhosis Vascular abnormalities Alterations caused by underlying disease	Normal architecture	Normal architecture	Frequently cirrhosis (up to 80%, chronic hepatitis, (non-) alcoholic liver damage, haemochromatosis	

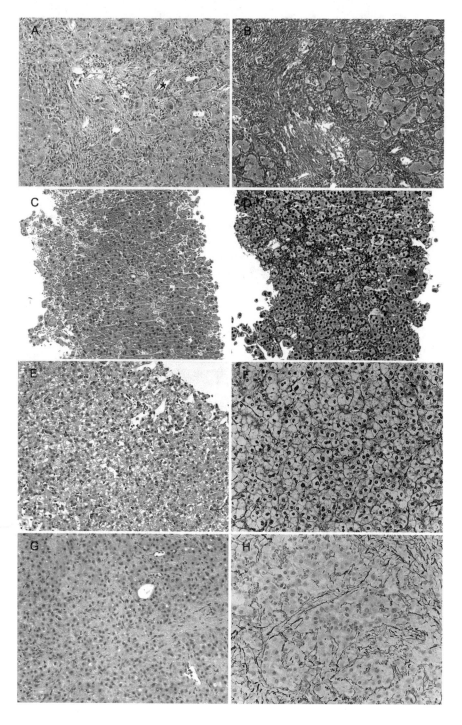

In contrast, teleangiectatic focal nodular hyperplasia (TFNH) is infrequent and differs from the solid type in the lack of a central scar and the presence of only a few fibrous septa. Little or even no ductular proliferation is seen, but sinusoids are widened, and in some cases, haemorrhagic or necrotic centres are observed[34]. Recently Paradis et al. performed comparative molecular-biological analyses of classical FNH, teleangiectatic variant and liver cell adenoma (LCA), and suggested that the teleangiectatic variant of FNH actually may be a variant of LCA, because in five of six cases protein profiles clustered with LCA instead of FNH[35]. Differential diagnosis of TFNH in biopsy specimens may include cavernous haemangioma.

LIVER CELL ADENOMA

In contrast to FNH, LCA represents a monoclonal neoplasia, which occurs as a solitary lesion in about 90% of cases. LCA is frequently observed in the setting of hormonal or metabolic stimulation of hepatocellular proliferation, e. g. long-term use of oral contraceptives, androgens or anabolics (treatment of Fanconi's anaemia, bodybuilding) as well as hormonal abnormalities such as Klinefelter's syndrome or steroid hormone-producing lesions[36-41]. Additionally, LCA occurs in metabolic disorders such as familial diabetes mellitus, glycogenosis, and haematological disorders such as beta-thalassaemia[42-45]. Association of LCA with prolonged carbamazepine therapy, Hurler's disease, and severe combined immunodeficiency has been described[46,47]. In general the incidence is much higher in women, but it is increasing in men due to the rising abuse of anabolic steroids. Diagnosis without a suggestive history should lead to the suspicion of alternative diagnoses such as FNH or HCC. The primary treatment option is the discontinuation of the causative agent, since many reports are published describing spontaneous regression of LCA after omission of the drug[48-51]. If cessation of the causative drug does not lead to regression, surgical resection or, in the case of liver adenomatosis (more than three adenomas), liver transplantation has to be considered, because LCA (especially of more than 5 cm in diameter) has an attributable risk of life-threatening, spontaneous rupture, and pregnancy is thought to increase this likelihood[3,52,53]. Malignant transformation of LCA to HCC is rare, but has been documented in some

---

Figure 1 **A**: Focal nodular hyperplasia with numerous ductular proliferations at the septal–parenchymal junction sometimes associated with inflammatory infiltration. Note the hyperplastic arteriole within the fibrous stroma (asterisk). **B**: Septa are composed of broad collagenous bands. The hepatocytes are surrounded by a regular reticulin framework. **C**: The hepatocytes of this liver cell adenoma are uniform without nuclear atypia. Portal tracts are not visible. Note focal hyperemia. **D**: The liver cell plates of the adenoma are up to two cells thick and are surrounded by a proper reticulin framework. **E**: The hepatocytes of this high-grade dysplatic nodule show microvesicular steatosis. They grow clonally expansive and the nuclei are partly peripherally aligned. **F**: The reticulin framework is intact. **G**: Well-differentiated HCC with nuclear crowding and pseudogland formation. **H**: The reticulin framework is focally absent and surrounds up to five cells-wide plates

cases. In contrast to HCC, LCA is extremely rare in cirrhotic livers (matrix diagnosis!) and it is widely accepted that LCA does not represent a common precursor lesion of HCC[27,54–56].

Histologically, LCA usually shows a solid, clonal growth pattern consisting of liver cell plates, which are up to two cells wide and are arranged in sheets and cords with compression of the sinusoids. In contrast to many (but not all) well-differentiated HCC, liver cell adenoma typically lacks a capsule. The hepatocytes are usually uniform, and in contrast to highly differentiated HCC, exhibit a regular nuclear–cytoplasmic ratio. The cell size is typically increased compared to normal hepatocytes. The cytoplasm may be normal or paler compared to normal hepatocytes due to glycogen or fat storage. In contrast to dysplastic nodules or well-differentiated HCC, increased cytoplasmic basophilia is not a typical feature. LCA associated with anabolic steroids may show some nuclear atypia as well as pseudogland formation with bile plugs within canaliculi[3,27]. Malignant transformation of liver cell adenoma should be diagnosed very carefully, especially in steroid hormone-associated LCA, since even complete regression after discontinuation of the drug has been observed (e.g. danazole). The hepatocytes of LCA are usually surrounded by a regular reticulin framework. LCA lack ductular proliferations and portal tracts, but sometimes pre-existing portal tracts may be entrapped at the periphery of the lesion (Figure 1C and 1D). The lack of portal tracts and ductular proliferation is an important diagnostic feature for differentiation from MRN and FNH. The presence of thin-walled arteriolar vessels, which are also not found in MRN and FNH, are quite characteristic for LCA, but may be seen incidentally in high-grade dysplastic nodules, hepatocellular carcinomas and even in a normal non-tumorous liver. Areas of infarction, haemorrhage or regression may be present and indicate an increased risk of spontaneous rupture.

DYSPLASTIC NODULES

Dysplastic nodules (DN), which have previously been called adenomatous hyperplasia, are nowadays accepted as the common premalignant lesions in human hepatocarcinogenesis[57–62]. In contrast to the classification systems of IWP and AFIP, the term adenomatous hyperplasia is still accepted in the WHO classification, although it is misleading in its close resemblance to LCA.

Both the IWP and the AFIP have defined clonal proliferations, which show small-cell dysplasia, nuclear crowding, and which are smaller than 0.1 cm as dysplastic foci. These foci have no direct diagnostic impact, but if they are incidentally found in a biopsy obtained for other purposes, such as chronic hepatitis, they should be mentioned as a risk indicator for malignant transformation. It has been shown by comparative genomic hybridization that hepatocytes of dysplastic foci carry genomic alterations, which are also present in adjacent HCC, but not in the peritumorous cirrhotic liver, and the prevalence of dysplastic foci is higher in cirrhotic livers with HCC than those without it[63,64]. Comparable lesions, which measure at least 1 mm in diameter, are called dysplastic nodules. The clonal character of these lesions has been shown at least in a few cases by analyses of HBV integration[65]. Dysplastic nodules show a clonal, expansive growth pattern and nuclear crowding (Figure

1E and 1F). In genetic haemochromatosis, dysplastic nodules may appear as iron-free foci. They are more or less arbitrarily divided into low- and high-grade DN, since a continuum exists. Low-grade DN (LGDN) show less atypia and structural changes than high-grade DN. The nuclear–cytoplasmic ratio may be mildly increased, the cytoplasm is usually eosinophilic and may be fatty; nuclear atypia is minimal and mitotic figures are absent. The plates are one or two cells thick. Staining for endothelial cell markers such as CD31 displays a peripheral staining pattern similar to cirrhotic nodules[22]. Additionally, the reticulin framework is regularly formed[4]. In contrast, high-grade DN (HGDN) show moderate nuclear atypia and may sometimes be indistinguishable from well-differentiated HCC in liver biopsy. The nuclear–cytoplasmic ratio is further increased and the nuclear contour may be mildly irregular. The cytoplasm is often more basophilic and, occasionally, peripheral nuclear alignment may occur. The plates are two or three cells thick and pseudoglands are rarely formed. Staining for CD31 may reveal diffuse capillarization and an increased number of so-called unpaired arteries (e.g. not accompanied by bile ducts) may be detected compared to the surrounding liver tissue[22,66]. HGDN lack interstitial or vascular invasion, which are definite criteria of malignancy. Dysplastic lesions normally do not exceed 2 cm in diameter and lesions of larger size are suggestive of an 'early HCC', even if they lack definite signs of malignancy in biopsy. Clinical follow-up has shown that the risk for malignant transformation is up to 50% in patients having DN compared to those without them, but these studies were based solely on biopsy diagnosis of DN, which is questionable[59,67]. Currently, there is no consensus as to whether these patients should be solely monitored or treated by percutaneous intervention or surgery[67–69]. Since human hepatocarcinogenesis represents a multi-step process, which presents itself as a morphological continuum for any lesion which at least represents a DN, surgical treatment should be recommended, since it is impossible to exclude malignant transformation of a DN by biopsy.

WELL-DIFFERENTIATED HCC

Diagnosis of moderately or poorly differentiated HCC is usually straightforward, because the differential diagnosis includes mainly metastatic lesions (e.g. endocrine carcinoma, mammary carcinoma), which can be differentiated immunohistochemically in the vast majority of cases (e.g. AFP, Hep Par 1)[70–72]. In contrast, biopsy assessment of early, well-differentiated HCC and its discrimination from DN may sometimes be impossible. In contrast to other cancer entities, well-differentiated HCC shows only subtle cytological and structural abnormalities. Experience with 'early' HCC is lower in Western countries compared to Eastern countries, where HCC reflects an endemic problem and screening and detection of such lesions is more sophisticated.

Malignant transformation is proven by interstitial or vascular invasion[73,74]. The term interstitial invasion refers to small tumour cell complexes invading fibrotic septa or portal tracts. Typically, these cells form arrow-like complexes, which frequently exhibit more pronounced cytological atypia. Vascular or interstitital invasion is, on the other hand, only infrequently encountered in liver biopsies. Therefore, additional structural and cytological criteria have been developed to facilitate the diagnosis of highly differentiated HCC in liver biopsies[58,75]. The most important biopsy criteria are increased cytoplasmic basophilia, nuclear crowding and trabecular disarrangement (Figure 1G and 1H). In most cases of well-differentiated HCC, cellularity, which represents the nuclear–cytoplasmic ratio, is at least doubled compared to non-tumorous liver. Trabecular disarrangement includes more than two cells-wide hepatocyte plates, pseudogland formation, so called 'floating' cross-sections of trabecula (blind or free ends), and (focal) loss of the reticulin network. In contrast, the measuring of the proliferation index and mitoses, which is of impact in other malignancies, is not of diagnostic help. Staining for endothelial cell markers (e.g. CD31, CD34) shows a more diffuse and uniform staining pattern of sinusoids compared to DN, but the patterns are overlapping[22]. A 'nodule-in-nodule' pattern, which means a distinct minute nodule of moderate- within well-differentiated HCC, is rarely found in biopsy specimens. Differential diagnoses of well-differentiated HCC include dysplastic nodules and multiacinar regenerative nodules, as well as liver cell adenoma and focal nodular hyperplasia. As mentioned above, assessment of the peritumorous liver tissue, together with the so-called matrix diagnosis, has an impact on the likelihood of an HCC (and DN) diagnosis. In general, peritumorous parenchyma displays alterations which are caused by the underlying chronic liver disease (e.g. chronic HBV/HCV hepatitis or cirrhosis, alcoholic cirrhosis or genetic haemochromatosis). Higher age, male sex, serological markers of past or present HBV or HCV hepatitis and the absence of predisposing conditions for hepatocellular adenoma also facilitate the diagnosis of HCC.

Considering the rising incidence of HCC, as well as the improved imaging-guided biopsy techniques, it seems likely that the assessment of well-differentiated hepatocellular tumours by biopsy will gain further importance. Therefore, expertise with regard to these lesions is essential and a detailed examination for subtle histological and cytological alterations is mandatory. So far, immunohistological analyses are of limited value in this field. Considering the increasing number of screening analyses such as cDNA arrays, it is reasonable to assume that new diagnostic markers or marker constellations will be developed in the future, which will improve assessment of well-differentiated liver lesions. Currently, liver biopsy has to be considered as one of the decisive diagnostic tools for interpretation of well-differentiated hepatocellular proliferations.

References

1. International Working Party. Terminology of nodular hepatocellular lesions. Hepatology. 1995;22:983–93.
2. Hamilton S, Aaltonen, L, editors. Pathology and Genetics of Tumours of the Digestive System. Lyon: IARC Press, 2000.
3. Ishak KG, Goodman ZD, Stocker JT. Benign hepatocellular tumors. In: Ishak KG, Goodman ZD, Stocker JT, editors. Tumors of the Liver and Intrahepatic Bile Ducts. Washington: Armed Forces Institute of Pathology; 2001:9–48.
4. Ishak KG, Goodman ZD, JT Stocker. Putative precancerous lesions. In: Ishak KG, Goodman ZD, Stocker JT, editors. Tumors of the Liver and Intrahepatic Bile Ducts. Washington: Armed Forces Institute of Pathology; 2001:185–96.

5. Ishak KG, Goodman ZD, JT Stocker. Hepatocellular carcinoma. In: Ishak KG, Goodman ZD, Stocker JT, editors. Tumors of the Liver and Intrahepatic Bile Ducts. Washington: Armed Forces Institute of Pathology; 2001:199–230.
6. Bruix J, Sherman M, Llovet JM et al. Clinical management of hepatocellular carcinoma. Conclusions of the Barcelona-2000 EASL conference. European Association for the Study of the Liver. J Hepatol. 2001;35:421–30.
7. Torzilli G, Minagawa M, Takayama T et al. Accurate preoperative evaluation of liver mass lesions without fine-needle biopsy. Hepatology. 1999;30:889–93.
8. Yu JS, Kim KW, Kim EK, Lee JT, Yoo HS. Contrast enhancement of small hepatocellular carcinoma: usefulness of three successive early image acquisitions during multiphase dynamic MR imaging. Am J Roentgenol. 1999;173:597–604.
9. Lim JH, Kim CK, Lee WJ et al. Detection of hepatocellular carcinomas and dysplastic nodules in cirrhotic livers: accuracy of helical CT in transplant patients. Am J Roentgenol. 2000;175:693–8.
10. Kim T, Murakami T, Takahashi S et al. Optimal phases of dynamic CT for detecting hepatocellular carcinoma: evaluation of unenhanced and triple-phase images. Abdom Imaging. 1999;24:473–80.
11. Baron RL, Brancatelli G. Computed tomographic imaging of hepatocellular carcinoma. Gastroenterology. 2004;127(5 Suppl. 2):S133–43.
12. Taouli B, Losada M, Holland A, Krinsky G. Magnetic resonance imaging of hepatocellular carcinoma. Gastroenterology. 2004;127(5 Suppl. 2):S144–52.
13. Giorgio A, Tarantino L, de Stefano G et al. Complications after interventional sonography of focal liver lesions: a 22-year single-center experience. J Ultrasound Med. 2003;22:193–205.
14. Weiss H, Duntsch U. Komplikationen der Feinnadelpunktion. DEGUM-Umfrage II. Ultraschall Med. 1996;17:118–30.
15. Durand F, Regimbeau JM, Belghiti J et al. Assessment of the benefits and risks of percutaneous biopsy before surgical resection of hepatocellular carcinoma. J Hepatol. 2001;35:254–8.
16. Huang GT, Sheu JC, Yang PM, Lee HS, Wang TH, Chen DS. Ultrasound-guided cutting biopsy for the diagnosis of hepatocellular carcinoma – a study based on 420 patients. J Hepatol. 1996;25:334–8.
17. Kim SH, Lim HK, Lee WJ, Cho JM, Jang HJ. Needle-tract implantation in hepatocellular carcinoma: frequency and CT findings after biopsy with a 19.5-gauge automated biopsy gun. Abdom Imaging. 2000;25:246–50.
18. Takamori R, Wong LL, Dang C, Wong L. Needle-tract implantation from hepatocellular cancer: is needle biopsy of the liver always necessary? Liver Transplant. 2000;6:67–72.
19. Navarro F, Taourel P, Michel J et al. Diaphragmatic and subcutaneous seeding of hepatocellular carcinoma following fine-needle aspiration biopsy. Liver. 1998;18:251–4.
20. Ferrell L, Wright T, Lake J, Roberts J, Ascher N. Incidence and diagnostic features of macroregenerative nodules vs. small hepatocellular carcinoma in cirrhotic livers. Hepatology. 1992;16:1372–81.
21. Theise ND, Schwartz M, Miller C, Thung SN. Macroregenerative nodules and hepatocellular carcinoma in forty-four sequential adult liver explants with cirrhosis. Hepatology. 1992;16:949–55.
22. Roncalli M, Roz E, Coggi G et al. The vascular profile of regenerative and dysplastic nodules of the cirrhotic liver: implications for diagnosis and classification. Hepatology. 1999;30:1174–8.
23. Quaglia A, Bhattacharjya S, Dhillon AP. Limitations of the histopathological diagnosis and prognostic assessment of hepatocellular carcinoma. Histopathology. 2001;38:167–74.
24. Schirmacher P, Prange W, Dries V, Dienes HP. Hochdifferenzierte hepatozelluläre Tumoren: Konzepte, Kriterien und Differenzialdiagnose. Pathologe. 2001;22:407–16.
25. Roncalli M. Hepatocellular nodules in cirrhosis: focus on diagnostic criteria on liver biopsy. A Western experience. Liver Transplant. 2004;10(Suppl. 2):S9–15.
26. Libbrecht L, Desmet V, Roskams T. Preneoplastic lesions in human hepatocarcinogenesis. Liver Int. 2005;25:16–27.
27. International Working Party. Terminology of nodular hepatocellular lesions. Hepatology. 1995;22:983–93.

28. Wanless IR, Mawdsley C, Adams R. On the pathogenesis of focal nodular hyperplasia of the liver. Hepatology. 1985;5:1194–200.
29. Hussain SM, Terkivatan T, Zondervan PE et al. Focal nodular hyperplasia: findings at state-of-the-art MR imaging, US, CT, and pathologic analysis. Radiographics. 2004;24:3–17; discussion 18–19.
30. Wanless IR, Albrecht S, Bilbao J et al. Multiple focal nodular hyperplasia of the liver associated with vascular malformations of various organs and neoplasia of the brain: a new syndrome. Mod Pathol. 1989;2:456–62.
31. Ohmoto K, Honda T, Hirokawa M et al. Spontaneous regression of focal nodular hyperplasia of the liver. J Gastroenterol. 2002;37:849–53.
32. Kleespies A, Settmacher U, Neuhaus P. Spontanruptur einer fokal nodulären Hyperplasie der Leber. Zentralbl Chir. 2002;127:326–8.
33. Butron Vila MM, Haot J, Desmet VJ. Cholestatic features in focal nodular hyperplasia of the liver. Liver. 1984;4:387–95.
34. Lepreux S, Laurent C, Le Bail B, Saric J, Balabaud C, Bioulac-Sage P. Multiple telangiectatic focal nodular hyperplasia: vascular abnormalities. Virchows Arch. 2003;442:226–30.
35. Paradis V, Benzekri A, Dargere D et al. Telangiectatic focal nodular hyperplasia: a variant of hepatocellular adenoma. Gastroenterology. 2004;126:1323–9.
36. Edmondson HA, Henderson B, Benton B. Liver-cell adenomas associated with use of oral contraceptives. N Engl J Med. 1976;294:470–2.
37. Creagh TM, Rubin A, Evans DJ. Hepatic tumours induced by anabolic steroids in an athlete. J Clin Pathol. 1988;41:441–3.
38. Bagia S, Hewitt PM, Morris DL. Anabolic steroid-induced hepatic adenomas with spontaneous haemorrhage in a bodybuilder. Aust NZ J Surg. 2000;70:686–7.
39. Velazquez I, Alter BP. Androgens and liver tumors: Fanconi's anemia and non-Fanconi's conditions. Am J Hematol. 2004;77:257–67.
40. Beuers U, Richter WO, Ritter MM, Wiebecke B, Schwandt P. Klinefelter's syndrome and liver adenoma. J Clin Gastroenterol. 1991;13:214–16.
41. Toso C, Rubbia-Brandt L, Negro F, Morel P, Mentha G. Hepatocellular adenoma and polycystic ovary syndrome. Liver Int. 2003;23:35–7.
42. Reznik Y, Dao T, Coutant R et al. Hepatocyte nuclear factor-1 alpha gene inactivation: cosegregation between liver adenomatosis and diabetes phenotypes in two maturity-onset diabetes of the young (MODY)3 families. J Clin Endocrinol Metab. 2004;89:1476–80.
43. Bianchi L. Glycogen storage disease I and hepatocellular tumours. Eur J Pediatr. 1993;152 (Suppl. 1):S63–70.
44. Alshak NS, Cocjin J, Podesta L et al. Hepatocellular adenoma in glycogen storage disease type IV. Arch Pathol Lab Med. 1994;118:88–91.
45. Shuangshoti S, Thaicharoen A. Hepatocellular adenoma in a beta-thalassemic woman having secondary iron overload. J Med Ass Thai. 1994;77:108–12.
46. Tazawa K, Yasuda M, Ohtani Y, Makuuchi H, Osamura RY. Multiple hepatocellular adenomas associated with long-term carbamazepine. Histopathology. 1999;35:92–4.
47. Resnick MB, Kozakewich HP, Perez-Atayde AR. Hepatic adenoma in the pediatric age group. Clinicopathological observations and assessment of cell proliferative activity. Am J Surg Pathol. 1995;19:1181–90.
48. Farrell GC, Joshua DE, Uren RF, Baird PJ, Perkins KW, Kronenberg H. Androgen-induced hepatoma. Lancet. 1975;1:430–2.
49. Buhler H, Pirovino M, Akobiantz A et al. Regression of liver cell adenoma. A follow-up study of three consecutive patients after discontinuation of oral contraceptive use. Gastroenterology. 1982;82:775–82.
50. Daldrup HE, Reimer P, Rummeny EJ, Fischer H, Bocker W, Peters PE. Regression eines hepatozellulären Adenoms nach Absetzen der hormonalen Kontrazeption. Rofo. 1995;163:449–51.
51. Aseni P, Sansalone CV, Sammartino C et al. Rapid disappearance of hepatic adenoma after contraceptive withdrawal. J Clin Gastroenterol. 2001;33:234–6.
52. Mueller J, Keeffe EB, Esquivel CO. Liver transplantation for treatment of giant hepatocellular adenomas. Liver Transplant Surg. 1995;1:99–102.
53. Yunta PJ, Moya A, San-Juan F et al. [A new case of hepatic adenomatosis treated with orthotopic liver transplantation]. Ann Chir. 2001;126:672–4.

54. Gyorffy EJ, Bredfeldt JE, Black WC. Transformation of hepatic cell adenoma to hepatocellular carcinoma due to oral contraceptive use. Ann Intern Med. 1989;110:489–90.
55. Foster JH, Berman MM. The malignant transformation of liver cell adenomas. Arch Surg. 1994;129:712–17.
56. Ito M, Sasaki M, Wen CY et al. Liver cell adenoma with malignant transformation: a case report. World J Gastroenterol. 2003;9:2379–81.
57. Nakanuma Y, Terada T, Ueda K, Terasaki S, Nonomura A, Matsui O. Adenomatous hyperplasia of the liver as a precancerous lesion. Liver. 1993;13:1–9.
58. Sakamoto M, Hirohashi S, Shimosato Y. Early stages of multistep hepatocarcinogenesis: adenomatous hyperplasia and early hepatocellular carcinoma. Hum Pathol. 1991;22:172–8.
59. Takayama T, Makuuchi M, Hirohashi S et al. Malignant transformation of adenomatous hyperplasia to hepatocellular carcinoma. Lancet. 1990;336:1150–3.
60. Maggioni M, Coggi G, Cassani B et al. Molecular changes in hepatocellular dysplastic nodules on microdissected liver biopsies. Hepatology. 2000;32:942–6.
61. Sun M, Eshleman JR, Ferrell LD et al. An early lesion in hepatic carcinogenesis: loss of heterozygosity in human cirrhotic livers and dysplastic nodules at the 1p36-p34 region. Hepatology. 2001;33:1415–24.
62. Tornillo L, Carafa V, Sauter G et al. Chromosomal alterations in hepatocellular nodules by comparative genomic hybridization: high-grade dysplastic nodules represent early stages of hepatocellular carcinoma. Lab Invest. 2002;82:547–53.
63. Marchio A, Terris B, Meddeb M et al. Chromosomal abnormalities in liver cell dysplasia detected by comparative genomic hybridisation. Mol Pathol. 2001;54:270–4.
64. Le Bail B, Bernard PH, Carles J, Balabaud C, Bioulac-Sage P. Prevalence of liver cell dysplasia and association with HCC in a series of 100 cirrhotic liver explants. J Hepatol. 1997;27:835–42.
65. Tsuda H, Hirohashi S, Shimosato Y, Terada M, Hasegawa H. Clonal origin of atypical adenomatous hyperplasia of the liver and clonal identity with hepatocellular carcinoma. Gastroenterology. 1988;95:1664–6.
66. Park YN, Yang CP, Fernandez GJ, Cubukcu O, Thung SN, Theise ND. Neoangiogenesis and sinusoidal 'capillarization' in dysplastic nodules of the liver. Am J Surg Pathol. 1998;22: 656–62.
67. Borzio M, Fargion S, Borzio F et al. Impact of large regenerative, low grade and high grade dysplastic nodules in hepatocellular carcinoma development. J Hepatol. 2003;39:208–14.
68. Lencioni R, Caramella D, Bartolozzi C, Mazzeo S, Di Coscio G. Percutaneous ethanol injection therapy of adenomatous hyperplastic nodules in cirrhotic liver disease. Acta Radiol. 1994;35:138–42.
69. Ishikawa M, Yogita S, Miyake H et al. Differential diagnosis of small hepatocellular carcinoma and borderline lesions and therapeutic strategy. Hepatogastroenterology. 2002; 49:1591–6.
70. Minervini MI, Demetris AJ, Lee RG, Carr BI, Madariaga J, Nalesnik MA. Utilization of hepatocyte-specific antibody in the immunocytochemical evaluation of liver tumors. Mod Pathol. 1997;10:686–92.
71. Leong AS, Sormunen RT, Tsui WM, Liew CT. Hep Par 1 and selected antibodies in the immunohistological distinction of hepatocellular carcinoma from cholangiocarcinoma, combined tumours and metastatic carcinoma. Histopathology. 1998;33:318–24.
72. Fan Z, van de Rijn M, Montgomery K, Rouse RV. Hep par 1 antibody stain for the differential diagnosis of hepatocellular carcinoma: 676 tumors tested using tissue microarrays and conventional tissue sections. Mod Pathol. 2003;16:137–44.
73. Kondo F, Kondo Y, Nagato Y, Tomizawa M, Wada K. Interstitial tumour cell invasion in small hepatocellular carcinoma. Evaluation in microscopic and low magnification views. J Gastroenterol Hepatol. 1994;9:604–12.
74. Tomizawa M, Kondo F, Kondo Y. Growth patterns and interstitial invasion of small hepatocellular carcinoma. Pathol Int. 1995;45:352–8.
75. Nagato Y, Kondo F, Kondo Y, Ebara M, Ohto M. Histological and morphometrical indicators for a biopsy diagnosis of well-differentiated hepatocellular carcinoma. Hepatology. 1991;14:473–8.

Section Liver II
Metabolic liver disease

Chair: H.E. BLUM and A. PIETRANGELO

16
Role of insulin resistance and extra-hepatic signalling in fatty liver disease

A. M. DIEHL

INTRODUCTION

Non-alcoholic fatty liver disease (NAFLD) is a spectrum of liver pathology that ranges from non-alcoholic fatty liver (NAFL, simple steatosis), on the most clinically benign end of the spectrum, to cirrhosis on the opposite extreme where most liver-related morbidity and mortality occurs. Non-alcoholic steatohepatitis (NASH) is an intermediate stage of liver damage that is characterized by overtly increased liver cell death in fatty livers. This sometimes triggers hepatic infiltration with inflammatory cells and accumulation of fibrous tissue[1]. Thus it is not surprising that the risk of progressing to cirrhosis is greater in individuals with NASH than in those with NAFL[2]. Over the past decade considerable progress has been made in delineating the mechanisms that cause NAFL and NASH. It remains less evident why only a minority of individuals with these 'early' stages of NAFLD progress to cirrhosis or develop liver cancer. The purpose of this chapter is to summarize current understanding of the role of insulin resistance and extrahepatic signalling in the pathogenesis of fatty liver disease.

PATHOGENESIS OF EARLY–INTERMEDIATE STAGES OF NAFLD

NAFLD is strongly associated with the metabolic syndrome, a constellation of disorders including obesity, dyslipidaemia, hypertension, and type 2 diabetes[3]. The metabolic syndrome is now known to reflect a state of insulin resistance that develops as a result of excessive production of inflammatory mediators. Stated another way, individuals with the metabolic syndrome overproduce proinflammatory factors relative to anti-inflammatory factors[4]. The metabolic syndrome is associated with obesity because adipose tissue itself is a major source of these inflammatory mediators (Figure 1).

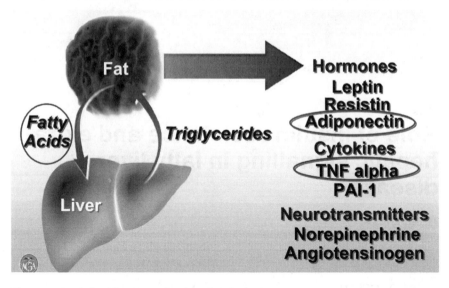

Figure 1   Fat-derived factors regulate hepatic inflammatory response

ROLE OF FAT-DERIVED FACTORS IN NAFL/NASH

Three of the best-characterized adipose-derived factors that modulate inflammatory responses in the liver are fatty acids, tumour necrosis factor alpha (TNF-α), and adiponectin. Interestingly, the latter two proteins regulate fatty acid turnover within hepatocytes. Adiponectin generally reduces lipid accumulation within hepatocytes by inhibiting fatty acid import and increasing fatty acid oxidation and export. It is also a potent insulin-sensitizing agent[5]. TNF-α antagonizes the actions of adiponectin, and thereby promotes hepatocyte steatosis and insulin resistance; therefore, situations that increase TNF-α relative to adiponectin promote hepatic steatosis and insulin resistance. TNF-α also increases mitochondrial generation of reactive oxygen species (ROS), promotes hepatocyte apoptosis, and recruits inflammatory cells to the liver[6]. Thus, it is not hard to imagine how protracted exposure to TNF-α might generate a state of oxidative and apoptotic stress that eventually overwhelms anti-oxidant and anti-apoptotic defences in individual hepatocytes, leading to NASH. Studies in at least two different strains of mice with genetic obesity and NASH (i.e. ob/ob mice and KKAy mice), as well as in wild-type mice with diet or ethanol-induced steatohepatitis prove that overproduction of TNF-α relative to adiponectin causes steatohepatitis, because treatments that inhibit TNF-α or that increase adiponectin improve NASH in all of these models[7–10]. In addition, studies in humans with NASH demonstrate that the relative risk of developing NASH correlates with increases in TNF-α or decreases in adiponectin levels[11].

ROLE OF LIVER-DERIVED INFLAMMATORY MEDIATORS IN SYSTEMIC INSULIN RESISTANCE

Given strong experimental and clinical evidence that unopposed TNF-α activity promotes NAFL/NASH, it is interesting that there is now compelling evidence that the simple accumulation of fatty acids within hepatocytes is sufficient to trigger these cells to produce TNF-α. Fatty acids induce signalling in hepatocytes that activates kinases, such as inhibitor kappa beta kinase (IKK) beta that activate the nuclear factor-kappa beta (NF-κB) transcription factor that increases hepatocyte synthesis of TNF-α and IL-6[10]. Recent studies in transgenic mice with hepatocyte-specific overexpression of IKKbeta demonstrate that hepatocyte-derived IL-6 is responsible for systemic insulin resistance[12]. Therefore, like adipose tissue, fatty livers (and specifically fatty hepatocytes) also make soluble factors that circulate to distant tissues and contribute to systemic insulin resistance (i.e. the metabolic syndrome).

ROLE OF INTESTINAL FACTORS IN NAFLD PATHOGENESIS

It is well accepted that non-obese individuals may also develop NAFL/NASH[13]. The mechanisms for liver damage in non-obese and obese individuals may be similar, and involve excessive hepatocyte exposure to fatty acids and fatty acid-inducible inflammatory mediators (i.e. TNF-α). In support of this concept, an important role for the intestinal microflora in regulating intestinal uptake of diet-derived lipids, as well as hepatic fatty acid synthesis, has been identified recently[14]. Thus, it is conceivable that the gut bacteria of some non-obese individuals might promote excessive hepatic accumulation of fatty acids, as well as exposure to other bacterial factors (e.g. lipopolysaccharide or other Toll-like receptor agonists) that trigger hepatic TNF production. As in obese individuals, increased TNF would antagonize adiponectin activity, and promote steatosis, steatohepatitis, and insulin resistance.

PATHOGENESIS OF CIRRHOSIS

It is generally believed that progression to cirrhosis is predominantly dictated by the severity of oxidant stress and consequent necroinflammation that occurs in individuals with NASH[15]. However, findings in animal models of NASH cast some doubt on this assumption. For example, mice that are genetically deficient in an enzyme that is required for the biosynthesis of S-adenosylmethionine (a key precursor of the antioxidant, glutathione) develop severe NASH but do not progress to cirrhosis[16]. Progression to cirrhosis is poorly predicted by the gravity of the injurious insult in many types of human liver disease. For example, although there is no doubt that alcohol is hepatotoxic, most lifelong heavy drinkers do not become cirrhotic[17]. Similarly, while it is evident that hepatitis C infection causes chronic hepatitis, there is no correlation between viral load and emmergence of cirrhosis[18].

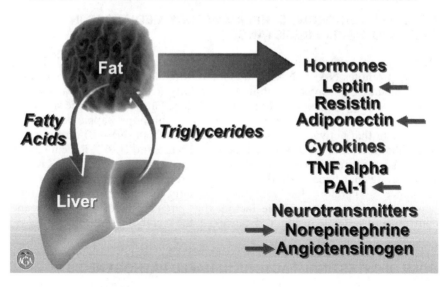

Figure 2   Fat-derived repair (fibrosis) regulators

Finally, although obesity clearly increases exposure to fat-derived inflammatory mediators, some morbidly obese individuals have normal livers at the time of gastric bypass surgery[19].

DEFECTIVE REPAIR MECHANISMS MIGHT PROMOTE PROGRESSIVE LIVER DAMAGE

These apparent paradoxes might be explained by the failure to acknowledge that liver damage is determined by the adequacy of liver repair mechanisms, as well as the severity of a particular noxious insult. Individuals who are 'poor repairers' suffer more net liver damage for any given level of injury than those who are 'average repairers', while those who are 'super repairers' may survive relatively unscathed, with little evidence of liver damage despite a significant noxious exposure. Viewed from this perspective, individuals who merely develop NAFL despite constant bombardment with proinflammatory factors might be 'super-repairers', while those who develop NASH have only 'average' repair capabilities, and the minority with 'poor repair' abilities develop cirrhosis.

ADIPOSE-DERIVED FACTORS MODULATE LIVER FIBROSIS

The possibility that differences in repair responses might contribute to liver disease outcome merits consideration in NAFLD because NAFLD is often associated with obesity and adipose tissue is an important source of various mediators that modulate wound-healing responses[5] (Figure 2).

Hepatic stellate cells (HSC) express receptors from several adipose-derived factors, including leptin, angiotensin, adiponectin and norepinephrine, that modulate HSC activation[20]. Studies in mice demonstrate that leptin, angiotensin and norepinephrine promote HSC proliferation, up-regulate HSC expression of pro-fibrogenic cytokines, such as transforming growth factor beta (TGF-β), and induce collagen gene expression. Conversely, adiponectin appears to inhibit HSC activation and decrease liver fibrosis[21]. It is likely that plasminogen activator inhibitor (PAI)-1 also regulates HSC since it has been shown to influence fibrosis in other tissues[22].

Studies of patients with NAFLD support a role for adipose-derived factors in progression to cirrhosis. For example, increases in adrenergic tone and angiotensin receptor activity mediate hypertension in individuals with the metabolic syndrome and hypertension has been identified as an independent risk factor for advanced liver fibrosis in some studies of NAFLD[3]. Consistent with this concept, a small open-label trial of losartan in individuals with NASH and hypertension suggested that losartan treatment for about a year decreased liver fibrosis and slowed NAFLD progression[23].

SUMMARY

NAFLD is a spectrum of liver damage that occurs in many obese individuals with the metabolic syndrome. The early–intermediate stages of the NAFLD (i.e. NAFL and NASH) are caused by excessive exposure to adipose-derived fatty acids and inflammatory cytokines that induce hepatocyte steatosis, threaten hepatocyte viability, and promote hepatic and systemic insulin resistance. Resultant increases in the rate of liver cell death trigger repair responses. The latter are also modulated by adipose-derived factors, including various factors that regulate the activation of hepatic stellate cells. In some individuals the net effect of these factors is 'unhealthy' repair, with resultant cirrhosis. More research is needed to clarify the molecular basis for inter-individual differences in repair responses that are triggered by chronic fatty liver injury. Improved understanding of such pathobiology should enhance identification of individuals who are at greatest risk for developing cirrhosis, as well as the development of effective treatments to abort disease progression.

References

1. Brunt EM. Nonalcoholic steatohepatitis. Semin Liver Dis. 2004;24:3–20.
2. Matteoni C, Younossi ZM, McCullough A. Nonalcoholic fatty liver disease: a spectrum of clinical pathological severity. Gastroenterology. 1999;116:1413–19.
3. Marchesini G, Bugianesi E, Forlani G et al. Nonalcoholic fatty liver, steatohepatitis, and the metabolic syndrome. Hepatology. 2003;37:917–23.
4. Lebovitz HE. The relationship of obesity to the metabolic syndrome. Int J Clin Pract Suppl. 2003:18–27.
5. Chaldakov GN, Stankulov IS, Hristova M, Ghenev PI. Adipobiology of disease: adipokines and adipokine-targeted pharmacology. Curr Pharm Des. 2003;9:1023–31.
6. Ruan H, Lodish HF. Insulin resistance in adipose tissue: direct and indirect effects of tumor necrosis factor-alpha. Cytokine Growth Factor Rev. 2003;14:447–55.

7. Uysal KT, Wiesbrock SM, Hotamisligil GS. Functional analysis of tumor necrosis factor (TNF) receptors in TNF-alpha-mediated insulin resistance in genetic obesity. Endocrinology. 1998;139:4832–8.
8. Li Z, Yang S, Lin H et al. Probiotics and antibodies to TNF inhibit inflammatory activity and improve nonalcoholic fatty liver disease. Hepatology. 2003;37:343–50.
9. Xu A, Wang Y, Keshaw H, Xu LY, Lam KS, Cooper GJ. The fat-derived hormone adiponectin alleviates alcoholic and nonalcoholic fatty liver diseases in mice. J Clin Invest. 2003;112:91–100.
10. Feldstein AE, Werneburg NW, Canbay A et al. Free fatty acids promote hepatic lipotoxicity by stimulating TNF-alpha expression via a lysosomal pathway. Hepatology. 2004;40:185–94.
11. Hui JM, Hodge A, Farrell GC, Kench JG, Kriketos A, George J. Beyond insulin resistance in NASH: TNF-alpha or adiponectin? Hepatology. 2004;40:46–54.
12. Cai D, Yuan M, Frantz DF et al Local and systemic insulin resistance resulting from hepatic activation of IKK-beta and NF-kappaB. Nat Med. 2005;11:183–90.
13. Adams LA, Lymp JF, St Sauver J et al. The natural history of nonalcoholic fatty liver disease: a population-based cohort study. Gastroenterology. 2005;129:113–21.
14. Backhed F, Ding H, Wang T et al. The gut microbiota as an environmental factor that regulates fat storage. Proc Natl Acad Sci USA. 2004;101:15718–23.
15. Chitturi S, Farrell GC. Etiopathogenesis of nonalcoholic steatohepatitis. Semin Liver Dis. 2001;21:27–41.
16. Lu SC, Alvarez L, Huang ZZ et al. Methionine adenosyltransferase 1A knockout mice are predisposed to liver injury and exhibit increased expression of genes involved in proliferation. Proc Natl Acad Sci USA. 2001;98:5560–5.
17. Tsukamoto H, Lu SC. Current concepts in the pathogenesis of alcoholic liver injury. FASEB J. 2001;15:1335–49.
18. Poupon RY, Serfaty LD, Amorim M, Galulal G, Chretien Y, Chazouilleres O. Combination of steatosis and alcohol intake is the main determinant of fibrosis progression in patients with hepatitis C. Hepatology. 1999;30:406A.
19. Beymer C, Kowdley KV, Larson A, Demonson P, Dellinger EP, Flum DR. Prevalence and predictors of asymptomatic liver disease in patients undergoing gastric bypass surgery. Arch Surg. 2003;138:1240–4.
20. Bataller R, Brenner DA. Liver fibrosis. J Clin Invest. 2005;115:209–18.
21. Kamada Y, Tamura S, Kiso S, Matsumoto H et al. Enhanced carbon tetrachloride-induced liver fibrosis in mice lacking adiponectin. Gastroenterology. 2003;125:1796–807.
22. Lijnen HR. Pleiotropic functions of plasminogen activator inhibitor-1. J Thromb Haemost. 2005;3:35–45.
23. Yokohama S, Yoneda M, Haneda M et al. Therapeutic efficacy of an angiotensin II receptor antagonist in patients with nonalcoholic steatohepatitis. Hepatology. 2004;40:1222–5.

17
Steatosis and hepatitis C

C. P. DAY

Hepatic steatosis (fatty liver) is extremely common in patients with hepatitis C virus (HCV) chronic infection and has been associated with both disease severity and more recently with response to antiviral therapy. It is therefore important to understand the basis for these associations to inform treatment strategies for the growing burden of patients with chronic HCV infection.

PREVALENCE OF STEATOSIS IN CHRONIC HCV INFECTION

The overall prevalence of steatosis in patients with HCV infection is approximately 56%, ranging from 35% to 81% in various studies[1]. This is approximately 2–3-fold higher than the prevalence of steatosis in other liver diseases and in the healthy background populations from which the patients are derived[2,3]. Importantly the prevalence of steatosis varies according to viral genotype with a prevalence of 70–80% in viral genotype 3 versus 45–50% in non-genotype 3 in studies reported thus far. Furthermore, the prevalence of severe, grade 3, steatosis (more than two-thirds of hepatocytes affected) is more than five times higher in patients with genotype 3 compared to those with other viral genotypes (30% versus 5.5%)[1].

MECHANISMS OF STEATOSIS IN CHRONIC HCV INFECTION

A considerable body of evidence suggests that steatosis in patients with chronic genotype 3 HCV infection is a direct effect of the viral infection, whereas in non-genotype 3 infection it occurs largely as a result of the 'normal' risk factors for steatosis – obesity, type 2 diabetes mellitus (T2DM) and insulin resistance[2]. Evidence supporting this concept comes from studies showing that hepatic/blood viral load is the most significant factor associated with steatosis in genotype 3 patients whereas in non-genotype 3 patients the degree of steatosis correlates with body mass index (BMI), the presence of T2DM and hypertension[2,4]. Further evidence supporting the notion of steatosis as a direct viral effect of genotype 3 HCV infection has come from several studies demonstrating that steatosis is reduced by successful antiviral treatment in patients infected with genotype 3 but not those infected with non-genotype 3. Castera et al. recently reported that almost all patients with genotype 3 who developed a sustained viral response (SVR) to standard antiviral therapy (interferon with or without ribavirin) had an improvement in their steatosis compared to less than 20% in non-responders, whereas in non-genotype 3-infected patients there was no difference in the proportion of patients who had an improvement in steatosis according to viral response[5]. Chronic genotype 3 HCV infection is closely associated with hypolipoproteinaemia and shares many phenotypic similarities with patients with familial heterozygous hypobetalipoproteinaemia (FHBL), strongly suggesting that, as in FHBL, steatosis in genotype 3 is due to an impairment of lipid export from hepatocytes[6,7]. Furthermore, serum cholesterol rises in patients with genotype 3 who develop a sustained viral response, further supporting the notion of a direct inhibitory effect of genotype 3 on lipid export[8]. Consistent with this latter concept, studies in HCV core protein transgenic mice have shown direct inhibition of microsomal triglyceride transfer protein (MTP) and very-low-density-lipoprotein (VLDL) secretion by the core protein. MTP is directly responsible for the assembly of VLDL particles from triglyceride and apolipoproteins. These *in-vivo* studies were performed using constructs from HCV genotype 1[9]; however, a recent *in-vitro* study expressing the HCV core protein from patients infected with different HCV genotypes in Huh7 cells has demonstrated conclusively that genotype 3a has the most profound steatogenic effect[10].

Further evidence supporting a 'metabolic' cause for the steatosis in non-genotype 3 patients compared to genotype 3 patients has been provided by a study demonstrating that patients with genotype 1 who had steatosis were markedly more insulin-resistant than patients without steatosis, whereas insulin resistance values did not differ between genotype 3 patients with and without steatosis and were uniformly within the normal range[11]. This would appear to suggest therefore that, while genotype 3 causes steatosis via a direct viral effect, the steatosis in non-genotype 3 patients is, as in classical non-alcoholic fatty liver disease (NAFLD) patients, due principally to obesity and associated insulin resistance with the proviso that evidence from the transgenic mice model suggests that there may be an additional direct viral effect.

HCV AS A CAUSE OF INSULIN RESISTANCE/T2DM

If we accept that the steatosis in non-genotype 3-infected patients is due principally to insulin resistance, the high prevalence of steatosis in non-genotype 3 patients (45–50%) suggests that there may be a direct effect of chronic HCV infection on insulin resistance. If this were not the case the prevalence of steatosis in non-genotype 3 patients would be expected to be no higher than in the background population, simply reflecting the underlying prevalence of obesity and the associated metabolic syndrome. In support of a direct effect of HCV infection on insulin resistance, HCV chronic hepatitis is undoubtedly associated with an increased risk of developing T2DM compared with chronic hepatitis due to other aetiologies[2], and the risk is independent of the presence of cirrhosis[12]. In addition, insulin resistance is frequently observed in chronic HCV-infected patients in the absence of the 'usual' risk factors – obesity, hypertension and dyslipidaemia[2].

Recent studies within and without the HCV field have provided persuasive evidence that chronic HCV infection can lead to impaired insulin signalling both directly and indirectly. Studies in liver biopsies from HCV patients have shown a profound impairment of insulin signalling, at the level of insulin receptor substrate (IRS)-1 tyrosine phosphorylation and PI3-kinase activation[13]. HCV core transgenic mice are also markedly insulin-resistant, and this has been linked to increased levels of TNF-α, which is known to act by impairing IRS-1 phosphorylation[14]. It has recently been demonstrated that hepatocyte inflammation (induced by hepatocyte-specific expression of the NF-κB activator I-κB kinase β) is associated with hepatic and systemic insulin resistance and with increased expression/levels of several hepatic and systemic cytokines capable of inducing insulin resistance including interleukin 6 and TNF-α[15]. Finally, chronic HCV infection can induce endoplasmic reticulum (ER) stress in hepatocytes which can result in steatosis, apoptosis and insulin resistance[16,17] and presumably accounts for the recently reported correlation between the extent of steatosis and serum caspase activity in patients with chronic HCV infection[18]. There are therefore at least three mechanisms whereby insulin signalling can be impaired in chronic HCV infection: (a) a direct effect of HCV core protein, (b) ER stress, and (c) hepatic inflammation with its associated increased cytokine levels. Direct evidence that chronic HCV infection *per se* plays a role in insulin resistance has come from a recent study by Romero-Gomez and colleagues[19] showing that patients who develop an SVR to antiviral therapy have a significant fall in insulin resistance (measured by homeostasis model assessment [HOMA]), whereas there is no change in non-responders and only a transient fall in treatment relapsers.

In summary, for genotype 3 patients steatosis is undoubtedly predominantly a viral effect on hepatic lipid export, whereas in non-genotype 3 patients it is predominantly due to insulin resistance, itself due both to non-viral effects (e.g. obesity) and almost certainly to an inhibitory effect of chronic HCV infection on insulin signalling.

STEATOSIS IN HCV AND DISEASE PROGRESSION

Several studies have shown a close correlation between the severity of steatosis and the severity of fibrosis on the same liver biopsy[1,2]. More recently, Castèra and colleagues showed a close correlation between the rate of steatosis change on paired biopsies and the change in fibrosis[20], and Fartoux and colleagues have shown a close correlation between the probability of fibrosis progression on follow-up biopsies and the severity of steatosis on the index biopsy[11]. In addition to an association with disease progression it has been convincingly shown that steatosis reduces the probability of an SVR to standard combination antiviral therapy[21,22]. The implications of these associations with steatosis in HCV depend critically on whether the associations with both disease progression and reduced SVR rate are due to steatosis playing a direct role in fibrosis progression or treatment resistance, or whether steatosis, viral response and disease progression are due to some other common factor leading to steatosis being attributed 'guilt-by-association'. This distinction is clearly important, since if steatosis plays a direct causal role it is a rational treatment target in HCV infection.

MECHANISMS OF ASSOCIATION BETWEEN STEATOSIS AND DISEASE PROGRESSION/TREATMENT RESPONSE

The most obvious explanation for the association between steatosis and disease progression is provided by the so-called 'two-hit' theory of steatohepatitis[23]. This states that steatosis is the 'first hit' sensitizing the liver to the second 'hits', oxidative stress and TNF-α. There is certainly a convincing body of evidence that oxidative stress and lipid peroxidation occur in livers infected with HCV[2] with the severity of oxidative stress and lipid peroxidation correlating with both the site and extent of fibrosis[24]. The antiviral inflammatory response clearly provides an excellent source of reactive oxygen species (ROS) and a direct effect of the HCV virus on mitochondria resulting in the production of ROS has also been demonstrated[25]. With respect to the other 'second hit', as discussed above, both elevated serum and intrahepatic levels of TNF-α have been demonstrated in HCV core expressing transgenic mice and increased serum levels of TNF-α have been demonstrated in patients with HCV[26]. Despite the attractions of the two-hit theory to explain the association between steatosis and disease progression, several lines of evidence argue against steatosis playing a direct causal role in the pathogenesis of fibrosis. First, genotype 3 patients undoubtedly have the worst steatosis, but there is no convincing evidence that they have the worst fibrosis. Second, as discussed above, it is clear that in non-genotype 3 patients steatosis is clearly linked to insulin resistance and in multivariate analysis it is insulin resistance and not steatosis that correlates with fibrosis in chronic HCV virus infection[27,28]. Insulin resistance is known to be profibrogenic, with insulin and glucose stimulating the release of connective tissue growth factor from hepatic stellate cells which has direct autocrine fibrogenic effects[29]. Similarly, ER stress and elevated levels of TNF-α, both known to be present in HCV infection, can both lead to steatosis *and* hepatocyte injury and fibrosis.

With respect to the association of steatosis with impaired treatment response, there is also evidence that this is not a direct causal effect. First, in multivariate analysis, insulin resistance, viral genotype and fibrosis score but not steatosis predict treatment response[19]. In patients infected with HCV genotype 1 the SVR rates range from over 60% in patients with normal levels of insulin sensitivity (HOMA <2) to only 20% in the most insulin-resistant patients (HOMA >4). Furthermore the SVR is reduced in obesity, cirrhosis, African Americans and type 2 diabetics, all conditions that are characterized by insulin resistance and in genotype 3, so-called 'viral' steatosis does not influence treatment response[22]. There has been preliminary evidence presented that insulin enhances HCV replication in an *in-vitro* model of the HCV replicon and inhibits the antiviral effects of interferon.

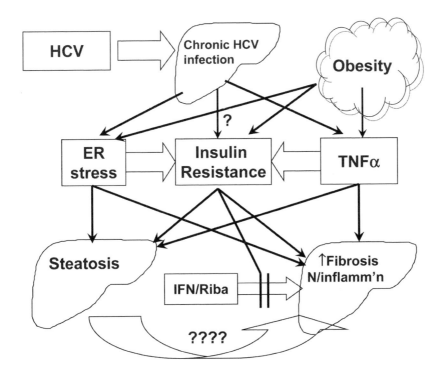

Figure 1   Potential links between chronic HCV infection, steatosis, liver disease progression and response to antiviral treatment. ER, endoplasmic reticulum; IFN, interferon

IMPLICATIONS FOR MANAGEMENT

In summary (Figure 1) it would appear that chronic HCV infection through either a direct effect of core protein, ER stress or hepatic inflammation leads to hepatic and systemic insulin resistance. This insulin resistance will be further enhanced by any coexistent obesity which is also associated with hepatic ER stress[30] and chronic inflammation[31]. Insulin resistance will lead to steatosis, increased fibrosis and inflammation and will directly impair the response to anti-viral therapy. ER stress and TNF-α are further mediators of both liver injury and steatosis. There is, as yet, little evidence that steatosis has any direct causal role in either disease progression or the response to antiviral therapy. The therapeutic implications of this scheme are clear. First, insulin resistance should be actively sought in patients with HCV. It should be particularly suspected in patients with non-genotype 3 who have steatosis. If insulin resistance is present, consideration should be given to adjusting the antiviral regime with consideration given to direct treatment of insulin resistance either with diet and exercise or with insulin sensitizers. Major trials are currently under way examining the role of insulin sensitizers in combination with antiviral therapy in patients with chronic HCV virus infection and insulin resistance. In future it seems likely that anti-TNF-α and anti-ER stress agents will be evaluated in patients with NAFLD and HCV. At present there is little justification for directing therapy solely at steatosis.

References

1. Lonardo A, Loria P, Adinolfi LE, Carulli, Rugiero G. Hepatitis C and steatosis: a reappraisal. J Viral Hepat. 2006;13:73–80.
2. Lonardo A, Adinolfi LE, Loria P, Carulli N, Ruggiero G, Day CP. Steatosis and hepatitis C virus: mechanisms and significance for hepatic and extrahepatic disease. Gastroenterology. 2004;126:586–97.
3. Cortez-Pinto H, Carneiro de Moura M, Day CP, Non-alcoholic steatohepatitis: from cell biology to clinical practice. J Hepatol. 2006;44:197–208.
4. Adinolfi LE, Gambardella M, Andreana A, Tripodi MF, Utili R, Ruggiero G. Steatosis accelerates the progression of liver damage of chronic hepatitis C patients and correlates with specific HCV and visceral obesity. Hepatology. 2001;33:1358–64.
5. Castera L, Hezode C, Roudot-Thoraval F et al. Effect of antiviral treatment on evolution of liver steatosis in patients with chronic hepatitis C: indirect evidence of a role of hepatitis C virus genotype 3 in steatosis. Gut. 2004;53:420–4.
6. Lonardo A, Lombardini S, Caglioni F et al. Hepatic steatosis and insulin reistance: does etiology make a difference? J Hepatol. 2006;44:190–6.
7. Rubbia-Brandt L, Quadri R, Abid K et al. Hepatocyte steatosis is a cytopathic effect of hepatitis C virus genotype 3. J Hepatol. 2000;33:106–15.
8. Hofer H, Bankl HC, Wrba F et al. Hepatocellular fat accumulation and low serum cholesterol in patients infected with HCV-3a. Am J Gastroenterol. 2002;97:2880–5.
9. Perlemuter G, Sabile A, Letteron P et al. Hepatitis C virus core protein inhibits microsomal triglyceride transfer protein activity and very low density lipoprotein secretion: a model of viral-related steatosis. FASEB J. 2002;16:185–94.
10. Abid K, Pazienza V, de Gottardi A et al. An *in vitro* model of hepatitis C virus genotype 3a-associated triglycerides accumulation. J Hepatol. 2005;42:744–51.
11. Fartoux L, Poujol-Robert A, Guechot J et al. Insulin resistance is a cause of steatosis and fibrosis progression in chronic hepatitis C. Gut. 2005;54:1003–8.
12. Mason AL, Lau JY, Hoang N et al. Association of diabetes mellitus and chronic hepatitis C virus infection. Hepatology. 1999;29:328–33.
13. Aytug S, Reich D, Sapiro LE, Bernstein D, Begum N. Impaired IRS-1/PI3-kinase signaling in patients with HCV: a mechanism for increased prevalence of type 2 diabetes. Hepatology. 2003;38:1384–92.
14. Shintani Y, Fujie H, Miyoshi H et al. Hepatitis C virus infection and diabetes: direct involvement of the virus in the development of insulin resistance. Gastroenterology. 2004;126:840–8.
15. Cai D, Yuan M, Frantz D, Melendez PA, Hansen L, Lee J, Shoelson SE. Local and systemic insulin resistance resulting from hepatic activation of IKK-β and NF-κβ. Nat Med. 2005; 11:183–90.
16. Ciccaglione AR, Costantino A, Tritarelli E et al. Activation of endoplasmic reticulum stress response by hepatitis C virus proteins. Arch Virol. 2005;150:1339–56.
17. Benali-Furet NL, Chami M, Houel L et al. Hepatitis C virus core triggers apoptosis in liver cells by inducing ER stress and ER calcium depletion. Oncogene. 2005;24:4921–33.
18. Seidel N, Volkmann X, Langer F et al. The extent of liver steatosis in chronic hepatitis C virus infection is mirrored by caspase activity in serum. Hepatology. 2005;42:113–20.
19. Romero-Gomez M, Del Mar Viloria M, Andrade RJ et al. Insulin resistance impairs sustained response rate to peginterferon plus ribavirin in chronic hepatitis C patients. Gastroenterology. 2005;128:636–41.
20. Castèra L, Hézode C, Roudot-Toraval F, Bastie A, Zafrani ES, Pawltowski JM. Worsening of steatosis is an independent factor of fibrosis progression in untreated patients with chronic hepatitis C and paired liver biopsies. Gut. 2003;52:288–92.

21. Zeuzem S, Hultcrantz R, Bourliere M et al. Peginterferon alfa-2b plus ribavirin for treatment of chronic hepatitis C in previously untreated patients infected with HCV genotypes 2 or 3. J Hepatol. 2004;40:993–9.
22. Poynard T, Ratziu V, McHutchison J et al. Effect of treatment with peginterferon or interferon alfa-2b and ribavirin on steatosis in patients infected with hepatitis C. Hepatology. 2003;38:75–85.
23. Day CP, James OF. Steatohepatitis: a tale of two 'hits'? Gastroenterology. 1998;114:842–5.
24. Paradis V, Mathurin P, Kollinger M et al. *In situ* detection of lipid peroxidation in chronic hepatitis C: correlation with pathological features. J Clin Pathol. 1997;50:401–6.
25. Okuda M, Li K, Beard MR et al. Mitochondrial injury, oxidative stress, and antioxidant gene expression are induced by hepatitis C virus core protein. Gastroenterology. 2002;122: 366–75.
26. Knobler H, Zhornicky T, Sandler A, Haran N, Ashur Y, Schattner A. Tumor necrosis factor α-induced insulin resistance may mediate the hepatitis C virus–diabetes association. Am J Gastroenterol. 2003;98:2751–6.
27. Hui JM, Sud A, Farrell GC et al. Insulin resistance is associated with chronic hepatitis C and virus infection fibrosis progression. Gastroenterology. 2003;125:1695–704.
28. Hickman IJ, Powell EE, Prins JB et al. In overweight patients with chronic hepatitis C, circulating insulin is associated with hepatic fibrosis: implications for therapy. J Hepatol. 2003;39:1042–8.
29. Paradis V, Perlemuter G, Bonvoust F et al. High glucose and hyperinsulinemia stimulate connective tissue growth factor expression: a potential mechanism involved in progression to fibrosis in nonalcoholic steatohepatitis. Hepatology. 2001;34:738–44.
30. Ozcan U, Cao Q, Yilmaz E et al. Endoplasmic reticulum stress links obesity, insulin action and type 2 diabetes. Science 2004;306;457–61.
31. Weisberg SP, McCann D, Desai M, Rosenbaum M, Leibel RL, Ferrante AW Jr. Obesity is associated with macrophage accumulation in adipose tissue. J Clin Invest. 2003;112:1796– 808.

18
Hereditary haemochromatosis: the genes and the disease

E. CORRADINI, F. FERRARA and A. PIETRANGELO

INTRODUCTION

In 1996 *HFE*, the long-awaited haemochromatosis gene, was discovered[1] and unprecedented progress in the field of iron genetics began, that eventually led to the identification of new iron genes and diseases. This advancement has now challenged many historical concepts of this disorder (such as its presumed monogenic nature or the intestinal origin of the primary defect; see below) and also complicated its definition and classification. Here, the term 'haemochromatosis' (HC) (synonymous with 'hereditary haemochromatosis') will be exclusively used to refer to a clinicopathological entity that, in spite of its multigenic nature, is characterized by distinguishing features as outlined in ref. 2 and summarized in Table 1. These features differentiate HC from other genetic iron-overload disorders (Table 2), which are, with the exception of the 'ferroportin disease'[3] and the hereditary iron-loading anaemias (e.g. thalassaemia or hereditary sideroblastic anaemias), much rarer.

Although the HC syndrome is unique, usually two basic phenotypes can be recognized based primarily on age at symptom onset and clinical severity: an adult and a juvenile form. In the adult form, the most common, iron overload and disease progression are gradual and hepatic involvement predominates. The vast majority of cases in this category are the result of pathogenic mutation of HFE[1], generally a single-base transition, 845G→A, that causes the substitution of tyrosine for cysteine at position 282 (C282Y) of the HFE protein. A smaller subgroup of subjects with adult-onset HC have mutations of the transferrin receptor 2 (*TfR2*) gene instead of *HFE* gene.

The juvenile form is more severe, and cardiac and endocrine involvement are much more pronounced. This form of HC is linked to mutation of a gene on chromosome 1 (haemojuvelin, *HJV*) or, in fewer cases, *HAMP,* the gene encoding hepcidin, a major regulator of iron traffic within the body. Intermediate phenotype may originate from inheritance of a heterozygote juvenile gene mutation (*HAMP* or HJV) in combination with a pathogenic mutations of HFE or TfR2[2]: in this case an earlier onset and more severe expression of an adult-onset HC form occurs.

Table 1 Distinguishing features of hemochromatosis

1. Hereditary (usually autosomal recessive) trait.
2. Early and progressive increase of circulatory iron (i.e. high transferrin saturation) that precedes iron accumulation in tissues (i.e. high serum ferritin).
3. Early and preferential iron deposition in parenchymal cells with potential for damage and diseases such as liver cirrhosis, cardiomiopathy, endocrinopathy, arthropathy.
4. Unimpaired erythropoiesis and optimal response to phlebotomy.
5. Inappropriate synthesis/activity of hepcidin

Table 2 Human iron overload disorders

Hereditary	Acquired	Miscellaneous
Hereditary haemochromatosis (*HFE*-, *TfR2*-, *HJ-V*-, *HAMP*-related) Ferroportin disease Aceruloplasminaemia Atransferrinaemia Hereditary iron-loading anaemias	Dietary Long-term haemodialysis Chronic liver disease Hepatitis C and B Alcoholic cirrhosis NASH Porphyria cutanea tarda Post-portacaval shunting Dysmetabolic iron overload syndrome	Neonatal haemochromatosis African siderosis

PATHOGENESIS

The haemochromatosis genes

The HFE gene, placed on the short arm of chromosome 6, is the most common HC gene. HFE is a major histocompatibility class-I-like protein whose ancestral peptide-binding groove is too narrow to allow antigen presentation[4]. The fact that it is incapable of binding iron[5] strongly implies that it does not act alone; in fact, interaction between HFE and the transferrin receptor 1, TfR1, which mediates transferrin-bound iron uptake by most cells[6], has been fully documented, although its biological effects are still uncertain. Recent findings now suggest that HFE might also bind to other uncharacterized proteins in the cell[7]. The C282Y mutation is associated with disruption of a disulphide bond in HFE that is critical for its binding to β_2-microglobulin[8]. The latter interaction is necessary for the stabilization, [intracytoplasmic] transport and expression of HFE on the cell surface and endosomal membranes where HFE interacts with TfR1. The H63D mutation, by contrast, does not impair HFE–TfR1 interaction.

In 1999 the gene for a second human transferrin receptor (TfR2) was cloned[9]. Unlike TfR1, the new receptor was found to be highly expressed in the liver, and it was not regulated by intracellular iron status[10]. TfR2 can mediate the uptake of transferrin-bound iron by hepatocytes[10], possibly through the mechanism of receptor-mediated endocytosis similar to that described for TfR1, but its *in-vitro* affinity for transferrin is 25–30-fold lower than that of TfR1[11]. These data, which suggest that TfR2 inactivation should impair tissue uptake of iron, are difficult to reconcile with reports of a haemochromatosis-like phenotype in humans with pathogenic mutations of TfR2[12] and in mice subjected to *TfR2* gene deletion[13]. *In-vitro* studies with soluble recombinant forms of TFR2 and HFE have revealed no direct interaction between the two[11].

Haemojuvelin has been identified very recently[14]. It is expressed is many tissues but particularly in the liver. Although the function of haemojuvelin is unknown, hepcidin levels are depressed in individuals with *HJV* mutations[14], suggesting that haemojuvelin is probably a hepcidin transcriptional modulator.

Hepcidin is an antimicrobial peptide produced by hepatocytes in response not only to inflammatory stimuli but also iron overload[15–17]. Evidence from transgenic mouse models indicates that hepcidin is the principal down-regulator of the absorption of iron in the small intestine, its transport across the placenta, and its release from macrophages (reviewed in ref. 18). The absence of circulating hepcidin has been shown to produce the rare and severe juvenile haemochromatosis in humans[19]. It is still unclear how hepcidin modulates iron egress from cells but its interaction with a main iron-export protein, ferroportin, has been recently postulated[20].

The common pathogenic basis for haemochromatosis

The common basis to all forms of haemochromatosis is the genetic predisposition for circulatory iron overload[2] (Figure 1). This iron is eventually deposited in parenchymal cells of the liver, pancreas and heart, where it can cause cytotoxicity and organ impairment. In normal individuals subjected to enteral or transfusion iron overload, iron excretion can exceed absorption by as much as 4 mg/day[21]. This elimination is largely based on the sloughing of senescent intestinal mucosal cells, where non-absorbed dietary iron is normally stored in the form of ferritin. In haemochromatosis the plasma iron pool increases as a result of altered iron traffic but the compensatory response fails, probably because the sloughed enterocytes contain little or no iron or ferritin, and total iron absorption generally exceeds loss by 2–3 mg/day[22]. This positive balance occurs from birth, but, at least in the HFE- and probably TfR2-related forms, marked tissue accumulation is generally not observed during childhood and adolescence due to high growth demands and, in females, the elimination of circulatory iron through menstruation. In early adulthood, however, iron build-up begins in parenchymal cells of the liver, pancreas, heart and other organs, and by middle age toxic cell damage and organ disease may develop[23].

The progressive expansion of the plasma iron pool in HC, which occurs at a much faster rate in the juvenile forms, is the result of an increased transfer of iron to the blood compartment from enterocytes (i.e. increased intestinal absorption), and in all probability from reticuloendothelial macrophages[2]. The latter cells are the principal source of iron in the blood stream (followed by enterocytes and hepatocytes)[24].

The main regulator of iron efflux from enterocytes and macrophages in humans is hepcidin. The extent and efficiency of the interaction between hepcidin with ferroportin, the main iron export protein in mammals, probably

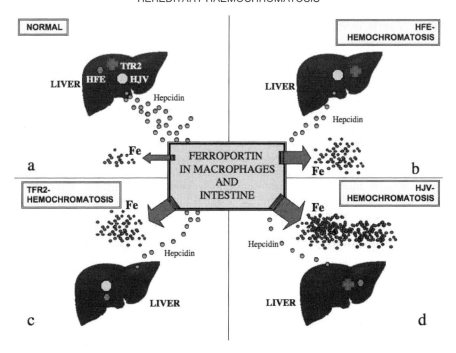

Figure 1 Hepcidin as a common pathogenic denominator in hemochromatosis. (**a**) In normal subjects circulatory iron sets a basal level of hepcidin synthesis by hepatocytes. Serum hepcidin modulates the amount of iron released from macrophages and enterocytes that contributes the pool of circulatory iron able, in a regulatory feedback loop, to control the hepatic production of hepcidin. HFE, TfR2 and HJV are probably required for hepcidin activation in response to the circulatory iron signal (**b**). If HFE is non-functional (i.e. HFE-related hereditary haemochromatosis) hepcidin synthesis by the hepatocytes is unregulated and inappropriately low, although a residual hepcidin activity will be still possible due to the presence of functional TfR2 and HJV: the consequent unrestricted release of iron from macrophages and enterocytes leads to progressive expansion of the plasma iron pool followed by tissue iron overload and organ damage. Circumstantial evidence indicates that TfR2 may also be required for iron sensing by the hepatocyte. Therefore, a similar pathogenic pathway may be shared by TfR2-related haemochromatosis (**c**). HJV is probably a more important regulator of hepcidin than HFE and TfR2; therefore a mutated HJV will lead to a more profound inhibitory effect on hepcidin synthesis, a more dramatic increase in circulatory iron and a more severe iron overload syndrome (**d**)

dictates the extent of iron release from various tissues into the circulation. In HFE, TfR2 and HJV-related HC, hepatic expression or serum/urine levels of this peptide are inappropriately low for the rate of iron overload[25,26]. Hepcidin expression in the liver is also significantly impaired in *HFE* and *TfR2* knockout mice[27,28] and hepatic deposition of iron in *HFE*-knockout animals can be prevented by hepcidin overexpression[29]. These findings suggest a unifying pathogenic model for all forms of HC[2] in which the inadequate production of hepcidin provokes an excessive influx of iron into the blood stream from macrophages and enterocytes[2] (Figure 1). The signal for appropriate hepcidin up-regulation in haemochromatosis might come from the blood stream (e.g. non-transferrin-bound iron levels) or from tissue macrophages. Macrophage activity (i.e. secretion of interleukin 6) seems to be a key event for hepcidin induction during infection, and other (currently uncharacterized) macrophage signal(s) important for up-regulated hepcidin expression during iron overload might conceivably be altered by mutant HFE. However, a recent study has shown that Kupffer cells and macrophages are not required for hepcidin response to iron[30]. As to a role for mutant TfR2, its high expression in hepatocytes raises the possibility that TfR2 might somehow regulate hepcidin synthesis, at least during iron overload. The fact that cases of severe juvenile haemochromatosis are associated with mutations of HJV suggests that haemojuvelin might be a major regulator of hepcidin synthesis. Recently, it has been reported that combination of HFE and TfR2 mutations in humans may lead to a severe juvenile haemochromatosis[31]. This reinforces the hypothesis that all three proteins, HFE, TfR2 and HJV, may be required more or less for controlling hepcidin expression and, if mutated, may cause an haemochromatotic phenotype[31].

GENETICS AND EPIDEMIOLOGY

HFE-related haemochromatosis is the most common form of HC and also the most frequently inherited metabolic disorder found in whites, with a prevalance ten times higher than that of cystic fibrosis. Genetic predisposition for this disease, i.e. C282Y homozygosity, is found in approximately 5/1000 of individuals of northern European descent[32]. HFE-HC is an excellent illustration of the 'founder effect', according to which a genetic disease can arise from a chance mutation occurring in a single individual, in this case a Celtic ancestor inhabiting northwestern Europe some 2000 years ago. The genetic defect, which caused no serious obstacle to reproduction and may even have conferred some advantages, was passed on and spread through population migration. The distribution of the C282Y mutation coincides with its northern European origin and with the presence of the disease[33].

Organ disease is highly unlikely in simple C282Y heterozygotes. The clinical impact of the H63D mutation on the second HFE allele appears to be limited[34], yet 1–2% of compound C282Y/H63D heterozygotes seem to be predisposed to expression of the disease[35]. The clinical significance of other seemingly rarer forms of compound heterozygosity, e.g. monoallelic C282Y or H63D mutation with substitution of cysteine for serine at amino-acid position 65 (S65C) or other rare changes on the second allele, and that of other rare changes observed in HFE, is still being debated[2], but undetected situations of this type might explain some cases of mild disease in individuals who appear to have only monoallelic HFE mutations.

The frequency of TfR2 mutations is low and so far they have been detected in a few pedigrees throughout the world. Apparently, TfR2 mutations do not appear to be restricted to northern Europeans. The *TFR2* gene is relatively large, spanning 21 kilobases and including 18 exons; thus, detection of new TFR2 mutations in single patients remains cumbersome. Analysis of TfR2 mutations should be especially considered in individuals with adult non-HFE haemochromatosis, particularly from families with high consanguinity.

The juvenile form of haemochromatosis is rare. Most cases are due to mutations of *HJV* located on chromosome 2^{14}. However, a small proportion of patients carry mutations in the gene encoding the iron regulatory peptide hepcidin on chromosome $19q13^{19}$. In the initial study on *HJV* 12 families were found to be homozygous or compound heterozygous for six mutations in *HJV*. To date 23 mutations have been identified in 43 juvenile HC families. One common mutation, G320V, has been reported in all studies; it is present in half of juvenile HC families.

CLINICAL ASPECTS

HFE-related haemochromatosis is a multifactorial disease characterized by stepwise progression from biochemical abnormality to organ toxicity[2]. The altered HFE protein plays an essential role in this process but its presence alone is insufficient to explain the broad spectrum of metabolic and pathological consequences ascribed to the disease. Expressivity of the genetic defect may lead to biochemical abnormalities, symptoms and signs or overt organ disease. Early diagnosis in haemochromatosis is especially important since treatment by venesection before irreversible end-organ damage has occurred can restore a normal life expectancy[36,37].

Haemochromatosis should be suspected in a middle-aged men presenting with cirrhosis of the liver, bronze skin, diabetes and other endocrine failure, or joint inflammation and heart disease. However, this classical syndromic presentation is rare. Today diagnosis is made at earlier stages as an effect of screening and enhanced case detection due to greater clinician awareness and higher index of suspicion. The most common presenting symptoms are now fatigue, malaise, and arthralgia, while hepatomegaly is one of the earliest physical signs. Elevated serum transferrin saturation iron, which precedes increased serum ferritin, and moderately increased transaminase levels are common biochemical abnormalities. Once the diagnosis of HFE-HC is established, all family members, particularly siblings, should be subjected to a thorough biochemical and clinical evaluation, and genetic testing is advisable for adult first-degree relatives.

As specified, while all patients with overt HFE-related HC (i.e. with organ damage) carry the C282Y mutation on both HFE alleles, some C282Y homozygotes present no evidence of organ disease or biochemical abnormalities, although they should still be considered to be at increased risk. It is currently impossible to predict whether (and to what extent) a C282Y homozygote will express the disease phenotype. At present we can only conclude that, while the majority of C282Y homozygotes have laboratory evidence of plasma and tissue iron overload (i.e. high transferrin saturation and ferritin levels, respectively), organ disease requiring medical treatment is today much less common[2].

Although clinical descriptions of TfR2-related HC are currently limited, patients with TfR2 mutations almost invariably present signs of significant hepatic iron overload and express a systemic iron loading syndrome almost indistinguishable from that of HFE haemochromatosis[38].

The rather vague term, 'juvenile haemochromatosis', has been used to refer to a form of hereditary iron overload with a development pattern resembling that of adult HC but more rapidly progressive. Because of the higher rate of iron loading associated with this disorder (and possibly differential tissue sensitivities to this massive toxic insult), cardiomyopathy and endocrinopathy, including reduced glucose tolerance, appear earlier than they do in adult HC, and death before the age of 30 is not uncommon[39]. The commonest symptom at presentation is hypogonadism, which, at the end of the second decade, may be present in all cases[39]. In sporadic cases, abdominal pain and cardiac disease also represent common findings, while liver cirrhosis is recognized at later stages although silent micronodular cirrhosis is part of the syndrome.

Increased risk of clinically expressed disease has already been documented in patients with heterozygous mutations of both HFE and HAMP[40]. Reports of uncharacteristically severe disease in patients who apparently have TfR2 mutations alone, or in combination with HFE variants, might also be accounted for by undetected mutations of other hereditary haemochromatosis genes. The variety of genotypes that can produce a hereditary haemochromatosis phenotype highlights the importance of defining and classifying this disease as a unique clinicopathological entity.

Therapeutic phlebotomy is the safest, most effective and most economical approach to treatment. It can normalize life expectancy if initiated before organ damage has occurred. One unit (400–500 ml) of blood (containing approximately 200–250 mg of iron) is removed weekly until serum ferritin is less than 20–50 µg/L and transferrin saturation drops below 30%. Maintenance therapy, which typically involves removal of 2–4 units a year, can then be initiated, and must be continued for the duration of the patient's life to keep transferrin saturation and ferritin normal. As noted above, phlebotomy has little effect if started after organ impairment has already developed: the hypogonadism, cirrhosis, destructive arthritis, and insulin-dependent diabetes associated with HC are usually irreversible.

FERROPORTIN DISEASE

Ferroportin disease (FD) (Table 2) is an hereditary iron storage disease distinct from HC. It is an autosomal dominant inherited disorder of iron metabolism which causes progressive iron retention predominantly in reticuloendothelial cells of the spleen and liver and is characterized by a steady increase of serum ferritin, inappropriately high as compared to the extent of serum transferrin saturation, marginal anaemia, and mild organ disease[3].

The disorder was described clinically in 1999[41] and associated with the A77D mutation of ferroportin (FPN) in 2001[42]. The disorder has been now reported in many countries and, at variance with the distribution of the HFE gene mutations that appear to be restricted to Caucasians of northern European ancestry, it appears to be spread worldwide in different ethnic groups[3].

FPN is the main iron export protein in mammals. It is expressed in several cell types that play critical roles in mammalian iron metabolism, including placental syncytiotrophoblasts, duodenal enterocytes, hepatocytes and reticuloendothelial macrophages[43-45]. *In vitro*, FPN has been found to be the cellular receptor for hepcidin: in cultured cells stably expressing FPN, hepcidin administration causes FPN internalization and degradation[20]. This implies decreased surface FPN amount, and reduced iron egress from cells such as enterocytes and macrophages, whenever circulating hepcidin levels are high; namely, inflammation and iron overload. The opposite would occur when hepcidin is low; namely, anaemia and hypoxia[18].

A current pathogenic model for the FD is that loss-of-function mutations of FPN cause a mild but significant impairment of iron recycling, particularly by reticuloendothelial macrophages[42], which normally must process and release a large quantity of iron derived from the lysis of senescent erythrocytes. As a consequence, iron retention by macrophages would lead to tissue iron accumulation (i.e. high serum ferritin) but decreased availability of iron for circulating transferrin (i.e. low transferrin saturation) and for bone marrow. At later stages, both iron retention in cells and activation of feedback mechanisms to increase intestinal absorption might contribute to more pronounced iron overload. This pathophysiological model is consistent with the finding that patients with mutations in FPN have much larger reticuloendothelial iron stores than do patients with HC. Although the patients are not anaemic in adulthood, indicating that adequate iron is available for normal erythropoiesis, they may show a reduced tolerance to phlebotomy and become anaemic on therapy in spite of persistently elevated serum ferritin values[41,42]. It is possible that different mutations along the protein may differently affect the function of FPN and indirectly lead to variability in clinical expressivity. In this context, recent *in-vitro* studies[46-48] and a clinical report[49] suggest that a subgroup of patients with FD may carry gain-of-function mutations that might lead to enhanced iron release from enterocytes and macrophages and a phenotype similar to classic HC. This latter hypothesis awaits validation by additional experimental and clinical studies.

The FD should be suspected in all cases of isolated hyperferritinaemia in the absence of known secondary causes (such as infection, inflammation and malignancy), or unexplained anaemia with normal/high serum ferritin, or familial hyperferritinaemia (see algorithm in ref. 3).

CONCLUSIONS

The basic features of the hereditary haemochromatosis syndrome, as we recognize it today, can be produced by pathogenic mutations of at least four different iron metabolism genes. Since the common pathogenic denominator of all forms of HC is the uncontrolled expansion of the plasma iron pool, mutations in other known or unknown genes affecting this iron compartment may very well lead to the same syndrome. Depending on the gene involved, and its physiological role in iron homeostasis, the hereditary haemochromatosis phenotype varies, ranging from massive early-onset iron loading with severe organ disease (e.g. associated with homozygous mutations of HAMP or HJV) to the milder late-onset phenotype characterizing classic HFE and TfR2-related forms. Phenotypes on the latter end of the spectrum are also particularly subject to the modifying effects of host-related and environmental factors, such as dietary iron, alcohol consumptions, and viral hepatitis. 'Intermediate phenotypes' could result from combined heterozygous or homozygous mutations of multiple haemochromatosis genes. For instance, the relatively mild phenotype associated with homozygotic mutation of HFE can be aggravated and accelerated by a coexistent heterozygotic mutation in a 'juvenile' gene, such as *HAMP*. The latter mutation combined with a normally silent heterozygotic HFE mutation could also result in unexpected disease expression. *In-vitro* and *in-vivo* studies will be needed to dissect the biochemical consequences of each hereditary haemochromatosis allele and increase our understanding of the precise contribution of each gene to the hereditary haemochromatosis phenotype.

References

1. Feder JN, Gnirke A, Thomas W et al. A novel MHC class I-like gene is mutated in patients with hereditary haemochromatosis. Nat Genet. 1996;13:399–408.
2. Pietrangelo A. Hereditary hemochromatosis – a new look at an old disease. N Engl J Med. 2004;350:2383–97.
3. Pietrangelo A. The ferroportin disease. Blood Cells Mol Dis. 2004;32:131–8.
4. Lebron JA, Bennett MJ, Vaughn DE et al. Crystal structure of the hemochromatosis protein HFE and characterization of its interaction with transferrin receptor. Cell. 1998;93:111–23.
5. Feder JN, Penny DM, Irrinki A et al. The hemochromatosis gene product complexes with the transferrin receptor and lowers its affinity for ligand binding. Proc Natl Acad Sci USA. 1998;95:1472–7.
6. Gross CN, Irrinki A, Feder JN, Enns CA. Co-trafficking of HFE, a nonclassical major histocompatibility complex class I protein, with the transferrin receptor implies a role in intracellular iron regulation. J Biol Chem. 1998;273:22068–74.
7. Davies PS, Zhang AS, Anderson EL et al. Evidence for the interaction of the hereditary haemochromatosis protein, HFE, with the transferrin receptor in endocytic compartments. Biochem J. 2003;373:145–53.
8. Waheed A, Parkkila S, Zhou XY et al. Hereditary hemochromatosis: Effects of C282Y and H63D mutations on association with beta(2)-microglobulin, intracellular processing, and cell surface expression of the HFE protein in COS-7 cells. Proc Natl Acad Sci USA. 1997; 94:12384–9.
9. Kawabata H, Yang R, Hirama T et al. Molecular cloning of transferrin receptor 2. A new member of the transferrin receptor-like family. J Biol Chem. 1999;274:20826–32.
10. Kawabata H, Germain RS, Vuong PT, Nakamaki T, Said JW, Koeffler HP. Transferrin receptor 2-alpha supports cell growth both in iron-chelated cultured cells and *in vivo*. J Biol Chem. 2000;275:16618–25.
11. West AP Jr, Bennett MJ, Sellers VM, Andrews NC, Enns CA, Bjorkman PJ. Comparison of the interactions of transferrin receptor and transferrin receptor 2 with transferrin and the hereditary hemochromatosis protein HFE. J Biol Chem. 2000;275:38135–8.
12. Camaschella C, Roetto A, Cali A et al. The gene TFR2 is mutated in a new type of haemochromatosis mapping to 7q22. Nat Genet. 2000;25:14–15.
13. Fleming RE, Ahmann JR, Migas MC et al. Targeted mutagenesis of the murine transferrin receptor-2 gene produces hemochromatosis. Proc Natl Acad Sci USA. 2002;99:10653–8.
14. Papanikolaou G, Samuels ME, Ludwig EH et al. Mutations in HFE2 cause iron overload in chromosome 1q-linked juvenile hemochromatosis. Nat Genet. 2004;36:77–82.
15. Krause A, Neitz S, Magert HJ et al. LEAP-1, a novel highly disulfide-bonded human peptide, exhibits antimicrobial activity. FEBS Lett. 2000;480:147–50.

16. Park CH, Valore EV, Waring AJ, Ganz T. Hepcidin, a urinary antimicrobial peptide synthesized in the liver. J Biol Chem. 2001;276:7806–10.
17. Pigeon C, Ilyin G, Courselaud B et al. A new mouse liver-specific gene, encoding a protein homologous to human antimicrobial peptide hepcidin, is overexpressed during iron overload. J Biol Chem. 2001;276:7811–19.
18. Ganz T. Hepcidin, a key regulator of iron metabolism and mediator of anemia of inflammation. Blood. 2003;102:783–8.
19. Roetto A, Papanikolaou G, Politou M et al. Mutant antimicrobial peptide hepcidin is associated with severe juvenile hemochromatosis. Nat Genet. 2003;33:21–2.
20. Nemeth E, Tuttle MS, Powelson J et al. Hepcidin regulates iron efflux by binding to ferroportin and inducing its internalization. Science. 2004;306:2090–3.
21. Finch S, Finch C. Idiopathic hemochromatosis, an iron storage disease: A. Iron metabolism in hemochromatosis. Medicine. 1955;34:381–430.
22. Crosby WH. The control of iron balance by the intestinal mucosa. Blood. 1963;22:441–9.
23. Pietrangelo A. Metals, oxidative stress, and hepatic fibrogenesis. Semin Liver Dis. 1996;16: 13–30.
24. Bothwell TH. Overview and mechanisms of iron regulation. Nutr Rev. 1995;53:237–45.
25. Bridle KR, Frazer DM, Wilkins SJ et al. Disrupted hepcidin regulation in HFE-associated haemochromatosis and the liver as a regulator of body iron homoeostasis. Lancet. 2003; 361:669–73.
26. Gehrke SG, Kulaksiz H, Herrmann T et al. Expression of hepcidin in hereditary hemochromatosis: evidence for a regulation in response to serum transferrin saturation and non-transferrin-bound iron. Blood. 2003;102:371–6.
27. Muckenthaler M, Roy CN, Custodio AO et al. Regulatory defects in liver and intestine implicate abnormal hepcidin and Cybrd1 expression in mouse hemochromatosis. Nat Genet. 2003;34:102–7.
28. Kawabata H, Fleming RE, Gui D et al. Expression of hepcidin is down-regulated in TfR2 mutant mice manifesting a phenotype of hereditary hemochromatosis. Blood. 2005;105: 376–81.
29. Nicolas G, Viatte L, Lou DQ et al. Constitutive hepcidin expression prevents iron overload in a mouse model of hemochromatosis. Nat Genet. 2003;34:97–101.
30. Montosi G, Corradini E, Garuti C et al. Kupffer cells and macrophages are not required for hepatic hepcidin activation during dietary iron overload. Hepatology. 2005;41:545–52.
31. Pietrangelo A, Caleffi A, Henrion J et al. Juvenile hemochromatosis associated with pathogenic mutations of adult hemochromatosis genes. Gastroenterology. 2005;128:470–9.
32. Merryweatherclarke AT, Pointon JJ, Shearman JD, Robson KJH. Global prevalence of putative haemochromatosis mutations. J Med Genet. 1997;34:275–8.
33. Rochette J, Pointon JJ, Fisher CA et al. Multicentric origin of hemochromatosis gene (HFE) mutations [published erratum appears in Am J Hum Genet. 1999;64:1491]. Am J Hum Genet. 1999;64:1056–62.
34. Gochee PA, Powell LW, Cullen DJ, Du Sart D, Rossi E, Olynyk JK. A population-based study of the biochemical and clinical expression of the H63D hemochromatosis mutation. Gastroenterology. 2002;122:646–51.
35. Mura C, Raguenes O, Ferec C. HFE mutations analysis in 711 hemochromatosis probands: evidence for S65C implication in mild form of hemochromatosis. Blood. 1999;93:2502–5.
36. Niederau C, Fischer R, Sonnenberg A, Stremmel W, Trampisch HJ, Strohmeyer G. Survival and causes of death in cirrhotic and in noncirrhotic patients with primary hemochromatosis. N Engl J Med. 1985;313:1256–62.
37. Wojcik JP, Speechley MR, Kertesz AE, Chakrabarti S, Adams PC. Natural history of C282Y homozygotes for hemochromatosis. Can J Gastroenterol. 2002;16:297–302.
38. Mattman A, Huntsman D, Lockitch G et al. Transferrin receptor 2 (TfR2) and HFE mutational analysis in non-C282Y iron overload: identification of a novel TfR2 mutation. Blood. 2002;100:1075–7.
39. De Gobbi M, Roetto A, Piperno A et al. Natural history of juvenile haemochromatosis. Br J Haematol. 2002;117:973–9.
40. Merryweather-Clarke AT, Cadet E, Bomford A et al. Digenic inheritance of mutations in HAMP and HFE results in different types of haemochromatosis. Hum Mol Genet. 2003; 12:2241–7.

41. Pietrangelo A, Montosi G, Totaro A et al. Hereditary hemochromatosis in adults without pathogenic mutations in the hemochromatosis gene [see comments]. N Engl J Med. 1999; 341:725–32.
42. Montosi G, Donovan A, Totaro A et al. Autosomal-dominant hemochromatosis is associated with a mutation in the ferroportin (SLC11A3) gene. J Clin Invest. 2001;108: 619–23.
43. Donovan A, Brownlie A, Zhou Y et al. Positional cloning of zebrafish ferroportin1 identifies a conserved vertebrate iron exporter. Nature. 2000;403:776–81.
44. McKie AT, Marciani P, Rolfs A et al. A novel duodenal iron-regulated transporter, IREG1, implicated in the basolateral transfer of iron to the circulation. Mol Cell. 2000;5:299–309.
45. Abboud S, Haile DJ. A novel mammalian iron-regulated protein involved in intracellular iron metabolism. J Biol Chem. 2000;275:19906–12.
46. Drakesmith H, Schimanski LM, Ormerod E et al. Resistance to hepcidin is conferred by hemochromatosis-associated mutations of ferroportin. Blood. 2005;106:1092–7.
47. Schimanski LM, Drakesmith H, Merryweather-Clarke AT et al. *In vitro* functional analysis of human ferroportin (FPN) and hemochromatosis-associated FPN mutations. Blood. 2005;105:4096–102.
48. De Domenico I, Ward DM, Nemeth E et al. The molecular basis of ferroportin-linked hemochromatosis. Proc Natl Acad Sci USA. 2005;102:8955–60.
49. Sham RL, Phatak PD, West C, Lee P, Andrews C, Beutler E. Autosomal dominant hereditary hemochromatosis associated with a novel ferroportin mutation and unique clinical features. Blood Cells Mol Dis. 2005;34:157–61.

19
Wilson disease: the impact of molecular advances

D. W. COX

INTRODUCTION

Wilson disease (WND) has been recognized as a disease entity for more than 100 years; however, the past decade has brought major advances both in our understanding and in improved diagnosis of this condition. C. Westphal (1983) and A. Strumpell (1898), in Germany, described an entity, referred to as Westphal–Strumpell pseudosclerosis, recognized later as a neurological form of Wilson disease. B. Kayser and B. Fleischer, respectively in 1902 and 1903, noted the unique brownish rings on the outer circumference of the cornea (Kayser–Fleischer ring) that we now recognize as copper deposition, and a characteristic feature in some WND patients. S.A.K. Wilson, in 1912, described a progressive lenticular degeneration, affecting both brain and liver[1]. However, it was not until 1948 that B.M. Mandelbrote and J.N. Cumings recognized WND as a disorder of copper transport and excess accumulation.

COPPER: BOTH ESSENTIAL AND TOXIC

Copper is an essential dietary component for simple and complex organisms, as a required component for enzymes such as cytochrome oxidase (electron transfer), lysyl oxidase (connective tissue and elastin crosslinking), superoxide dismutase (free radical scavenging), dopamine β-mono-oxgenase (neurotransmission) and tyrosinase (pigment production). The human diet contains approximately 1.5–3 mg copper daily. Copper is absorbed in the upper intestine and is transferred to plasma where it is bound to albumin. Albumin and copper histidine transport the copper to tissues, with the majority being transported to the liver. Copper is never free within cells. Within the hepatocyte there are a series of low molecular weight metallochaperones, each of which delivers copper to a specific target molecule[2].

Entry into the cells is facilitated by the protein CTR1 (copper transporter 1). In the liver, copper is incorporated into the protein apo-caeruloplasmin, producing copper-containing caeruloplasmin (also called holocaeruloplasmin). ATOX1 is the chaperone delivering copper into ceruloplasmin. The majority of copper is eliminated from the hepatocyte via the bile. Copper remaining in the hepatocytes is bound to low molecular weight proteins, metallothioneins, which store excess copper in a non-toxic form (see review ref. 3). The characteristic feature of Wilson disease is the storage of excess copper in the tissues, which can lead to the production of free radicals, and to subsequent tissue destruction.

FEATURES OF WILSON DISEASE

Wilson disease is an autosomal recessive disorder, occurring in most populations with an incidence of about one in 30 000. In certain populations, such as those of China and Sardinia, the frequency is reported to be as high as one in 10 000. In spite of the long history of recognition of Wilson disease as an entity, this condition remains a diagnostic challenge. Recent reviews, with references, provide details of the clinical and biochemical features[4–7].

Clinical features

The clinical features are highly variable. Hepatic disease can be acute or chronic. Neurological manifestations include tremor and/or rigidity[8]. Patients can have hepatic or neurological features only, or a combination of both. Psychiatric disorders and kidney malfunction can also be features of the disease. A less frequent but acute presentation of the disease is haemolytic anaemia, as increased copper in the blood leads to haemolysis[9]. The onset of disease symptoms can occur as early as 3 years of age[10], or even into the seventh decade[11,12], but most commonly between approximately 8 and 45 years of age. Three reported cases of WND with an onset of greater than 65 years are shown in Table 1. With such a wide range of clinical features and age of onset, it is not surprising that this disease presents a diagnostic challenge.

Biochemical features

Biochemical assays reflecting copper status have traditionally been used for diagnosis; however none is specific[13]. Serum caeruloplasmin is often decreased from its normal level of 200–400 mg/L, rising from a very low level at birth, to a peak of 300–500 mg/L by about 3 years of age[14]. However, caeruloplasmin is an acute-phase protein, elevated by pregnancy, oestrogen, and inflammation. Hepatic copper overload can probably also increase the concentration of serum copper. Up to 40% of patients with hepatic manifestations of WND[15], and perhaps 10% of patients with neurological manifestations, have a normal concentration of serum caeruloplasmin. A decreased serum caeruloplasmin cannot, therefore, provide a reliable diagnostic sign. The non-caeruloplasmin component of serum may be increased, as a reflection of copper overload. The 24-h urinary copper value is almost always increased, at least two to three times the normal level of <0.6 μmol/24 h, but may be borderline in patients in the

Table 1 Unusual patients with late onset of Wilson disease symptoms: variants found: Glu1064Ala (E1064A) + His1069Gln (H1069Q)[11,12]

Patient	Onset	Sex	Clinical	Urine Cu (24 h) (n < 40 μg/24 h)	Liver Cu (n < 50 μg/g)
1	72 years	Female	Normal serum Cp (37 mg/dl) KF rings	39 μg/24 h After penicillamine challenge: 9390 μg/24 h	
2 (sibling to patient 1)	70 years	Male	Mild hand tremor, age 45 years Mild gait dyscoordination (69 years) Cp 20 mg/dl KF rings	218 μg/24 h	671 μg/g dry weight
3	60 years	Female	Normal LFT Minimally abnormal Cp No KF rings	> 120 μg/24 h	1021 μg/g dry weight

Cp, caeruloplasmin; KF, Kayser–Fleischer; LFT, liver function test.

early phase of the disease. Hepatic copper concentration is almost always increased to >250 µg/g of dry weight, but distribution of copper throughout the liver may be variable[16]. Patients with typical clinical features, including Kayser–Fleischer rings, as well as clear abnormalities of all of the biochemically based copper assays, are infrequent. Because of this variability a diagnosis is not necessarily made. Since the disease is one of the metabolic disorders that is treatable by removing copper, or preventing its absorption, diagnosis as early as possible in the course of the disease is critical.

Another diagnostic problem is that heterozygotes sometimes have features that overlap with patients, causing some heterozygotes to be treated as patients[17]. They can have a markedly decreased serum caeruloplasmin, borderline or slight increased urinary copper, and borderline or slightly increased hepatic copper. In spite of such copper abnormalities, heterozygotes are not known to develop clinical symptoms or to need treatment.

THE BASIC DEFECT IN WILSON DISEASE: GENE DISCOVERY

The discovery of the causative gene for WND in 1993[18,19] has not only increased our understanding of the biological basis of the disease, but has created new opportunities for reliable diagnosis. The gene (*ATP7B*) encodes a copper-transporting P-type ATPase, with eight transmembrane domains (Figure 1). While a similar gene in yeast has only one copper-binding domain, the WND copper transporter, ATP7B, has six copper-binding domains that probably fold in a specific conformation. The copper chaperone ATOX11, binds to the coppers in the CXXC motif of the copper-binding domain. A TEG motif is responsible for the transduction of energy. A phosphorylated aspartate residue in the DKTG motif is typical of P-type ATPases. The ATP binding domain is similar to that of a number of other ion transporters. The characteristic feature is a conserved CPC motif in transmembrane domain six[18].

MUTATIONS IN THE COPPER TRANSPORTER ATP7B

More than 280 mutations have been described throughout the length of *ATP7B*, and in the promoter region, with specific mutations characteristic to specific ethnic groups. Mutations, detected mostly by single-stand conformation polymorphism (SSCP) and/or sequencing, have been reported in numerous populations. The reported mutations, with references, are listed in a database maintained in the Department of Medical Genetics at the University of Alberta: http://www.medicalgenetics.med.ualberta.ca/wilson/index.php. Most mutations identified in *ATP7B* to date are missense mutations (59%). Small deletions (21%) and insertions (8%) usually result in a frameshift that is predicted to disrupt gene function. Nonsense mutations (7%) cause premature truncation of the protein. Splice site mutations (8%) occur throughout the gene and are predicted to generally produce a non-functional protein. The mutation spectrum for the similar Menkes gene, *ATP7A*, is

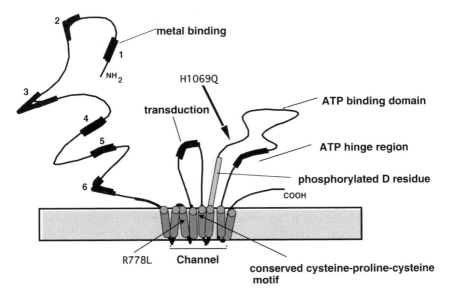

Figure 1 Model of the predicted product of the Wilson disease gene, *ATP7B*. Functional domains conserved in the Menkes disease copper transporter, ATP7A, are indicated. Two mutations common in European (H1069Q) and Asian (R778L) populations are shown. Model modified from the original proposed by Bull and Cox[18]

different from that of *ATP7B*[20]. In addition, large gene deletions in the *ATP7A* gene are found in about 20% of patients with Menkes disease, but appear rarely in WND. Only one such large deletion, of exon 20, has been reported[21]. Insertions, deletions, and nonsense mutations occur throughout the gene. Missense mutations are more highly focused in the important functional regions.

With such a large number of mutations within the gene, the prospect of diagnosis by DNA analysis appears daunting. However, in the past few years, high-throughput methods for mutation analysis have now made molecular diagnosis feasible. New equipment for mutation detection is continually being introduced (e.g. high-performance liquid chromatography and methods based on heteroduplex melting curves) allowing relatively inexpensive screening of all 21 exons, plus the promoter, of *ATP7B*. An alternative currently preferred in this laboratory is complete sequencing of the gene, beginning with exons most likely to contain mutations. Using Variant Sequencer (Applied Biosystems™), we have been able to obtain results in 2 days if needed. Thus the technicalities of mutation detection are no longer a deterrent to mutation testing. However, the current problem is in deciding which mutations are disease causing and which are rare normal variants. For small deletions and insertions causing frameshifts, or for nonsense mutations, function of the protein will be disrupted in most cases[22,23], although exon skipping to produce a functional protein is always a consideration. Splice site mutations cannot be assumed to affect splicing in all cases, and need to be functionally tested[24]. Only 17% of such mutations listed in the Wilson Disease Database have been tested. In Menkes disease the splice site mutations frequently show a more mild disease, occipital horn syndrome[25,26]. A large number of missense mutations, of which less than 20% have been tested for function, now pose the greatest problem for molecular diagnosis.

Population variation

Very few mutations in ATP7B are common. The spectrum of mutations found in different ethnic groups varies considerably. The histidine1069glutamine (H1069Q) mutation[19] is the only mutation found relatively frequently in populations of European origin. Among 115 Caucasian patients we have studied, with origins in various parts of Europe, exon 14 carries the highest proportion of mutations (Cox, unpublished). The high frequency in exon 14 reflects the presence of H1069Q. Exon 8, followed by 13, 18, and 20, also had more mutations than other exons. The frequency of the H1069Q mutation is about 35–45% in mixed European populations, and is even higher in eastern Europe[27]. Each ethnic group has its specific mutations and frequencies. The arginine778leucine (R778L) mutation[22] is a relatively frequent mutation in Asian populations, accounting for over 50% of WND alleles in this population. A 15 base pair deletion in the promoter region is common in the Sardinian population[28]. Interestingly, this is the only disease mutation identified to date in the promoter region[29]. In selected populations, targeted screening of the common mutations by low-cost methods is effective for a large proportion of the patient mutations – such as those in eastern Germany[30] and Sardinia[31]. The differences between the exon location of mutations in populations from the eastern region of Germany, the Canary Islands and Sardinia are shown in Figure 2. Even with complete sequencing of all exons there are about 2% of patients in whom we cannot identify a mutation (Cox, unpublished). No doubt, in rare cases, a mutation lies within an intron. Examination of the RNA would therefore be required.

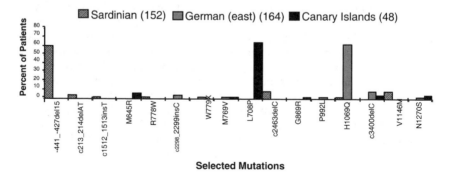

Figure 2 Specific mutations differ between populations. These results show the percent of patients that carry the mutations indicated, as tested in Sardinia (152 patients)[28] East Germany (164 patients)[27] and Canary Islands (48 patients)[62]

Functional assessment of mutations

ATP7B serves two functions: one is a transport function, in which copper is incorporated into caeruloplasmin and transported through the cell membrane. A second feature, that of trafficking within the cell, is required for normal function. This trafficking within the cell was first identified for the related copper transporter, ATP7A[32]. ATP7B traffics from the trans Golgi/late endosome compartment, to cytoplasmic vesicles, and then to the apical membrane of the hepatocyte and other polarized cells[33,34]. Testing of the transport function can be effectively carried out in yeast[35-37]. The yeast *Saccharomyces cerevisiae* has a copper transport system similar to that found in humans and other higher organisms. The *ATP7B* counterpart, *CCC2*, can be knocked out in yeast and a normal or variant human gene substituted. CCC2, like its counterpart in humans, obtains its copper from outside the cell through CTR1, carried by the metallochaperone ATOX1, to CCC2/ATP7B (Figure 3). FET3 is the yeast counterpart of caeruloplasmin. Caeruloplasmin and FET3 are both required for cellular iron transport. The normal yeast, yeast with a normal human *ATP7B*, or mutant *ATP7B*, is then grown in appropriate media to test function. Yeasts with a functioning *CCC2* gene do not require the addition of iron and copper to their media, while a defective mutant has this

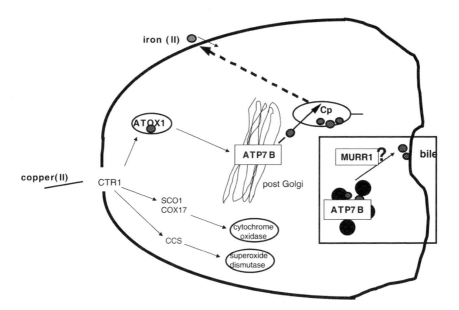

Figure 3 Diagram of a hepatocyte, showing major proteins in the copper transport pathway, highlighting ATP7B. Low molecular weight copper 'chaperones' (ATOX1, SCO1 and COX17, and CCS) deliver copper to specific target proteins (ATP7B, cytochrome oxidase, and superoxide dismutase, respectively). SCO1 transports copper across the mitochondrial membrane. ATP7B incorporates copper into ceruloplasmin, which facilitates iron transport, and traffics from the trans Golgi network (TGN) to cytoplasmic vesicles that deliver copper to the bile canaliculus. MURR1 may be involved in excretion into bile

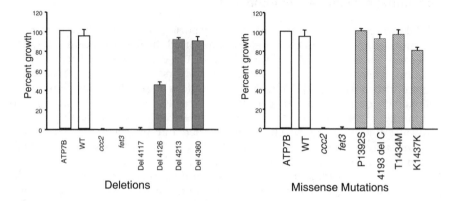

Figure 4 A yeast assay to assess transport function. The yeast copper transporter, CCC2, similar to ATP7B, has been 'knocked out' (ccc2) and cannot transport copper in copper deficient growth medium. The wild type (WT) transport activity is indicated as 100% growth. Missense mutation and deletion constructs are shown in gray or shaded. Growth of the mutants in this assay varies from zero to 100 percent of normal growth. Adapted from ref. 39

requirement. This laboratory, and others, have used various cells in culture to examine the ability of mutant ATP7B to traffick within the cell. In this laboratory we have successfully used CHO cells[36,38,39]. An example of the results is shown in Figure 4. Those mutants tested for functional activity have been indicated in the Wilson Disease Database.

In addition to functional assessment, the properties of the mutant ATP7B can be compared with those of the normal ATP7B. These properties include hydrophobicity, size, and conservation in the ATP7B or Menkes protein (ATP7A) in other species. Most reports of new mutations include such analyses. For example, my colleagues and I have recently reported 24 new mutations with comparison of these properties in the mutant with the normal ATP7B[40]. A three-dimensional model has been proposed[41,42], based on protein structure of the calcium transporter, SCRCA1, which has been crystallized. We have used this to examine mutations that lie within the ATP loop (G Macintyre, unpublished).

DIAGNOSTIC ISSUES

In a patient with characteristic clinical features, and at least some abnormalities of copper biochemistry, the identification of one of the two gene mutations may be adequate. However, this one mutation must be well established as a mutation with no uncertainty regarding its status (disease-causing vs normal). For a patient with atypical clinical features the potential overlap with heterozygotes in some cases needs to be kept in mind.

Gene discovery has brought the opportunity for accurate diagnosis of WND. The identification of mutations has demonstrated that the typical clinical and biochemical features are not always reliable for the diagnosis. The potential diagnosis of WND needs to be kept in mind for patients with any of the hepatic, common neurological, psychiatric or haematological features suggestive of this disease. Technically, the mutations can be readily detected. However, functional studies are needed to ensure the best use of the new mutation detection technologies.

DIAGNOSIS OF SIBS OF A PATIENT

Another area in which molecular approaches are invaluable is in the correct diagnosis of asymptomatic sibs of WND patients with the secure diagnosis of WND. In some families the heterozygotes cannot be distinguished from affected homozygotes[17,43]. The use of dinucleotide repeat markers, or microsatellites, is important in all cases for correct diagnosis of sibs, where both mutations in the patients are not known. This is particularly essential because of the overlap in biochemical features between presymptomatic patients and heterozygotes. An example of such diagnosis is shown in Figure 5. My colleagues and I have now demonstrated in several families that individuals with biochemical abnormalities (low caeruloplasmin, borderline increased urinary copper) were incorrectly considered to be presymptomatic patients (Cox, unpublished).

Molecular analysis clearly identifies such people as heterozyotes. Appropriate copper analyses can be carried out to confirm the diagnosis of presymptomatic patients as made by marker studies. In populations in which there is a possibility for distant relationships, as in geographical isolates or in communities that have originated from a small number of ancestors, carrier testing in the family is recommended. In this laboratory we have recently had a family in which a first cousin twice removed of two patients who died in childhood has now been identified with WND. Her relatively rare presentation as haemolytic anaemia was recognized as WND because testing had been carried out in the grandmother in a large previous family study (Cox, unpublished). Haplotype analysis is of course not required if both mutations are identified in the patient, and testing of relatives can be carried out directly by mutation analysis.

Accurate diagnosis by haplotype analysis requires confidence that the copper storage in the initial patient is in fact due to WND.

MURR1 (COMMD1) AND COPPER STORAGE

Bedlington terriers develop a copper storage disorder, copper toxicosis, that can lead to liver disease. Through linkage analysis, copper toxicosis was identified as linked to a specific marker, C0147, on canine chromosome 10[44]. Further linkage studies led to the identification of a deletion of an exon in a gene MURR1 (now called COMMD1) as a potential causative gene for this disease[45]. However, while it was found that most affected dogs are homozygous for this deletion, at least some are heterozygous or do not carry the deletion at all[46].

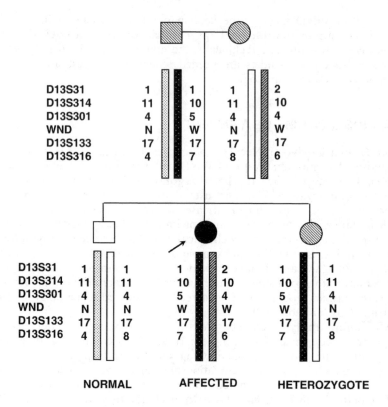

Figure 5 Diagnostic use of polymorphic DNA microsatellite markers for non-symptomatic sibs of a confirmed patient in a pedigree. Highly variable markers (microsatellites) allow tracking of the chromosome region containing the WND (ATP7B) gene, or its normal counterpart. DNA markers are listed in centromeric to telomeric order. Three markers are usually sufficient for an unambiguous result: D13S314, D13S301, and D13S316. Numbers represent alleles of each marker listed. Markers indicate the genotype of each sib: one normal (clear) and one a heterozygote, like the parents (shaded)

MURR1 (recently renamed COMMD1) interacts with the amino terminus of ATP7B, and could therefore be involved in the transport function[47], as shown in Figure 3. MURR1 has been reported to have many additional functions, including: regulation of the sodium channel that regulates blood pressure and salt balance through interaction with subunit EnaC[48], interaction with XIAP, an X-linked suppressor of apoptosis[49], and restriction of HIV-1 replication in lymphocytes through inhibition of NF-κB activity[50]. However, it is not yet clear whether this is the main cause of Bedlington copper toxicosis or a modifier. An important question is whether MURR1 could be responsible for copper storage disease in humans. In a study examining children with copper storage and liver disease early in childhood[51], no mutations in the MURR1 gene were identified. MURR1 was sequenced in patients from ages 6 to 66

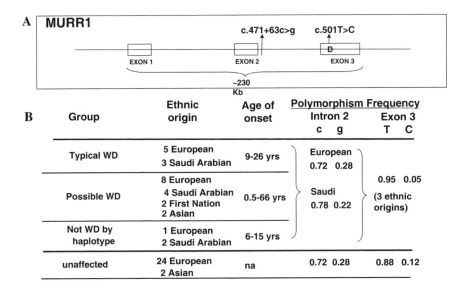

Figure 6 **A**: Gene structure of MURR1 (COMMD1), showing the position of two common polymorphisms. **B**: Results of sequence analysis of *MURR1* in patients with evidence of copper storage, but with no ATP7B mutation identified. Data are from ref. 52

years who show some evidence of copper storage, in some cases at least in part suggestive of WND[52]; results are shown in Figure 6. Again, no disease-related mutations were found, but two common polymorphisms were identified. One of these polymorphisms has been suggested to modify the course of WND[53].

TREATMENT

Availability of effective treatment for WND reinforces the need for appropriate early diagnosis. Treatment continues throughout the patient's lifetime. The treatments fall into two categories: removal of copper by a chelating agent (penicillamine, trientine) or prevention of absorption of copper through the use of a high intake of oral zinc. Penicillamine has been widely used since described by J.M. Walshe in 1956[54], and trientene, or 'trien', since 1982[55]. Zinc sulphate, used extensively in Europe since the 1970s[56], and later in North America[57,58] interferes with intestinal absorption of copper. A combination of penicillamine or trientine with zinc is experimental at present and has not been adequately assessed. The combination of trientine and zinc has been used successfully for rapid initiation of treatment in a patient with decompensated liver disease[59]. However, there is a requirement for a strict timing of trientine with respect to zinc, requiring medication every few hours, so that the two medications, that act in different ways, do not neutralize each other. This requirement can influence compliance. Ammonium tetrathyol molybdate is extremely effective at removing copper, but is still considered an experimental treatment.

Treatment has been discussed extensively in current references, including American Association for the Study of Liver Disease Practice Guidelines[5]. The goal of all treatment is to prevent tissue damage from the accumulation of copper. In addition to removal of copper or prevention of its absorption, the use of an antioxidant such as vitamin E can be useful to counteract the free radicals produced by copper in tissues. Patients have been shown to have a low level of serum antioxidants[54,60]. Given the effective treatments for WND, liver transplantation should seldom be required. However, in cases of fulminant hepatic failure this is the only option.

CONCLUSION

The identification of ATP7B as a causative gene in WND has made possible accurate and early diagnosis by DNA technologies. Current technologies make this approach feasible. DNA diagnosis is essential for sibs of known patients and does not require the identification of both mutations in the patient. Finally, new treatments are under evaluation to add to the well-established treatments that have been available for almost 50 years.

My personal hope and dream is that all patients with this treatable disease will be recognized early, so they may live normal and productive lives.

Acknowledgements

Mutation analysis for these studies was carried out by Lisa Prat Davies, computer molecular modelling by Georgina Macintyre, MURR1 studies by Veronica Coronado, ATP7B functional assays by Gloria Hsi, sequencing by Susan Kenney and Lynn Podemski. The copper studies are supported by CIHR (Canadian Institutes for Health Research) and NSERC (National Science and Engineering Research Council of Canada.

References

1. Wilson SAK. Progressive lenticular degeneration: a familial nervous disease associated with cirrhosis of the liver. Brain. 1912;34:295–309.
2. Field LS, Luk E, Culotta VC. Copper chaperones: personal escorts for metal ions. J Bioenerg Biomembr. 2002;34:373–9.
3. Mercer JF, Llanos RM. Molecular and cellular aspects of copper transport in developing mammals. J Nutr. 2003;133(Suppl 1):1481S–4.
4. Cox DW, Roberts EA. Wilson disease. In: Feldman M, Friedman LS, Brandt LJ editors. Sleisinger and Fordtran's Gastrointestinal and Liver Disease, 8th edn. Philadelphia: Elsevier, 2006 (In press).
5. Roberts EA, Schilsky ML. A practice guideline on Wilson disease. Hepatology. 2003;37: 1475–92.
6. Ferenci P. Wilson's disease. Clin Gastroenterol Hepatol. 2005;3:726–33.
7. Roberts EA, Cox DW. Wilson disease. In: Boyer TD, Manns M, Wright TL, editors. Zakim and Boyer's Hepatology, 5th edn. Philadelphia: Elsevier, 2006 (In press).
8. Oder W, Prayer L, Grimm G. Wilson's disease: evidence of subgroups derived from clinical findings and brain lesions. Neurology. 1993;43:120–4.

9. Hoshino T, Kumasaka K, Kawano K. Low serum alkaline phosphatase activity associated with severe Wilson's disease. Is the breakdown of alkaline phosphatase molecules caused by reactive oxygen species? Clin Chim Acta. 1995;238:91–100.

10. Wilson DC, Phillips MJ, Cox DW, Roberts EA. Severe hepatic Wilson's disease in preschool-aged children. J Pediatr. 2000;137:719–22.

11. Ala A, Borjigin J, Rochwarger A, Schilsky M. Wilson disease in septuagenarian siblings: raising the bar for diagnosis. Hepatology. 2005;41:668–70.

12. Perri RE, Hahn SH, Ferber MJ, Kamath PS. Wilson disease – keeping the bar for diagnosis raised. Hepatology. 2005;42:974.

13. Sallie R, Katsiyiannakis L, Baldwin D. Failure of simple biochemical indexes to reliably differentiate fulminant Wilson's disease from other causes of fulminant liver failure. Hepatology. 1992;16:1206–11.

14. Cox DW. Factors influencing serum ceruloplasmin in normal individuals. J Lab Clin Med. 1966;68:893–904.

15. Steindl P, Ferenci P, Dienes HP et al. Wilson's disease in patients with liver disease: a diagnostic challenge. Gastroenterology. 1998;113:212–18.

16. Faa G, Nurchi V, Demelia L et al. Uneven hepatic copper distribution in Wilson's disease. J Hepatol. 1995;22:303–8.

17. Lyon TD, Fell GS, Gaffney D et al. Use of a stable copper isotope (65Cu) in the differential diagnosis of Wilson's disease. Clin Sci. 1995;88:727–32.

18. Bull PC, Thomas GR, Rommens JM, Forbes JR, Cox DW. The Wilson disease gene is a putative copper transporting P-type ATPase similar to the Menkes gene Nat Genet. 1993;5: 327–37.

19. Tanzi RE, Petrukhin KE, Chernov I et al. The Wilson disease gene is a copper transporting ATPase with homology to the Menkes disease gene. Nat Genet. 1993;5:344–50.

20. Hsi G, Cox DW. A comparison of the mutation spectra of Menkes disease and Wilson disease. Hum Genet. 2004;114:165–72.

21. Moller LB, Ott P, Lund C, Horn N. Homozygosity for a gross partial gene deletion of the C-terminal end of ATP7B in a Wilson patient with hepatic and no neurological manifestations. Am J Med Genet A. 2005;138:340–3.

22. Thomas GR, Forbes JR, Roberts EA, Walshe JM, Cox DW. The Wilson disease gene: spectrum of mutations and their consequences [published erratum appears in Nat Genet 1995;9:451]. Nat Genet. 1995;9:210–17.

23. Panagiotakaki E, Tzetis M, Manolaki N et al. Genotype-phenotype correlations for a wide spectrum of mutations in the Wilson disease gene (ATP7B). Am J Med Genet. 2004;131A: 168–73.

24. Loudianos G, Lovicu M, Dessi V et al. Abnormal mRNA splicing resulting from consensus sequence splicing mutations of ATP7B. Hum Mutat. 2002;20:260–6.

25. Proud VK, Mussell HG, Kaler SG, Young DW, Percy AK. Distinctive Menkes disease variant with occipital horns: delineation of natural history and clinical phenotype. Am J Med Genet. 1996;65:44–51.

26. Kaler SG, Gallo LK, Proud VK et al. Occipital horn syndrome and a mild Menkes phenotype associated with splice site mutations at the MNK locus. Nat Genet. 1994;8: 195–202.

27. Caca K, Ferenci P, Kuhn HJ et al. High prevalence of the H1069Q mutation in East German patients with Wilson disease: rapid detection of mutations by limited sequencing and phenotype-genotype analysis. J Hepatol. 2001;35:575–81.

28. Loudianos G, Dessi V, Lovicu M et al. Molecular characterization of Wilson disease in the Sardinian population – evidence of a founder effect. Hum Mutat. 1999;14:294–303.

29. Cullen LM, Prat L, Cox DW. Genetic variation in the promoter and 5′ UTR of the copper transporter, ATP7B, in patients with Wilson disease. Clin Genet. 2003;64:429–32.

30. Huster D, Weizenegger M, Kress S, Mossner J, Caca K. Rapid detection of mutations in Wilson disease gene ATP7B by DNA strip technology. Clin Chem Lab Med. 2004;42:507–10.

31. Lovicu M, Dessi V, Zappu A, De Virgiliis S, Cao A, Loudianos G. Efficient strategy for molecular diagnosis of Wilson disease in the sardinian population. Clin Chem. 2003;49: 496–8.

32. Petris MJ, Voskoboinik I, Cater M et al. Copper-regulated trafficking of the Menkes disease copper ATPase is associated with formation of a phosphorylated catalytic intermediate. J Biol Chem. 2002;277:46736–42.
33. Schaefer M, Hopkins RG, Failla ML, Gitlin JD. Hepatocyte-specific localization and copper-dependent trafficking of the Wilson's disease protein in the liver. Am J Physiol. 1999;276:G639–46.
34. Roelofsen H, Wolters H, Van Luyn MJA, Miura N, Kuipers F, Vonk RJ. Copper-induced apical trafficking of ATP7B in polarized hepatoma cells provides a mechanism for biliary copper excretion. Gastroenterology. 2000;119:782–93.
35. Payne AS, Kelly EJ, Gitlin JD. Functional expression of the Wilson disease protein reveals mislocalization and impaired copper-dependent trafficking of the common H1069Q mutation. Proc Natl Acad Sci USA. 1998;95:10854–9.
36. Forbes JR, Cox DW. Copper-dependent trafficking of Wilson disease mutant ATP7B proteins. Hum Mol Genet. 2000;9:1927–35.
37. Payne AS, Gitlin JD. Functional expression of the menkes disease protein reveals common biochemical mechanisms among the copper-transporting p-type atpases. J Biol Chem. 1998;273:3765–70.
38. Forbes JR, Cox DW. Functional characterization of missense mutations in ATP7B: Wilson disease mutation or normal variant? Am J Hum Genet. 1998;63:1663–74.
39. Hsi G, Cullen LM, Moira Glerum D, Cox DW. Functional assessment of the carboxy-terminus of the Wilson disease copper-transporting ATPase, ATP7B. Genomics. 2004;83:473–81.
40. Cox DW, Prat L, Walshe JM, Heathcote J, Gaffney D. Twenty-four novel mutations in Wilson disease patients of predominantly European ancestry. Hum Mutat. 2005;26:280–5.
41. Fatemi N, Sarkar B. Structural and functional insights of Wilson disease copper-transporting ATPase. J Bioenerg Biomembr. 2002;34:339–49.
42. Morgan CT, Tsivkovskii R, Kosinsky YA, Efremov RG, Lutsenko S. The distinct functional properties of the nucleotide-binding domain of ATP7B, the human copper-transporting ATPase: analysis of the Wilson disease mutations E1064A, H1069Q, R1151H, and C1104F. J Biol Chem. 2004;279:36363–71.
43. Gaffney D, Walker JL, O'Donnell JG et al. DNA-based presymptomatic diagnosis of Wilson disease. J Inher Metab Dis. 1992;15:161–70.
44. Yuzbasiyan-Gurkan V, Blanton SH, Cao Y et al. Linkage of a microsatellite marker to the canine copper toxicosis locus in Bedlington terriers. Am J Vet Res. 1997;58:23–7.
45. van de Sluis B, Rothuizen J, Pearson PL, Van Oost BA, Wijmenga C. Identification of a new copper metabolism gene by positional cloning in a purebred dog population. Hum Mol Genet. 2002;11:165–73.
46. Coronado VA, Damaraju D, Kohijoki R, Cox DW. New haplotypes in the Bedlington terrier indicate complexity in copper toxicosis. Mamm Genome. 2003;14:483–91.
47. Tao TY, Liu F, Klomp L, Wijmenga C, Gitlin JD. The copper toxicosis gene product Murr1 directly interacts with the Wilson disease protein. J Biol Chem. 2003;278:41593–6.
48. Biasio W, Chang T, McIntosh CJ, McDonald FJ. Identification of Murr1 as a regulator of the human delta epithelial sodium channel. J Biol Chem. 2004;279:5429–34.
49. Burstein E, Ganesh L, Dick RD et al. A novel role for XIAP in copper homeostasis through regulation of MURR1. EMBO J. 2004;23:244–54.
50. Ganesh L, Burstein E, Guha-Niyogi A et al. The gene product Murr1 restricts HIV-1 replication in resting CD4$^+$ lymphocytes. Nature. 2003;426:853–7.
51. Muller T, van de Sluis B, Zhernakova A et al. The canine copper toxicosis gene MURR1 does not cause non-Wilsonian hepatic copper toxicosis. J Hepatol. 2003;38:164–8.
52. Coronado VA, Bonneville JA, Nazer H, Roberts EA, Cox DW. COMMD1 (MURR1) as a candidate in patients with copper storage disease of undefined etiology. Clin Genet. 2005;68:548–51.
53. Stuehler B, Reichert J, Stremmel W, Schaefer M. Analysis of the human homologue of the canine copper toxicosis gene MURR1 in Wilson disease patients. J Mol Med. 2004;82:629–34.
54. Walshe JM. The story of penicillamine: a difficult birth. Mov Disord. 2003;18:853–9.
55. Walshe JM. Treatment of Wilson's disease with trientine (triethylenetetramine) dihydro-chloride. Lancet. 1982;1:643–7.

56. Hoogenraad TU, Van Haltum J, Van der Hamer CJA. Management of Wilson's disease with zinc sulphate. J Neurol Sci. 1987;77:137–46.

57. Brewer GJ, Hill GM, Prasad AS, Cossack ZT, Rabbani P. Oral zinc therapy for Wilson's disease. Am Intern Med. 1983;99:314–19.

58. Brewer GJ, Dick RD, Johnson VD, Brunberg JA, Kluin KJ, Fink JK. Treatment of Wilson's disease with zinc: XV long-term follow-up studies. J Lab Clin Med. 1998;132: 264–78.

59. Askari FK, Greenson J, Dick RD, Johnson VD, Brewer GJ. Treatment of Wilson's disease with zinc. XVIII. Initial treatment of the hepatic decompensation presentation with trientine and zinc. J Lab Clin Med. 2003;142:385–90.

60. von Herbay A, de Groot H, Hegi U, Stremmel W, Strohmeyer G, Sies H. Low vitamin E content in plasma of patients with alcoholic liver disease, hemochromatosis and Wilson's disease. J Hepatol. 1994;20:41–6.

61. Ogihara H, Ogihara T, Miki M, Yasuda H, Mino M. Plasma copper and antioxidant status in Wilson's disease. Pediatr Res. 1995;37:219–26.

62. Garcia-Villarreal L, Daniels S, Shaw SH et al. High prevalence of the very rare wilson disease gene mutation Leu708Pro in the island of Gran Canaria (Canary islands, spain): a genetic and clinical study. Hepatology. 2000;32:1329–36.

Section Liver III
Viral hepatitis

Chair: W.O. BÖCHER and G. GERKEN

20
Immune pathogenesis of hepatitis B and C

R. THIMME, C. NEUMANN-HAEFELIN, T. BOETTLER,
H.-C. SPANGENBERG and H. E. BLUM

INTRODUCTION

More than 500 million people are persistently infected with the hepatitis B virus (HBV) or hepatitis C virus (HCV) and are at risk of developing chronic liver disease, cirrhosis and hepatocellular carcinoma. The host immune response has a unique role in viral hepatitis because it contributes not only to viral control, clinical recovery and protective immunity but also to chronic hepatitis and liver cirrhosis. Although the determinants of HBV and HCV clearance and persistence have only been poorly defined, it is widely accepted that cellular immune responses play an important role in viral clearance and disease pathogenesis of both viral infections. Indeed, spontaneous elimination of HBV and HCV during acute infection is associated with multispecific and strong virus-specific CD4$^+$ and CD8$^+$ T cell responses that accumulate in the infected liver. The central role for T cell responses in HBV and HCV clearance has recently been directly demonstrated in the chimpanzee model. The mechanisms that lead to the failure of the virus-specific T cell response and thus to viral persistence are only poorly defined. Various mechanisms of virus-specific T cell failure, such as primary T cell failure, T cell exhaustion and emergence of viral escape mutations, have been suggested. A detailed and better understanding of the immunological mechanisms of the virus–host interactions will be central for the development of a vaccine against HCV infection and immunotherapies that eliminate persistent HBV and/or HCV infection.

HEPATITIS B VIRUS

Hepatitis B virus (HBV), the prototype member of the Hepadnaviridae family, is a non-cytopathic, hepatotropic virus. The prevalence of HBV infection varies in different geographical regions of the world, ranging from 0.1% in the

Western world up to 15% in Asian and African countries. HBV is parenterally transmitted via blood or blood products or by sexual or perinatal exposure. HBV infection occurs in regions with high prevalence mostly in early childhood via horizontal transmission, but also in rare cases by vertical transmission. Persistence of HBV infection is much greater in infants (90%) than in adults $(<5\%)$[1].

Immune response to HBV

Viral clearance and disease pathogenesis of HBV infection are largely mediated by the immune response that is composed of the innate and adaptive immune response[2]. Of note, microarray analysis of serial liver biopsies of experimentally infected chimpanzees revealed that HBV does not induce any detectable changes in the expression of intrahepatic genes in the first weeks of infection[3]. These results indicate that HBV may evade the innate immune response by just not inducing it. In contrast, the adaptive immune response is clearly induced by HBV. Indeed, it is generally accepted that the virus-specific CD8+ T cell response plays a major role in the outcome of HBV infection. Several studies have shown that the peripheral blood cytotoxic T lymphocyte (CTL) response to HBV is polyclonal and multispecific in patients with acute viral hepatitis[4,5] and persists indefinitely after recovery, when it is maintained by continued antigenic stimulation by residual virus that persists, apparently harmlessly, in healthy convalescent individuals[6]. In contrast, the CTL response to HBV is relatively weak in patients with chronic HBV infection, except during spontaneous disease flares or interferon (IFN)-induced recovery, when it is readily detectable[6]. These observations suggest an important role of the virus-specific T cell response in viral clearance. A causal role for CD8+ T cell responses in HBV clearance and disease pathogenesis has only recently been proven in the chimpanzee model. Indeed, by performing depletion studies of CD4+ and CD8+ cells in acutely infected chimpanzees, it was shown that CD8-depletion greatly prolonged the infection and delayed the onset of viral clearance and liver disease until CD8+ T cells reappeared in the circulation and virus-specific CD8+ T cells entered the liver[7]. In the absence of CD8+ cells the duration of peak infection was prolonged and the time of onset of the initial decrease in HBV DNA levels and increase in serum ALT activity was delayed. The reappearance of CD8+ cells correlated with the appearance of interferon gamma (IFN-γ) producing virus-specific CD8+ T cells in the liver, the onset of a mild liver disease, the appearance of IFN-γ mRNA in the liver and a 50-fold reduction in total liver HBV DNA. These results suggest that HBV replication is inhibited early non-cytopathically in a CD8-dependent and probably IFN-γ-associated manner. The final elimination of the virus occurred several months later and was associated with a rebound of CD8+ T cells to baseline levels, a surge of the intrahepatic CD8+ T cell response, a surge in intrahepatic IFN-γ mRNA and a surge in sALT activity[7]. Thus, these results have clearly demonstrated that intrahepatic HBV-specific CD8+ T cells are required for rapid viral clearance during acute HBV infection and they have suggested the existence of dual antiviral functions that overlap temporally during natural infection but can be clearly separated by CD8 depletion: a primarily non-

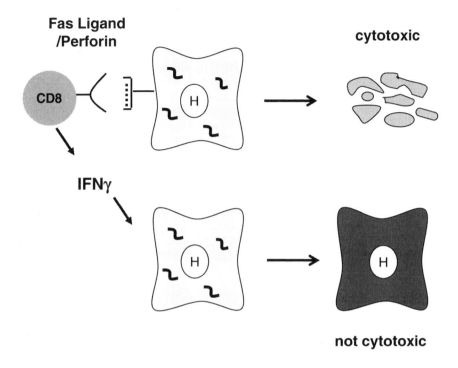

Figure 1 Virus-specific CD8[+] T cells perform two different antiviral effector functions during viral hepatitis. They either kill the infected cell (cytotoxic) or they secrete cytokines that clear the virus without killing the cell (non-cytotoxic)

cytolytic CD8[+]-dependent mechanism that may be mediated by IFN-γ and a primarily cytolytic mechanism that clears the remaining infected cells (Figure 1).

Importantly, the non-cytolytic effect of CD8[+] T cells has first been described in the HBV transgenic mouse. Indeed, several studies in this model have shown that, in addition to causing viral hepatitis, virus-specific T cells as well as NK and NKT cells can abolish HBV expression and replication without killing the hepatocytes, and that this antiviral activity is mediated by IFN-γ and tumour necrosis factor alpha (TNF-α)[2].

Thus, the combined results from the transgenic mouse model, the chimpanzee model and acutely infected patients point to an important role of the immune response, especially the cellular immune response, in successful control of HBV.

Mechanisms of viral persistence during HBV infection

Several mechanisms contribute to viral persistence during HBV infection. Chronic HBV infection is characterized by absent, weak, narrowly focused or dysfunctional T cell responses. T cell deletion, anergy, exhaustion or ignorance have all been reported to occur in HBV infection and to contribute to HBV-specific T cell failure[6]. Of note, HBV establishes chronic hepatitis mainly by vertical transmission from HBsAg and HBeAg-positive mothers to neonates. Immunomodulatory roles of HBV proteins, such as HBeAg, might play a role in this setting. For example, it has been shown that the HBeAg suppresses the T cell response in transgenic mice[8]. Another possible mechanism of T cell failure is the development of viral escape mutations. HBV variants with mutations in dominant T cell epitopes have been demonstrated to arise during acute HBV infection[9]. However, they do not often develop, do not necessarily affect clinical recovery and are even uncommon in chronic HBV infection consistent with the weak T cell response[6]. Thus, viral escape is clearly not a universal mechanism of viral persistence in HBV infection. Clearly, additional studies are needed to better define the pathways to viral persistence in HBV infection.

HEPATITIS C VIRUS

HCV is a small enveloped, single-stranded RNA virus that belongs to the family of flaviviruses. The HCV genome is approximately 9600 nucleotides long and contains a single ORF that encodes a large viral polypeptide precursor of 3010–3033 amino acids. The cleavage of the protein by viral and cellular proteases results in the structural and non-structural viral proteins. Viral replication is very rapid and it is estimated that 10^{10}–10^{12} virions are produced per day. The lack of a proofreading function of the viral polymerase in part accounts for the fact that the HCV RNA genome mutates frequently. As a result, HCV circulates as a population of quasispecies with individual viral genomes differing by 1–5% in nucleotide sequence, presenting a major challenge to the immune-mediated control of HCV infection. HCV is transmitted by percutaneous (e.g. blood transfusion, needle-stick inoculation) or non-percutaneous (e.g. sexual contact or perinatal) exposure to infectious blood or blood-derived body fluids[10].

Immune response to HCV

In contrast to HBV, HCV leads to the rapid induction of the innate immune response after infection. Indeed, microarray analysis of liver biopsies from infected chimpanzees revealed transcriptional changes in type I IFN-response genes within 1 week of infection[11–13]. Of note, these rapid type I IFN-responses do not correlate with the outcome of infection, suggesting that HCV might not be very sensitive to the antiviral effects of this cytokine.

Virus-specific T cell responses are usually detectable within 5–12 weeks after infection. Importantly, very similar to HBV infection, there is strong evidence for an important role of both virus-specific CD4+ and CD8+ T cells in viral control as well as liver injury[14,15]. Several studies of acutely HCV-infected patients revealed that a strong, multispecific, broad and sustained HCV-specific CD4$^+$ T cell response is associated with a self-limited course of infection[16-20]. The virus-specific CD8$^+$ T cell response in acute resolving HCV infection is also vigorous and multispecific, targeting up to eight to twelve epitopes[21,22]. In the acute phase of infection, virus-specific CD8$^+$ T cells were demonstrated that do not produce IFN-γ, a property also referred to as stunned[22,23]. In a later phase, CD8$^+$ T cells recover their ability to produce IFN-γ, coinciding with a significant drop in viraemia and resolution of liver disease. This implies that virus-specific CD8$^+$ T cells might contribute to viral clearance by cytolytic as well as non-cytolytic mechanisms, as described in HBV infection, and that both mechanisms overlap in the course of acute infection (Figure 1). The important role of IFN-γ in viral clearance is further supported by the finding that IFN-γ inhibits the replication of HCV in the replicon model[24]. In addition, genomic analysis of acutely infected chimpanzees revealed that transient or sustained viral clearance was associated with the up-regulation of IFN-γ-induced genes in the liver[11,12].

Studies in experimentally HCV-infected chimpanzees showed that virus-specific CD4$^+$ and CD8$^+$ T cells accumulate in the liver about 8–14 weeks after infection, and that this coincides with viral clearance and liver disease[13,25]. The relative contribution of CD4$^+$ and CD8$^+$ T cell responses to viral clearance in acutely HCV-infected patients has not been fully defined. However, depletion studies in chimpanzees have demonstrated a crucial role for both, CD4$^+$ and CD8$^+$ T cells, in mediating protective immunity[26,27].

Importantly, even after HCV clearance, virus-specific CD4$^+$ and CD8$^+$ T cell responses remain detectable[15]. In a cohort of women accidentally exposed to the same HCV strain, HCV-specific CD4$^+$ and CD8$^+$ T cells were still detectable two decades after recovery, whereas circulating HCV-specific antibodies were undetectable in several of these patients[28].

VIRAL EVASION STRATEGIES

Being a persistently infecting virus, HCV was forced to evolve sophisticated escape strategies for both the innate and the adaptive immune system. These countermeasures appear to be quite efficient, since 85% of HCV-infected patients develop a chronic infection. For example, HCV is astonishingly efficient in disturbing the IFN response at multiple levels[6].

The mechanisms responsible for the evasion of HCV from the adaptive immune response are still only partially understood. Various mechanisms of virus-specific T cell failure leading to HCV persistence have been suggested (Table 1), but so far most of them are poorly defined[14,15]. Several studies have shown that HCV-infected patients who develop chronic infection typically have only weak, oligo- /mono-specific or no virus-specific CD4$^+$ and CD8$^+$ T cell responses in the acute and chronic phase of infection[14,15,29]. In addition, the direct loss (exhaustion) of HCV-specific CD4$^+$ T and CD8$^+$ cell responses in acute hepatitis has been demonstrated in acutely infected patients that transiently controlled the virus but subsequently progressed to viral persistence[17,30]. The mechanisms responsible for primary T cell failure or T cell exhaustion are unclear, although it has been suggested that antigen presentation by dendritic cells (DC) and macrophages might be impaired in HCV infection[31–33]. This may result in ineffective priming of T cells or impaired maintenance of antigen-experienced T cells. However, other studies have not been able to confirm the dysfunctions of the antigen-presenting cells[34]. Another explanation for T cell exhaustion might be the deletion of virus-specific T cells in the presence of continuous high viral load or the rapid induction of activation-induced cell death, e.g. in the liver[35]. In this context it is interesting to note that, in some chronically infected chimpanzees, virus-specific T cells were detectable in the blood but not in the liver[13], supporting the concept of rapid loss of HCV-specific T cells from the liver. However, it is also possible that a failure of T cells to home to the infected organ is responsible for this observation.

As in HBV infection, mutational escape from the adaptive immune response has been suggested as one of the major viral evasion strategies. Infection outcome in humans was predicted by sequence changes in the hypervariable region of the E2 envelope glycoprotein, a major target of the antibody response, that occurred at the time of antibody seroconversion[36]. Thus, these sequence changes have been suggested to represent escape mutations within possible B cell epitopes. Viral amino acid substitutions that inhibit $CD4^+$ and $CD8^+$ T cell recognition have initially been observed in chronically HCV-infected patients[37] and chimpanzees[38]. Interestingly, escape mutations detected in chronically infected patients did not diversify further during several years of follow-up[37]. Consequently, it was suggested that T cell escape occurs early during infection. This hypothesis has been subsequently confirmed by an analysis of the early T cell–virus interactions in acutely infected chimpanzees[39] and humans[40–43]. Population-based approaches have provided support for T cell-driven HCV evolution[43,44]. Interestingly, variant-specific virus-specific T cell responses are usually undetectable in these patients. The failure to generate variant-specific $CD8^+$ T cell responses can be explained by the lack of sufficient $CD4^+$ T cell help or a variant epitope-mediated expansion of wild-type-specific $CD8^+$ T cells, a phenomenon known as original antigenic sin[45]. It should be noted, however, that the importance of viral escape mutations for the development of HCV persistence is still not completely understood. Indeed, viral escape occurs typically in the presence of a CTL response that is focused on a single viral epitope. This type of T cell response is unusual, however, during acute HCV infection. Accordingly, the loss of a single epitope would probably not be sufficient for the survival of viral escape mutants. In addition, most studies have clearly shown that the development of viral escape mutations is not universal. For example, viral clearance can occur with minimal epitope variation prior to resolution, and studies in chronically HCV-infected chimpanzees and humans have shown that not all epitopes restricted by class I alleles undergo variations to produce escape mutations[37,39]. The virological (e. g. viral fitness cost) and immunological (e.g. genetically restricted T cell repertoire or TCR diversity) factors that determine the occurrence of escape mutations in HCV infection are currently not well defined[40,46,47]. It is also still not clear whether escape may be the result rather than the cause of viral persistence. Additional studies are needed to resolve this interesting question.

Another important possible mechanism of immune evasion is functional anergy of virus-specific T cells. Several studies using the tetramer technique have shown that dysfunction of CD8[+] T cells occurs in acute as well as chronic HCV infection[23,30,48,49]. Indeed, HCV-specific CD8[+] T cells may be impaired in their proliferative capacity, cytotoxicity, and ability to secrete TNF-α and IFN-γ upon stimulation, referred to as stunned phenotype. Interestingly, T cell dysfunction was observed in the early phase of acute HCV infection in all patients irrespective of virological outcome. In patients with a self-limited course of infection, however, the recovery of CD8[+] T cell function was temporally associated with a sharp decline of viraemia and resolution of disease[23,30]. In contrast, CD8[+] T cell function remained suppressed in patients who progressed to chronic infection[50]. Interestingly, the impaired effector functions of HCV specific CD8[+] T cells are also associated with an immature differentiation phenotype of these HCV-specific CD8[+] T cells[51]. Of note, HCV-specific CD8[+] T cells are also impaired in their antiviral effector functions in the infected organ, the liver. A recent study showed that intrahepatic HCV, but not Flu-specific CD8[+] T cells are impaired in their ability to secrete IFN-γ despite the accumulation of these cells in the liver[52]. It is tempting to speculate that the different mechanisms of CD8[+] T cell failure are a direct result of weak and dysfunctional virus-specific CD4[+] T cell help that is common in persistent HCV infection[53–55]. The important role of CD4[+] T cells is further strengthened by a recent CD4[+] T cell depletion study in the chimpanzee model where incomplete control of HCV replication by memory CD8[+] T cell responses in the absence of CD4[+] T cells was associated with the emergence of viral escape mutations in class I epitopes and a failure to resolve the infection[26]. Growing evidence also suggests an important role of regulatory CD4[+]CD25[+] T cells in the suppression of HCV-specific CD8[+] T cells. These cells have been found to be enriched in chronically HCV-infected patients when compared with recovered or uninfected subjects, and in-vitro depletion studies and co-culture experiments revealed that peptide specific IFN-γ production as well as proliferation of HCV-specific CD8[+] T cells were inhibited by CD4[+]CD25[+] T cells in a dose-dependent manner and by direct cell–cell contact[56–59]. In addition, intrahepatic IL-10-producing regulatory CD8[+] T cells have also been recently described[60]. Although these results point to an important role of regulatory T cells in HCV persistence, several important questions, such as antigen specificity and liver compartmentalization of regulatory T cells, still need to be addressed.

In sum, several different mechanisms seem to contribute to the failure of the adaptive immune response with mutational escape and functional anergy probably playing the most important role (Figure 2). As shown in Figure 2, a lack of CD4[+] T cell help and/or the action of regulatory T cells contribute to the failure of the virus-specific CD8[+] T cells. Clearly, a better understanding of the evasion strategies determining the outcome of HCV infection is required for the development of effective vaccines.

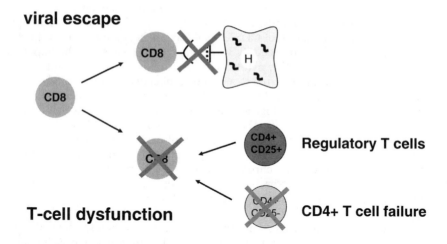

Figure 2 Mechanisms of T cell failure. Viral escape and T cell dysfunctions contribute to the failure of the virus-specific T cell response. T cell dysfunction may be caused by a lack of CD4$^+$ T cell help or the action of regulatory T cells

SUMMARY

In sum, much new important information has been forthcoming concerning the role of the immune response in HBV and HCV infection. HBV seems to be relatively invisible to the innate immune system and spreads until the onset of the adaptive immune response. Of note, depletion studies in acutely infected chimpanzees have clearly demonstrated that virus-specific CD8$^+$ T cells cause viral clearance as well as disease pathogenesis. HBV-specific CD8$^+$ cells perform two antiviral functions that overlap temporally: an early primarily non-cytolytic mechanism that may be mediated by IFN-γ and a primarily cytolytic mechanism that clears the remaining infected cells (Figure 1). In contrast, CD4$^+$ cells probably do not function as effector cells in the control of HBV since depletion of CD4$^+$ cells had little or no effect on the duration of the infection. However, since CD4$^+$ cells may play an early immunoregulatory role, it is impossible to make a final statement about the role of CD4$^+$ cells in the outcome of HBV infection. Clearly, additional studies are required to define the role of CD4$^+$ T cells in HBV infection. The mechanisms that lead to HBV persistence are only poorly understood and include the development of viral escape mutation, T cell anergy and tolerance induction.

In contrast to HBV, HCV strongly induces the innate immune response since significant levels of type I IFN induction are detectable in the liver as early as 1 week after infection. However, HCV is able to evade the antiviral effects of IFN and to persist in most infected subjects. Like HBV, HCV can be sufficiently controlled by virus-specific T cells. The presence of an intrahepatic HCV-specific T cell response is clearly associated with the control of acute HCV infection. Most likely HCV is also controlled by non-cytolytic effector mechanisms, such as IFN-γ. Of note, viral clearance can occur in the absence of liver disease but in the presence of IFN-γ in the liver, suggesting that IFN-γ might perform direct antiviral effector functions during acute HCV infection, similar to its ability to control HBV replication. These cytokines are probably secreted by virus-specific T cells that accumulate in the liver.

Studies in acutely infected humans and chimpanzees also revealed that different mechanisms contribute to the development of viral persistence, such as the development of viral escape mutations, the failure of T cells to accumulate in the liver or T cell dysfunction and deletion. However, much more work is needed before the mechanisms responsible for viral clearance and persistence are fully understood. That knowledge is essential for the rational development of effective immunotherapy for chronic HBV and HCV infection.

Acknowledgements

The work described in this chapter was supported by grants from the Deutsche Forschungsgemeinschaft (Th719 2-1, 2-2 and 2-3 (Emmy Noether Programm) and SFB 620, C6)), HepNet, and the Wilhelm Sander Foundation.

References

1. Ganem D, AM Prince. Hepatitis B virus infection – natural history and clinical consequences. N Engl J Med. 2004;350:1118–29.
2. Guidotti LG, Chisari FV. Noncytolytic control of viral infections by the innate and adaptive immune response. Annu Rev Immunol. 2001;19:65–91.
3. Wieland S, Thimme R, Purcell RH, Chisari FV. Genomic analysis of the host response to hepatitis B virus infection. Proc Natl Acad Sci USA. 2004;20:20.
4. Maini MK, Boni C, Ogg GS et al. Direct *ex vivo* analysis of hepatitis B virus-specific CD8 (+) T cells associated with the control of infection. Gastroenterology. 1999;117:1386–96.
5. Webster GJ, Reignat S, Maini MK et al. Incubation phase of acute hepatitis B in man: dynamic of cellular immune mechanisms. Hepatology. 2000;32:1117–24.
6. Rehermann B, Nascimbeni M. Immunology of hepatitis B virus and hepatitis C virus infection. Nat Rev Immunol. 2005;5:215–29.
7. Thimme R, Wieland S, Steiger C et al. CD8(+) T cells mediate viral clearance and disease pathogenesis during acute hepatitis B virus infection. J Virol. 2003;77:68–76.
8. Chen MT, Billaud JN, Sallberg M et al. A function of the hepatitis B virus precore protein is to regulate the immune response to the core antigen. Proc Natl Acad Sci USA. 2004;101: 14913–18.
9. Bertoletti A, Sette A, Chisari FV et al. Natural variants of cytotoxic epitopes are T-cell receptor antagonists for antiviral cytotoxic T cells. Nature. 1994;369:407–10.
10. Lauer GM, Walker BD. Hepatitis C virus infection. N Engl J Med. 2001;345:41–52.
11. Bigger CB, Brasky KM, Lanford RE. DNA microarray analysis of chimpanzee liver during acute resolving hepatitis C virus infection. J Virol. 2001;75:7059–66.
12. Su AI, Pezacki JP, Wodicka L et al. Genomic analysis of the host response to hepatitis C virus infection. Proc Natl Acad Sci USA. 2002;99:15669–74. Epub: 2002 Nov 19.
13. Thimme R, Bukh J, Spangenberg HC et al. Viral and immunological determinants of hepatitis C virus clearance, persistence, and disease. Proc Natl Acad Sci USA. 2002;99: 15661–8.
14. Bowen DG, Walker CM. Adaptive immune responses in acute and chronic hepatitis C virus infection. Nature. 2005;436:946–52.
15. Neumann-Haefelin C, Blum HE, Chisari FV, Thimme R. T cell response in hepatitis C virus infection. J Clin Virol. 2005;32:75–85.

16. Diepolder HM, Zachoval R, Hoffmann RM et al. Possible mechanism involving T-lymphocyte response to non-structural protein 3 in viral clearance in acute hepatitis C virus infection. Lancet. 1995;346:1006–7.

17. Gerlach JT, Diepolder HM, Jung MC et al. Recurrence of hepatitis C virus after loss of virus-specific CD4(+) T-cell response in acute hepatitis C. Gastroenterology. 1999;117:933–41.

18. Gerlach JT, Ulsenheimer A, Gruner NH et al. Minimal T-cell-stimulatory sequences and spectrum of HLA restriction of immunodominant CD4$^+$ T-cell epitopes within hepatitis C virus NS3 and NS4 proteins. J Virol. 2005;79:12425–33.

19. Missale G, Bertoni R, Lamonaca V et al. Different clinical behaviors of acute hepatitis C virus infection are associated with different vigor of the anti-viral cell-mediated immune response. J Clin Invest. 1996;98:706–14.

20. Schulze Zur Wiesch J, Lauer GM, Day CL et al. Broad repertoire of the CD4$^+$ Th cell response in spontaneously controlled hepatitis C virus infection includes dominant and highly promiscuous epitopes. J Immunol. 2005;175:3603–13.

21. Gruner NH, Gerlach TJ, Jung MC et al. Association of hepatitis C virus-specific CD8$^+$ T cells with viral clearance in acute hepatitis C. J Infect Dis. 2000;181:1528–36.

22. Lechner F, Wong DK, Dunbar PR et al. Analysis of successful immune responses in persons infected with hepatitis C virus. J Exp Med. 2000;191:1499–512.

23. Thimme R, Oldach D, Chang KM, Steiger C, Ray SC, Chisari FV. Determinants of viral clearance and persistence during acute hepatitis C virus infection. J Exp Med. 2001;194:1395–406.

24. Frese M, Schwarzle V, Barth K et al. Interferon-gamma inhibits replication of subgenomic and genomic hepatitis C virus RNAs. Hepatology. 2002;35:694–703.

25. Cooper S, Erickson AL, Adams EJ et al. Analysis of a successful immune response against hepatitis C virus. Immunity. 1999;10:439–49.

26. Grakoui A, Shoukry NH, Woollard DJ et al. HCV persistence and immune evasion in the absence of memory T cell help. Science. 2003;302:659–62.

27. Shoukry NH, Grakoui A, Houghton M et al. Memory CD8$^+$ T cells are required for protection from persistent hepatitis C virus infection. J Exp Med. 2003;197:1645–55.

28. Takaki A, Wiese M, Maertens G et al. Cellular immune responses persist and humoral responses decrease two decades after recovery from a single-source outbreak of hepatitis C. Nat Med. 2000;6:578–82.

29. Lauer GM, Barnes E, Lucas M et al. High resolution analysis of cellular immune responses in resolved and persistent hepatitis C virus infection. Gastroenterology. 2004;127:924–36.

30. Lechner F, Gruener NH, Urbani S et al. CD8$^+$ T lymphocyte responses are induced during acute hepatitis C virus infection but are not sustained. Eur J Immunol. 2000;30:2479–87.

31. Bain C, Fatmi A, Zoulim F, Zarski JP, Trepo C, Inchauspe G. Impaired allostimulatory function of dendritic cells in chronic hepatitis C infection. Gastroenterology. 2001;120:512–24.

32. Lee CH, Choi YH, Yang SH, Lee CW, Ha SJ, Sung YC. Hepatitis C virus core protein inhibits interleukin 12 and nitric oxide production from activated macrophages. Virology. 2001;279:271–9.

33. Sarobe P, Lasarte JJ, Casares N et al. Abnormal priming of CD4(+) T cells by dendritic cells expressing hepatitis C virus core and E1 proteins. J Virol. 2002;76:5062–70.

34. Longman RS, Talal AH, Jacobson IM, Albert ML, Rice CM. Presence of functional dendritic cells in patients chronically infected with hepatitis C virus. Blood. 2004;103:1026–9. Epub: 2003 Oct 2.

35. Nuti S, Rosa D, Valiante NM et al. Dynamics of intra-hepatic lymphocytes in chronic hepatitis C: enrichment for Valpha24$^+$ T cells and rapid elimination of effector cells by apoptosis. Eur J Immunol. 1998;28:3448–55.

36. Farci P, Shimoda A, Coiana A et al. The outcome of acute hepatitis C predicted by the evolution of the viral quasispecies. Science. 2000;288:339–44.

37. Chang KM, Rehermann B, McHutchison JG et al. Immunological significance of cytotoxic T lymphocyte epitope variants in patients chronically infected by the hepatitis C virus. J Clin Invest. 1997;100:2376–85.

38. Weiner A, Erickson AL, Kansopon J et al. Persistent hepatitis C virus infection in a chimpanzee is associated with emergence of a cytotoxic T lymphocyte escape variant. Proc Natl Acad Sci USA. 1995;92:2755–9.

39. Erickson AL, Kimura Y, Igarashi S et al. The outcome of hepatitis C virus infection is predicted by escape mutaions in epitopes targeted by cytotoxic T lymphocytes. Immunity. 2001;15:885–95.

40. Bowen DG, Walker CM. Mutational escape from CD8$^+$ T cell immunity: HCV evolution, from chimpanzees to man. J Exp Med. 2005;201:1709–14.

41. Cox AL, Mosbruger T, Mao Q et al. Cellular immune selection with hepatitis C virus persistence in humans. J Exp Med. 2005;201:1741–52.

42. Tester I, Smyk-Pearson S, Wang P et al. Immune evasion versus recovery after acute hepatitis C virus infection from a shared source. J Exp Med. 2005;201:1725–31.

43. Timm J, Lauer GM, Kavanagh DG et al. CD8 epitope escape and reversion in acute HCV infection. J Exp Med. 2004;200:1593–604.

44. Ray SC, Fanning L, Wang XH, Netski DM, Kenny-Walsh E, Thomas DL. Divergent and convergent evolution after a common-source outbreak of hepatitis C virus. J Exp Med. 2005;201:1753–9.

45. Klenerman P, Zinkernagel RM. Original antigenic sin impairs cytotoxic T lymphocyte responses to viruses bearing variant epitopes. Nature. 1998;394:482–5.

46. McKiernan SM, Hagan R, Curry M et al. Distinct MHC class I and II alleles are associated with hepatitis C viral clearance, originating from a single source. Hepatology. 2004;40:108–14.

47. Meyer-Olson D, Shoukry NH, Brady KW et al. Limited T cell receptor diversity of HCV-specific T cell responses is associated with CTL escape. J Exp Med. 2004;200:307–19.

48. Gruener NH, Lechner F, Jung MC et al. Sustained dysfunction of antiviral cd8(+) t lymphocytes after infection with hepatitis c virus. J Virol. 2001;75:5550–8.

49. Wedemeyer H, He XS, Nascimbeni M et al. Impaired effector function of hepatitis C virus-specific CD8$^+$ T cells in chronic hepatitis C virus infection. J Immunol. 2002;169:3447–58.

50. Urbani S, Boni C, Missale G et al. Virus-specific CD8$^+$ lymphocytes share the same effector-memory phenotype but exhibit functional differences in acute hepatitis B and C. J Virol. 2002;76:12423–34.

51. Appay V, Dunbar PR, Callan M et al. Memory CD8$^+$ T cells vary in differentiation phenotype in different persistent virus infections. Nat Med. 2002;8:379–85.

52. Spangenberg HC, Viazov S, Kersting N et al. Intrahepatic CD8(+) T-cell failure during chronic hepatitis C virus infection. Hepatology. 2005;42:828–37.

53. Day CL, Seth NP, Lucas M et al. *Ex vivo* analysis of human memory CD4 T cells specific for hepatitis C virus using MHC class II tetramers. J Clin Invest. 2003;112:831–42.

54. Semmo N, Day CL, Ward SM et al. Preferential loss of IL-2-secreting CD4$^+$ T helper cells in chronic HCV infection. Hepatology. 2005;41:1019–28.

55. Ulsenheimer A, Gerlach JT, Gruener NH et al. Detection of functionally altered hepatitis C virus-specific CD4 T cells in acute and chronic hepatitis C. Hepatology. 2003;37:1189–98.

56. Boettler T, Spangenberg HC, Neumann-Haefelin C et al. T cells with a CD4$^+$CD25$^+$ regulatory phenotype suppress *in vitro* proliferation of virus-specific CD8$^+$ T cells during chronic hepatitis C virus infection. J Virol. 2005;79:7860–7.

57. Cabrera R, Tu Z, Xu Y et al. An immunomodulatory role for CD4(+)CD25(+) regulatory T lymphocytes in hepatitis C virus infection. Hepatology. 2004;40:1062–71.

58. Rushbrook SM, Ward SM, Unitt E et al. Regulatory T cells suppress *in vitro* proliferation of virus-specific CD8$^+$ T cells during persistent hepatitis C virus infection. J Virol. 2005;79:7852–9.

59. Sugimoto K, Ikeda F, Stadanlick J, Nunes FA, Alter HJ, Chang KM. Suppression of HCV-specific T cells without differential hierarchy demonstrated *ex vivo* in persistent HCV infection. Hepatology. 2003;38:1437–48.

60. Accapezzato D, Francavilla V, Paroli M et al. Hepatic expansion of a virus-specific regulatory CD8(+) T cell population in chronic hepatitis C virus infection. J Clin Invest. 2004;113:963–72.

21
Therapeutic vaccination strategies in chronic hepatitis B

M. LU and M. ROGGENDORF

INTRODUCTION

According to WHO estimates there were over 5.2 million cases of acute hepatitis B infection in 2000. More than 2 billion people have been infected worldwide and, of these, 360 million suffer from chronic hepatitis B virus (HBV) infection[1]. Thus, HBV is the most prevalent among the known hepatitis viruses causing chronic infections in humans worldwide, and represents a global public health problem. Chronic hepatitis B may progress to cirrhosis and death from liver failure and is the major cause of hepatocellular carcinoma (HCC) worldwide. HCC prevalence is known to vary widely among the world population, and those areas with higher prevalence of chronic HBV infections present the highest HCC rates. HBV causes 60–80% of the world's HCC, one of the three major causes of death in Africa and Asia.

The development of effective strategies to control chronic HBV infection is an area of considerable interest. Therapeutic interventions that boost specific T-cell responses and lower the viral load may not only prevent the progression of infection but also reduce the rate of transmission of HBV. Furthermore, the principles of effective therapeutic vaccination may apply not only to chronic viral infections but also to preventing development of HCC. Thus, it is important to evaluate how to elicit a successful immune response in chronically HBV-infected patients by therapeutic intervention. Several studies have examined the potential benefits of therapeutic vaccination in chronic hepatitis B. Some of reports have demonstrated enhanced immune responses following therapeutic vaccination.

THE CRUCIAL ROLE OF AN APPROPRIATE T-CELL RESPONSE TO HBV FOR THE CONTROL OF HBV INFECTION

Acute HBV infections follow a self-limited course in 95% of adult subjects, with complete virus elimination in these patients. The innate and adaptive immune responses cooperate and lead to the elimination of virus. Yet the role of the innate immune response for control of HBV infection has not been investigated in detail. The adaptive immune response, especially the function of cytotoxic T cells (CTL), has been shown to be crucial for the control of HBV infection. Thimme et al. demonstrated that the depletion of CD8-positive cells in an acutely HBV-infected chimpanzee led to prolonged virus persistence[2]. The suppression of HBV replication in this chimpanzee occurred with the recovery of CD8-positive cells. These results are consistent with the hypothesis that the low specific T-cell response to HBV in chronically infected patients has a causal relationship with persistent HBV infection. Additionally, it became evident that antiviral cytokines such as interferon gamma (IFN-γ) or tumour necrosis factor alpha (TNF-α) secreted by CTL can efficiently reduce viral replication in hepatocytes without killing. This direct antiviral potential of cytokines produced by CTL was first demonstrated in HBV transgenic mice[3]. In a recent study in acutely HBV-infected chimpanzees the non-cytolytic antiviral mechanism has been shown to contribute to HBV clearance[4]. The major part of HBV DNA disappeared from the liver of acutely infected chimpanzees, concomitantly with intrahepatic appearance of IFN-γ but before the onset of liver disease. Furthermore, the appearance of IFN-γ in the liver preceded the peak of T cell infiltration, suggesting that IFN-γ might be produced initially by cells other than CTL, perhaps by NK or NKT cells. It is proposed, based on these data, that the elimination of HBV from hepatocytes in hepatitis B occurs in two steps. First, the HBV replication is down-regulated by cytokines secreted from NK, NKT cells, and shortly after by specific CTL. The second step is the killing of infected hepatocytes by specific CTL, causing elevation of liver enzymes such as ALT. Consequently, the restoration of specific T-cell responses in chronically HBV-infected patients is considered as the key for a successful therapeutic vaccination approach.

CURRENT APPROACHES IN THERAPEUTIC VACCINATION IN PATIENTS WITH CHRONIC HEPATITIS B

The currently available therapy with interferon may lead to virus elimination, but is successful only for a minority of patients, and is associated with severe side-effects[5]. The interferon therapy against chronic HBV infection has not been improved during the recent years, in constrast to the rapid progress in the treatment of chronic hepatitis C virus infection. The introduction of pegylated IFN-α alone, or in combination with nucleoside analogues, did not significantly change the situation[6,7]. A series of new nucleoside analogues such as lamivudine, adefovir, and entacavier are effective in patients in terms of suppression of reverse transcription of the pregenomic RNA and blocking of the HBV replication cycle[8,9]. Treatment with nucleoside analogues may improve the clinical conditions of chronically HBV-infected patients, e.g. delaying the progress of liver cirrhosis, but does not lead to the complete elimination of HBV. However, resistant HBV mutants may emerge during long-term treatment. Thus, therapeutic vaccines against chronic HBV infection are of general interest, both in basic science and clinical use. Several studies have been performed in patients with chronic hepatitis B (Table 1).

Table 1 Clinical trials for therapeutic vaccination in patients with chronic hepatitis B

	Patients	Application	Response to vaccinations			References
			Reduction of viraemia	T-cell responses	Anti-HBs antibody	
Protein vaccine						
HBsAg/anti-HBs immune complex		i.m.	Yes		No	22
HBsAg[1]	32	5 × i.m.	Yes	Yes		15
HBsAg[1,2]	118	s.c.	Yes/No			12
Peptide vaccine: CTL epitope	19	3 × i.m.	No	Yes		27
HBsAg[3]	22			Yes		18
glyco gp26 and preS2	13	3 × p.o.	Yes	Yes		15
HBsAg/preS1/preS2	42	3 × i.m.	Yes	Yes		16
PreS2/S[1]	31	3 × i.m.	No			17
HBsAg[2]	43	3 × i.m.	No		No	14
DNA vaccine						
HBsAg	10	3–4 × i.m.	Yes	Yes		29
Combination nucleoside analogues and vaccine						
HBsAg	72	12 × i.d.	Yes			21

[1] presS2/S genHevac B (Pasteur Mérieux).

[2] S vaccine RecombiVax (Merck); s.c. = subcutaneous.

[3] presS1/preS2/Sag.

i.d. = intradermal; p.o. = per os; i.m., intramuscular; s.c., subcutaneous.

Pol et al. reported that specific vaccine therapy by a standard anti-HBV vaccination may reduce HBV replication in chronic carrier patients[10,11]. However, subsequent studies failed to convincingly demonstrate a therapeutic effect of standard HBV vaccines. A controlled study showed the efficacy and limitation of standard vaccine therapy in chronic HBV infection[12]. A total of 118 patients who had received no previous HBV therapy were immunized five times with 20 μg of presS2/S vaccine (Ggenehevac B) or S vaccine (Recombivax) or placebo as control. There was no significant difference in the copy numbers of HBV DNA between vaccinated and unvaccinated subjects during 12 months follow-up after five vaccine injections. Nevertheless, in the first 6 months following vaccination patients treated with either vaccine were significantly more likely to clear serum HBV DNA and seroconverted to anti-HBV than untreated controls. These differences lost significance at month 12 due to the increased seroconversion rate in the placebo group. In a few similar studies, no or little effect on the viral replication and seroconversion was archived by therapeutic vaccinations with HBsAg vaccines[13-17]. However, the vaccinations appeared to enhance specific CD4-positive T-cell responses that might contribute to transient suppression of HBV replication[13,15,18].

A reduction of viraemia in patients with chronic hepatitis B by nucleoside analogues for several logs may help to overcome unresponsiveness to therapeutic vaccination with surface or core protein of HBV[19,20]. Horiike et al. treated 72 patients with chronic hepatitis B with lamivudine at a dose of 100 μg daily for 12 months[21]. Fifteen patients received vaccine containing 20 μg of HBsAg intradermally once every 2 weeks; 12 months after the start of therapy HBV DNA became negative in all nine patients receiving combination therapy and in 15 of 31 patients receiving lamivudine monotherapy. The rate of seroconversion from HBeAg to anti-HBe was also significantly higher in patients receiving combination therapy (56%) versus monotherapy (16%). Breakthrough of HBV DNA was found in 10 patients; but in none of the patients receiving combination therapy. This study shows for the first time that a combination therapy with nucleoside analogues and vaccination may be a useful therapy option for chronically HBV-infected patients. In this study intradermal vaccination was given 12 times, which may have induced a strong T-cell response in those patients. Unfortunately, T-cell response has not been investigated in this study to clarify whether CTL have been induced.

Overall, immunizations of chronic HBV-infected patients with standard HBsAg vaccines did not achieve a satisfactory result. Standard HBV vaccines are supposed to potently stimulate CD4-positive cells, as consistently reported by several studies. However, standard HBV vaccines are designed mainly to prime humoral responses to HBsAg and are not suitable for the enhancement of cell-mediated immune responses. Aimed to stimulate specific T-cell responses, three different approaches have been tested in clinical trials so far.

Wen et al. demonstrated that immunizations with immune complexes of HBsAg and anti-HBs antibodies reduced viraemia in patients with chronic hepatitis B and also induced anti-HBs in transgenic mice expressing HBsAg[22,23]. The immune complexes of HBsAg and anti-HBs are supposed to be taken up by antigen-presenting cells in a facilitated way, and may enhance the priming of specific T-cell responses. The immune complex has passed the clinical trial phase I and phase IIa in China[24]. It could effectively induce HBsAg-specific immune responses in healthy persons.

Vitiello et al. constructed a lipopeptide vaccine (CY1899) consisting of HBcAg peptide 18 to 27 as a CTL epitope, the T helper peptide derived from tetanus toxoid, and two palmitic acid molecules[25]. Immunization trials in 26 healthy subjects showed that this type of vaccine was safe and was able to induce an HBV-specific CTL response[26]. However, this T-cell vaccine only slightly enhanced CTL responses in chronically HBV-infected patients and failed to show any impact on viral replication in the liver and viral load in the serum[27].

DNA vaccines against HBV have been tested in a pilot study[28]. In a phase I clinical trial healthy volunteers received DNA including the surface antigen of HBV with a dose of 1, 2, or 4 µg. The vaccine was safe and well tolerated. All volunteers developed a productive antibody response. An antigen-specific CD8[+] T cell response could be detected in HLA-A2-positive volunteers. These results demonstrated the ability of DNA vaccine to induce productive antibody and cell-mediated immune response in humans. Mancini-Bourgin et al. immunized 10 chronically HBV-infected patients with DNA vaccines[29]. DNA vaccinations appeared to enhance T-cell responses in these patients. Five patients had reduced viraemia after 3 injections. Further studies on DNA vaccines are needed to improve their achievement in chronically HBV-infected patients.

TESTING NEW APPROACHES FOR THERAPEUTIC VACCINATION IN THE WOODCHUCK MODEL

It appears that the conventional HBV vaccines consisting of recombinant HBsAg absorbed to alum adjuvant are not suitable for therapeutic vaccination, possibly due to their preference to stimulate Th2-biased immune responses. Thus, the recent approaches are mainly directed by the idea that the stimulation of cell-mediated immune responses may be the key to reach control over HBV. Rapid developments in basic immunology bring more and more opportunities for the improvement of vaccines. For example, genetic vaccines based on plasmid DNA provide a series of new features and seem to be the most promising candidate for future development.

Woodchucks with chronic WHV infection provide excellent opportunities to test the effectiveness of new vaccination strategies. Through progress on the characterization of the woodchuck immune system and the development of specific immunological assays, the woodchuck model became an informative animal model for the development of HBV vaccines[30–32]. The woodchuck is an excellent model to assess prototype prophylactic or therapeutic vaccines as efficacy can be tested by challenge experiments or viral elimination in chronic carriers (Table 2).

Based on the assumption that the specific T-cell responses to hepadnaviral nucleocapsid protein are important for viral control, immunizations of chronic carrier woodchucks with WHcAg in incomplete Freund's adjuvant were carried out. However, no antiviral effects were achieved in chronically WHV-infected

Table 2 Therapeutic vaccinations in the woodchuck model

Vaccines	Application	Outcome	Reference
WHcAg	i.m.	Viral elimination in one of six animals	33
WHsAg and Th-peptide	i.m.	Transient anti-WHs antibody response, two woodchucks died	52, 53
WHsAg in combination with L-FMAU	i.m.	Stimulation of T-cell responses to WHV proteins, anti-WHs antibody response	36, 37
WHsAg with MPL as adjuvant	i.m.	Antibodies to WHsAg	30
WHsAg-anti-WHs immune complex and DNA vaccines in combination with lamivudine	i.m.	Stimulation of anti-WHs antibody and suppression of WHV viraemia	Lu et al. (unpublished results)

woodchucks with WHcAg only, or in combination with famciclovir[33,34]. Probably, such immunization procedures were not sufficient to overcome the T-cell unresponsiveness.

Subsequent experiments in the woodchuck model have demonstrated the feasibility to induce specific immune responses to WHV in chronic carriers. For example, chronically WHV-infected woodchucks were able to produce anti-WHsAg antibodies in response to vaccination with plasma-derived WHV surface antigens (WHsAg) adsorbed to aluminium salt with monophosphoryl lipid A[35]. Anti-WHsAg antibodies were detected in all immunized woodchucks and persisted for a time period of up to 2 years after immunization. Despite the induction of anti-WHsAg antibodies, neither WHV DNA nor WHsAg titres in immunized woodchucks changed significantly. These results indicate that the partial induction of specific B-cell responses to WHV proteins is not sufficient to control WHV infection. Additional components for the stimulation of T-cell responses are necessary to achieve therapeutic effects against chronic hepatitis B.

The T-cell response to HBV was successfully restored in patients treated with lamivudine or IFN-α, as published by Boni et al.[19,20]. Thus, a reduction of the viral load by antiviral treatments may enhance the effect of therapeutic vaccines. A combination of an antiviral treatment using a potent drug L-FMAU and immunization with WHsAg induces WHV-specific lymphoproliferation in chronic carriers[36,37]. Though immunizations with WHsAg were already sufficient to induce lymphoproliferative responses to WHV proteins in both treated and untreated woodchucks, the antiviral treatment led to a broader spectrum of specific T-cell responses to different WHV proteins including core and X proteins.

The available data from the experiments in the woodchuck model suggest that a combination of antiviral treatments and vaccinations with multiple components may be necessary to induce vigorous and sustained immune responses, leading to an effective control of HBV infection. Any single component vaccine may be potent to prime a partial response, either T- or B-cell response. However, such a partial response is not able to suppress HBV replication. Multiple, vigorous immune responses to HBV, as seen during acute self-limiting HBV infection, are required to reduce HBV replication and finally completely clear HBV in infected patients.

Based on this idea a triple combination of antiviral treatment with lamivudine and therapeutic vaccination with DNA vaccines and antigen–antibody complexes was carried out in the woodchuck model to evaluate the efficacy (Lu et al., unpublished). DNA immunization is a powerful method to induce protective immune responses to viral infection, particularly with the option to induce cellular immune responses[38,39]. DNA vaccination has been tested in different animal models including mouse, duck, woodchuck, and chimpanzees[40–51]. The novel prototype therapeutic vaccine based on antigen–antibody complexes was developed by the group of Wen et al.[22] and tested in HBV transgenic mice[23]. Ten woodchucks chronically infected with WHV were treated with 15 mg of lamivudine/day for 4 months. At 8 weeks after starting lamivudine treatment one group of woodchucks were immunized with pWHsIm, a plasmid-expressing WHsAg and a second group with WHsAg–

anti-WHsAg complex and pWHsIm. Two woodchucks treated with lamivudine only served as controls. The treatment with lamivudine led to a marginal decrease of WHV DNA concentrations in woodchucks. Interestingly, three woodchucks immunized with WHsAg–anti-WHs complexes and pWHsIm developed anti-WHs antibodies and showed a further decrease of serum WHV DNA and WHsAg concentrations. The anti-WHs antibodies persisted in two woodchucks for a period of 8 weeks. These results indicated that this triple combination therapy was an effective treatment against chronic hepadnaviral infection. Further efforts should focus on the induction of sustained immune responses to maintain control over viral replication.

The present work done in the woodchuck model proved the feasibility of therapeutic vaccination against chronic HBV infection. It became clear that the induction of antibodies to WHsAg could be achieved in chronically infected individuals while the control of viral replication needs multiple branches of immune responses, especially T-cell branches. Particularly, immunizations with immune complexes appear to be an effective method to stimulate antibody responses with antiviral action. The future investigations will take the major advantages in the woodchuck model as an authentic infection model. No other animal model is available to mimic the chronic course of hepadnaviral infection and present the features in pathogenesis and virus–host interaction in such a satisfactory way as the woodchuck model.

PERSPECTIVES

The rapid progress in immunology has opened many important aspects of HBV immunopathogenesis and given directions for future vaccine development. On the assumption that the improvement of specific CTL responses is most crucial for therapeutic vaccination, reagents stimulating T-cell responses, particularly new adjuvants, are under investigation. Though there are many approaches suitable to prime specific CTL responses, their ability to break the immune tolerance mechanisms in chronically HBV-infected patients is poorly understood. Therefore, the tolerance mechanisms leading to chronic HBV infection need to be analysed to provide rationales for design of therapeutic vaccines. It is assumed that a high level of viral replication may overwhelm host immune responses. Thus future approaches of therapeutic vaccination will include a vigorous antiviral treatment to reduce viral replication. Preferably, the expression of viral proteins should be reduced or completely inhibited as viral proteins represent important players to maintain tolerance mechanisms. The newly potent antivirals could even gradually lower the level of cccDNA that is mainly responsible for the persistence of HBV. The new development of RNA interference may provide suitable tools to contribute to antiviral treatments.

A specific CTL response requires the cooperation of other components of the immune system. It is clear that a CTL response could not be maintained without Th cells. Further, humoral responses, particularly the anti-HBs antibody response, are crucial to terminate HBV infection by clearing circulating HBV virions. As we understand that an immune response including multiple effectors is necessary to control primary HBV infection, therapeutic vaccines should stimulate all these effectors involved. Directed by this concept, experiments in the woodchuck model are designed to combine different components like DNA, proteins, cytokines, and adjuvants. Priming–boosting protocols using different components will provide additional options to target specific branches of the immune system.

References

1. World Health Organization, 1996. The World Health Report 1996. Geneva.
2. Thimme R, Wieland S, Steiger C et al. CD8(+) T cells mediate viral clearance and disease pathogenesis during acute hepatitis B virus infection. J Virol. 2003;77:68–76.
3. Guidotti LG, Ishikawa T, Hobbs MV, Matzke B, Schreiber R, Chisari FV. Intracellular inactivation of the hepatitis B virus by cytotoxic T lymphocytes. Immunity. 1996;4:25–36.
4. Guidotti LG, Rochford R, Chung J, Shapiro M, Purcell R, Chisari FV. Viral clearance without destruction of infected cells during acute HBV infection. Science. 1999;284:825–9.
5. Hoofnagle JH, Peters M, Mullen KD et al. Randomized controlled trial of recombinant human alpha-interferon in patients with chronic hepatitis B. Gastroenterology. 1988;95: 1318–25.
6. Janssen HL, van Zonneveld M, Senturk H et al. and HBV 99-01 Study Group; Rotterdam Foundation for Liver Research. Pegylated interferon alfa-2b alone or in combination with lamivudine for HBeAg-positive chronic hepatitis B: a randomised trial. Lancet. 2005;365: 123–9.
7. Lau GK, Piratvisuth T, Luo KX et al. Peginterferon Alfa-2a HBeAg-Positive Chronic Hepatitis B Study Group. Peginterferon Alfa-2a, lamivudine, and the combination for HBeAg-positive chronic hepatitis B. N Engl J Med. 2005;352:2682–95.
8. Dienstag JL, Perrillo RP, Schiff ER, Bartholomew M, Vicary C, Rubin M. A preliminary trial for chronic hepatitis B infection. N Engl J Med. 1995;333:1657–61.
9. Doong SL, Tsai CH, Schinazi RF, Liotta DC, Chen YC. Inhibition of the replication of hepatitis B virus *in vitro* by 2′,3′-dideoxy-3′-thiacytidine and related analogues. Proc Natl Acad Sci USA. 1991;88:8495–9.
10. Pol S, Driss F, Michel ML, Nalpas B, Berthelot P, Brechot C. Specific vaccine therapy in chronic hepatitis B infection. Lancet. 1994;344:342.
11. Pol S, Couillin I, Michel ML et al. Immunotherapy of chronic hepatitis B by anti-HBV vaccine. Acta Gastroenterol Belg. 1998;61:228–33.
12. Pol S, Nalpas B, Driss F et al. Efficacy and limitations of a specific immunotherapy in chronic hepatitis B. J Hepatol. 2001;34:917–21.
13. Couillin I, Pol S, Mancini M et al. Specific vaccine therapy in chronic hepatitis B: induction of T cell proliferative responses specific for envelope antigens. J Infect Dis. 1999;180:15–26.
14. Dikici B, Kalayci AG, Ozgenc F et al. Therapeutic vaccination in the immunotolerant phase of children with chronic hepatitis B infection. Pediatr Infect Dis J. 2003;22:345–9.
15. Ren F, Hino K, Yamaguchi Y et al. Cytokine-dependent anti-viral role of CD4-positive T cells in therapeutic vaccination against chronic hepatitis B viral infection. J Med Virol. 2003;71:376–84.
16. Safadi R, Isreali E, Papo O et al. Treatment of chronic hepatitis B virus infection via oral immune regulatione toward hepatitis B virus proteins. Am J Gastroenterology. 2003;98: 2505–15.
17. Yalcin K, Acar M, Degertekin H. Specific hepatitis B vaccine therapy in inactive HBsAg carriers: a randomized controlled trial. Infection. 2003;31:221–5.
18. Jung MC, Gruner N, Zachoval R et al. Immunological monitoring during therapeutic vaccination as a prerequisite for the design of new effective therapies: induction of a vaccine-specific CD4$^+$ T-cell proliferation response in chronic hepatitis B carriers. Vaccine. 2002;20:3598–612.
19. Boni C, Bertoletti A, Penna A et al. Lamivudine treatment can restore T cell responsiveness in chronic hepatitis B. J Clin Invest. 1998;102:968–76.

20. Boni C, Penna A, Ogg GS et al. Lamivudine treatment can overcome cytotoxic T-cell hyporesponsiveness in chronic hepatitis B: new perspectives for immune therapy. Hepatology. 2001;33:963–71.
21. Horiike N, Fazle Akbar SM, Michitaka K et al. *In vivo* immunization by vaccine therapy following virus suppression by lamivudine: a novel approach for treating patients with chronic hepatitis B. J Clin Virol. 2005;32:156–61.
22. Wen YM, Wu XH, Hu DC, Zhang QP, Guo SQ. Hepatitis B vaccine and anti-HBs complex as approach for vaccine therapy. Lancet. 1995;345:1575–6.
23. Zheng BJ, Ng MH, He LF et al. Therapeutic efficacy of hepatitis B surface antigen–antibodies–recombinant DNA composite in HBsAg transgenic mice. Vaccine 2001;19:4219–2.
24. Xu DZ, Huang KL, Zhao K et al. Vaccination with recombinant HBsAg-HBIG complex in healthy adults. Vaccine. 2005;23:2658–64.
25. Vitiello A, Ishioka G, Grey HM et al. Development of a lipopeptide-based therapeutic vaccine to treat chronic HBV infection. I. Induction of a primary cytotoxic T lymphocyte response in humans. J Clin Invest. 1995;95:341–9.
26. Livingston BD, Crimi C, Grey H et al. The hepatitis B virus-specific CTL responses induced in humans by lipopeptide vaccination are comparable to those elicited by acute viral infection. J Immunol. 1997;159:1383–92.
27. Heathcote J, McHutchison J, Lee S et al. A pilot study of the CY-1899 T-cell vaccine in subjects chronically infected with hepatitis B virus. CY1899 T Cell Vaccine Study Group. Hepatology. 1999;30:531–6.
28. Roy MJ, Wu MS, Barr LJ et al. Induction of antigen-specific CD8+ T cells, T helper cells, and protective levels of antibody in humans by particle-mediated administration of a hepatitis B virus DNA vaccine. Vaccine. 2000;19:764–78.
29. Mancini-Bourgine M, Fontaine H, Scott-Algara D, Pol S, Brechot C, Michel ML. Induction or expansion of T-cell responses by a hepatitis B DNA vaccine administered to chronic HBV carriers. Hepatology. 2004;40:874–82.
30. Lu M, Roggendorf M. Evaluation of new approaches to prophylactic and therapeutic vaccinations against hepatitis B viruses in the woodchuck model. Intervirology. 2001;44:124–31.
31. Roggendorf M, Lu M. The woodchuck: a model for studies on immunopathogenesis and therapy of hepadnaviral infection. In: F von Weizäcker, Roggendorf M, editors. Models for Viral Heptitis. Basel Karger: Monogr Virol, 2005:1–27.
32. Roggendorf M, Lu M. Woodchuck hepatitis virus. In: Thomas TH, Zuckermann A, Lemon S, editors. Viral Hepatitis, 3rd edn. Oxford: Blackwell Publishing, 2005:210–24.
33. Roggendorf M, Tolle TK. The woodchuck: an animal model for hepatitis B virus infection in man. Intervirology. 1995;38:100–12.
34. Roos S, Fuchs K, Roggendorf M. Protection of woodchucks from infection with woodchuck hepatitis virus by immunization with recombinant core protein. J Gen Virol. 1989;70:2087–95.
35. Lu M, Klaes R, Menne S et al. Induction of antibodies to the PreS region of surface antigens of woodchuck hepatitis virus (WHV) in chronic carrier woodchucks by immunizations with WHV surface antigens. J Hepatol. 2003;39:405–13.
36. Korba BE, Cote PJ, Menne S et al. Clevudine therapy with vaccine inhibits progression of chronic hepatitis and delays onset of hepatocellular carcinoma in chronic woodchuck hepatitis virus infection. Antivir Ther. 2004;9:937–52.
37. Menne S, Roneker CA, Korba BE, Gerin JL, Tennant BC, Cote PJ. Immunization with surface antigen vaccine alone and after treatment with 1-(2-fluoro-5-methyl-beta-L-arabinofuranosyl)-uracil (L-FMAU) breaks humoral and cell-mediated immune tolerance in chronic woodchuck hepatitis virus infection. J Virol. 2002;76:5305–14.
38. Donnelly JJ, Ulmer JB, Shiver JW, Liu MA. DNA vaccines. Ann Rev Immunol. 1997;15:617–48.
39. Ulmer JB, Sadoff JC, Liu MA. DNA vaccines. Curr Opin Immunol. 1996;8:531–36.
40. Davis HL, McCluskie MJ, Gerin JL, Purcell RH. DNA vaccine for hepatitis B: evidence for immunogenicity in chimpanzees and comparison with other vaccines. Proc Natl Acad Sci USA. 1996;93:7212–18.

41. Garcia-Navarro R, Blanco-Urgoiti B, Berraondo P et al. Protection against woodchuck hepatitis virus (WHV) infection by gene gun coimmunization with WHV core and interleukin-12. J Virol. 2001;75:9068–76.
42. Kuhrober A, Wild J, Pudollek HP, Chisari FV, Reimann J. DNA vaccination with plasmids encoding the intracellular (HBcAg) or secreted (HBeAg) form of the core protein of hepatitis B virus primes T cell responses to two overlapping Kb- and Kd-restricted epitopes. Int Immunol. 1997;9:1203–12.
43. Lu M, Hilken G, Kruppenbacher J et al. Immunization of woodchucks with plasmids expressing woodchuck hepatitis virus (WHV) core antigen and surface antigen suppresses WHV infection. J Virol. 1999;73:281–9.
44. Michel ML, Davis HL, Schleef M, Mancini M, Tiollais P, Whalen RG. DNA-mediated immunization to the hepatitis B surface antigen in mice: aspects of the humoral response mimic hepatitis B viral infection in humans. Proc Natl Acad Sci USA. 1995;92:5307–11.
45. Pancholi P, Lee DH, Liu Q et al. DNA prime/canarypox boost-based immunotherapy of chronic hepatitis B virus infection in a chimpanzee. Hepatology. 2001;33:448–54.
46. Prince AM, Whalen R, Brotman B. Successful nucleic acid based immunization of newborn chimpanzees against hepatitis B virus. Vaccine. 1997;15:916–19.
47. Rollier C, Sunyach C, Barraud L et al. Protective and therapeutic effect of DNA-based immunization against hepadnavirus large envelope protein. Gastroenterology. 1999;116: 658–65.
48. Schirmbeck R, Bohm W, Ando K, Chisari FV, Reimann J. Nucleic acid vaccination primes hepatitis B virus surface antigen-specific cytotoxic T lymphocytes in nonresponder mice. J Virol. 1995;69:5929–34.
49. Siegel F, Lu M, Roggendorf M. Coadministration of gamma interferon with DNA vaccine expressing woodchuck hepatitis virus (WHV) core antigen enhances the specific immune response and protects WHV infection. J Virol. 2001;75:5036–42.
50. Thermet A, Rollier C, Zoulim F, Trepo C, Cova L. Progress in DNA vaccine for prophylaxis and therapy of hepatitis B. Vaccine. 2003;21:659–62.
51. Triyatni M, Jilbert AR, Qiao M, Miller DS, Burrell CJ. Protective efficacy of DNA vaccines against duck hepatitis B virus infection. J Virol. 1998;72:84–94.
52. Hervas-Stubbs S, Lasarte JJ, Sarobe P et al. Therapeutic vaccination of woodchucks against chronic woodchuck hepatitis virus infection. J Hepatol. 1997;27:726–37.
53. Hervas-Stubbs S, Lasarte JJ, Sarobe P et al. T-helper cell response to woodchuck hepatitis virus antigens after therapeutic vaccination of chronically-infected animals treated with lamivudine. J Hepatol. 2001;35:105–11.

Section Liver IV
Hepatocellular carcinoma

Chair: M. GEISSLER and J.M. LLOVET

22
Gene expression profiling of hepatocellular carcinoma: past, present and future

J.-S. LEE and S. S. THORGEIRSSON

INTRODUCTION

Hepatocellular carcinoma (HCC) is one of the most common cancers in the world, accounting for an estimated 600 000 deaths annually[1]. Although much is known about both the cellular changes that lead to HCC and the aetiological agents (i.e. HBV, HCV infection, and alcohol) for the majority of HCC, the molecular pathogenesis of HCC is not well understood[2]. Patients with HCC have a highly variable clinical course[3], indicating that HCC comprises several biologically distinctive subgroups. The prognostic variability probably reflects a molecular heterogeneity that has not been appreciated from methods traditionally used to characterize HCC. Improving the classification of HCC patients into groups with homogeneous prognosis, as well as a more comprehensive understanding of the underlying biology of HCC development at the molecular level, would improve the application of currently available treatment modalities. To accomplish this goal, investigation of HCC at the molecular level is under way through functional genomic approaches including DNA microarray technology that can simultaneously detect the expression levels of thousands of genes. This new technology has been successfully used to predict the clinical outcome and survival, as well as to classify different types of HCC.

PAST; GENE EXPRESSION PATTERNS ASSOCIATED WITH CLINICOPATHOLOGICAL FEATURES

As conventional approaches for the prognostic classification of HCC largely rely on the single or multiple clinicopathological variables such as the severity of the liver function and characteristics of tumour (i.e. size, number of nodules, vascular invasion, distant metastasis, and tumour grade), the majority of DNA-microarray studies in human HCC have focused on uncovering differences in gene-expression patterns among tissues that are clinically or histologically well defined. As expected, prediction models based on gene expression profiles successfully discriminate HCC from non-tumour livers with expected high accuracy[4–6]. Many studies have identified differentially expressed gene sets in HCC that differ according to aetiological factors[7], mutations of tumour-suppressor genes[8], rate of recurrence[9], intrahepatic metastasis[10], and different stages[5]. The results from these studies demonstrate that genomic scale gene expression profiles recapitulate the well-known morphological distinctions of the tissues, and suggest that the differences in gene expression patterns might be biologically relevant. However, most of these studies have identified genes that are associated with limited aspects of the tumour pathogenesis, but do not necessarily reflect the underlying biological properties that probably drive tumour behaviour.

PRESENT; NOVEL SUBCLASS OF HCC AND COMPARATIVE FUNCTIONAL GENOMICS

In our recent study[11], an unbiased analytical approach was applied on gene expression data from human HCC to investigate the possibility that variations in gene expression of HCC would permit the identification of distinct subclasses of HCC patients with different prognoses. Two independent but complementary approaches (unsupervised and supervised methods) were applied for data analysis to uncover subclasses of HCC and the underlying biological differences in molecular level between the subclasses (subclasses A and B). The study shows that gene expression profiling analysis can identify previously unrecognized, clinically relevant subclasses of HCC in a robust and reproducible manner.

Despite facts showing that transgenic and knockout mouse models have significantly enhanced our understanding of human cancers, in most cases we still rely on casual correlation between human and mouse models due to lack of methods for direct comparisons[12]. In an effort to identify the best-fit mouse HCC models that mimic the human condition our laboratory has recently integrated gene expression data from human and mouse HCC[13]. Gene expression patterns of mouse HCC were obtained from seven HCC mouse models. Orthologous human and mouse genes from both data sets were selected, and the gene expression data were integrated and analysed together. In hierarchical clustering analysis of integrated data, gene expression patterns of HCC from *Myc*, *E2f1*, and *Myc/E2f1* mice had the highest similarity with those of the better survival group of human HCC, while the expression patterns of *Myc/Tgfa* and DENA-induced mouse HCC were most similar to those of the poorer survival group of human HCC. These results suggest that these two classes of mouse models might closely recapitulate the molecular patterns of the two subclasses of human HCC. The similarity of gene expression profiles between human and mouse models is in good agreement with the phenotypic characteristics of the tumours. The human tumours with increased proliferation, decreased apoptosis and worse prognosis are paired with the mouse models with the same characteristics. Although the precise molecular mechanism driving hepatocarcinogenesis is yet to be discovered, the relative similarity of *Myc/Tgfa* mice to the human poor survival group (subclass A) HCC indicates the role of the EGFR, receptor of TGFA[14], or related signalling pathways in prognosis of human HCC. These results strongly suggest that well-defined gene expression signatures from experimental condition or animal models can be used to stratify human cancer patients into more homogeneous groups at the molecular level. We can anticipate that unique molecular identities of each subclass of HCC uncovered by comparative analysis of a genome-wide survey of gene expression from human and animal models will provide new therapeutic strategies to maximize the efficiency of treatments.

FUTURE; INTEGRATIVE FUNCTIONAL GENOMICS

Gene expression profiling studies of various cancers have discovered consistent gene expression patterns associated with a histological or clinical phenotype and discovering subtypes of cancers previously unidentified with conventional technologies. The research focus has now shifted towards identifying genetic determinants that are components of the specific regulatory pathways altered in cancers, leading to the discovery of novel therapeutic targets. However, it is not easy to select few candidate genes for further studies from the lengthy gene lists generated from gene expression profiling studies, largely because too many confounding factors (i.e. ages, hospital care, different protocols of treatments, non-parallel progression of cancer, and unspecified environmental factors which are irrelevant to HCC development) are embedded in the gene expression profile data from human cancer tissues. However, this limitation has been overcome by applying cross-comparison of multiple gene expression data sets from human HCC and animal models, uncovering evolutionarily conserved gene expression patterns during HCC progression[13]. The success of the new experimental and analytical approach, comparative functional genomics, suggests that more integration of independent data sets will enhance our ability to identify key regulatory elements during HCC development.

In recent studies[15–18], gene expression signatures from an experimental condition mimicking the wound-healing process was used to calculate how much tumours may be like wounds and to develop a model to predict cancer progression based on the wound-healing gene expression signature. Patients carrying the wound-healing signature had a significantly increased risk of metastasis when compared with patients who lacked the signature, indicating that genomic data from the normal physiological condition can help to predict the prognosis of cancer patients. It is therefore important to obtain, in addition to the gene expression data from human HCC and mouse HCC models, gene expression signatures from experimental animals and humans unique for different normal physiological conditions, such as liver development and regeneration, as well as hepatic stem cells that can be integrated into the gene expression patterns from human HCC.

It is important to realize that we can obtain better biologically and clinically significant inference of genomic data by integrating gene expression data with diverse genomic data such as genomic sequence information in promoters, array-based CGH data, and non-coding gene (i.e. micro-RNA) expression data. Recent advances in translating cancer genomics into clinical oncology strongly indicate that, rather than relying on the current modelling of population risk assessment and empirical treatment of patients, it is essential to move to predictive personalized models based on molecular classification and targeted therapy. There can be little doubt that the future will bring a shift away from population risk assessment and empirical treatment of patients with HCC to the predictive personalized care based on molecular classification and targeted therapy. Serological molecular markers that are identified by gene expression profile studies and non-invasive imaging probes will be used for screening or early detection. Defined specific gene expression signatures of tumours will be used to identify altered genetic elements or pathways that point to the most beneficial therapy or combination of therapies. In parallel, new targeted therapies will emerge as gene expression profiling and other genome-wide screening technologies uncover pathways or interactions of pathways that are most vulnerable for therapeutic intervention.

References

1. Parkin DM, Bray F, Ferlay J, Pisani P. Global cancer statistics, 2002. CA Cancer J Clin. 2005;55:74–108.
2. Thorgeirsson SS, Grisham JW. Molecular pathogenesis of human hepatocellular carcinoma. Nat Genet. 2002;31:339–46.
3. Llovet JM, Burroughs A, Bruix J. Hepatocellular carcinoma. Lancet. 2003;362:1907–17.
4. Kim BY, Lee JG, Park S et al. Feature genes of hepatitis B virus-positive hepatocellular carcinoma, established by its molecular discrimination approach using prediction analysis of microarray. Biochim Biophys Acta. 2004;1739:50–61.
5. Nam SW, Park JY, Ramasamy A et al. Molecular changes from dysplastic nodule to hepatocellular carcinoma through gene expression profiling. Hepatology. 2005;42:809–18.
6. Neo SY, Leow CK, Vega VB et al. Identification of discriminators of hepatoma by gene expression profiling using a minimal dataset approach. Hepatology. 2004;39:944–53.
7. Okabe H, Satoh S, Kato T et al. Genome-wide analysis of gene expression in human hepatocellular carcinomas using cDNA microarray: identification of genes involved in viral carcinogenesis and tumor progression. Cancer Res. 2001;61:2129–37.
8. Chen X, Cheung ST, So S et al. Gene expression patterns in human liver cancers. Mol Biol Cell. 2002;13:1929–39.
9. Iizuka N, Oka M, Yamada-Okabe H et al. Oligonucleotide microarray for prediction of early intrahepatic recurrence of hepatocellular carcinoma after curative resection. Lancet. 2003;361:923–9.
10. Ye QH, Qin LX, Forgues M et al. Predicting hepatitis B virus-positive metastatic hepatocellular carcinomas using gene expression profiling and supervised machine learning. Nat Med. 2003;9:416–23.
11. Lee JS, Chu IS, Heo J et al. Classification and prediction of survival in hepatocellular carcinoma by gene expression profiling. Hepatology. 2004;40:667–76.
12. Lee JS, Grisham JW, Thorgeirsson SS. Comparative functional genomics for identifying models of human cancer. Carcinogenesis. 2005;26:1013–20.
13. Lee JS, Chu IS, Mikaelyan A et al. Application of comparative functional genomics to identify best-fit mouse models to study human cancer. Nat Genet. 2004;36:1306–11.
14. Yarden Y, Sliwkowski MX. Untangling the ErbB signalling network. Nat Rev Mol Cell Biol. 2001;2:127–37.
15. Chang HY, Sneddon JB, Alizadeh AA et al. Gene expression signature of fibroblast serum response predicts human cancer progression: similarities between tumors and wounds. PLoS Biol. 2004;2:E7.

16. Chang HY, Nuyten DS, Sneddon JB et al. Robustness, scalability, and integration of a wound-response gene expression signature in predicting breast cancer survival. Proc Natl Acad Sci USA. 2005;102:3738–43.
17. Ellwood-Yen K, Graeber TG, Wongvipat J et al. Myc-driven murine prostate cancer shares molecular features with human prostate tumors. Cancer Cell. 2003;4:223–38.
18. Sweet-Cordero A, Mukherjee S, Subramanian A et al. An oncogenic KRAS2 expression signature identified by cross-species gene-expression analysis. Nat Genet. 2005;37:48–55.

23
Hepatocellular carcinoma: a cancer of developed countries

S. KUBICKA

WORLDWIDE EPIDEMIOLOGY AND COMMON RISK FACTORS

Hepatocellular carcinoma (HCC) is one of the main complications of liver cirrhosis and a serious health problem worldwide. Estimates from the year 2000 indicate that liver cancer remains the fifth most common malignancy in men and the eighth in women worldwide[1]. The incidence of HCC in Western countries is low ($< 10/100\,000$), while in some regions of Africa and Asia HCC is the major cause of death among malignant diseases with an incidence up to $100/100\,000$[1–3].

These epidemiological data reflect the influence and the distribution of risk factors for HCC in high and low incidence areas. A causal relationship between liver cirrhosis and the development of HCC is obvious: worldwide over 80% of HCC occur in liver cirrhosis[4]. Emerging data indicate that the mortality rate of HCC associated with cirrhosis is rising in some developed countries[5–7], whereas mortality from non-HCC complications of cirrhosis is decreasing or stable[8,9]. Recent studies indicate that HCC is currently the major cause of liver-related deaths (54–70%) in patients with compensated liver cirrhosis[10,11].

Although cirrhosis *per se* appears to be the prime risk factor for HCC, hepatocarcinogenesis strongly depends also on the causative agents of the underlying cirrhosis and on secondary risk factors. Related to the cause of liver cirrhosis patients with high risk (viral hepatitis, haemochromatosis, tyrosinaemia) moderate risk (alcohol, α_1-antitrypsin deficiency, autoimmune hepatitis) and low risk for HCC (M. Wilson, PBC, PSC) can be distinguished[4,12–21]. Secondary risk factors for HCC among patients with chronic liver diseases are male sex, age and cigarette smoking[4,18].

Only few risk factors are known which may induce hepatocarcinogenesis in patients without liver cirrhosis. The best studied and most potent carcinogens inducing HCC are aflatoxin B1, a natural product of the *Aspergillus* fungus, and thorotrast[95]. Although oestrogens are capable of causing HCC in laboratory animals as promoting factors, the epidemiological association between steroids and human hepatocarcinogenesis is still debatable. Eight case–control studies showed in non-endemic hepatitis regions a higher risk for

HCC among women who were users of contraceptives. The results were consistent across the studies, showing a summary OR of 2.5 (95% CI 1.7–3.5) in ever- versus never-users of oral contraceptives and a summary of 5.8 (95% CI 3.0–11.0) for the longest duration of use[22]. In contrast to non-endemic regions, among endemic hepatitis populations no association between contraceptives and HCC was observed[4,23–26]. In these case–control studies only few patients were enrolled and probably larger sample sizes are required to detect an additional risk in oral contraceptive users against the very high background relative risk in HBV carriers. As a result it can be assumed, if any relationship between steroids and human HCC development does exist, that the ability of these agents inducing hepatocarcinogenesis is low.

The risk for development of liver cirrhosis and HCC increases when alcohol consumption exceeds 80 g/day for more than 10 years. Compared to patients with lifetime daily alcohol intake of 0–40 g, patients with a lifetime daily alcohol intake of 41–80 g had a 1.5-fold increased odds ratio for HCC, and the odds ratio increased to 7.3 in patients with a lifetime daily alcohol intake of greater than 80 g[27]. Alcohol use is common in the population of America and Western Europe. In the United States approximately 7% of adults meet the definition of alcohol abuse[28] and in several series from northern Europe, alcohol-induced cirrhosis accounted for more than one-third to one-half of the cases of HCC[29–33]. Alcohol is not only inducing HCC as a single agent by the development of liver cirrhosis, but is also a cofactor for the development of HBV-associated HCC[34,35] and HCV-associated HCC[27,36].

Hepatitis B and C virus infection are closely associated with the development of HCC. The geographic variation in the prevalence of HCC actually provides some of the most convincing evidence linking the disease and chronic hepatitis C and B infection. There is a striking correspondence between areas where HCC is common and where hepatitis B or C virus is hyperendemic. A second line of evidence linking HCC and viral hepatitis infection is the high rate of serological markers for hepatitis C and B in patients with this tumour. In China and Korea 85–95% of patients with HCC are HbsAg-positive, whereas in Japan, Spain and Italy 94.4%, 75% and 65% of the patients with this tumour were positive for anti-HCV[37–41].

A prospective study of more than 22 000 male government workers in Taiwan has shown the incidence of HCC to be more than 100 times higher in HBs-Ag positive than in HBs-Ag negative persons[42]. A prospective study on 917 patients revealed that the 3-year cumulative risk of HCC was 12.5% for 240 patients with liver cirrhosis and 3.8% for 677 patients with chronic hepatitis. Among patients with chronic liver diseases the risk of HCC was increased seven-fold in patients with HBs-Ag and four-fold in patients with hepatitis C antibody[18]. Although both viruses appear to be capable of inducing HCC in non-cirrhotic livers[43,44], epidemiological data suggest that HBV-associated HCC does not require cirrhosis as much as the HCV-associated counterpart does. HBV-associated HCC tends to evolve more frequently in younger patients than HCV-related HCC, and vice-versa HCV-associated HCC emerges more often in advanced cirrhotic liver in older patients[45].

MOLECULAR PATHOGENESIS WITH IMPLICATIONS TO EPIDEMIOLOGY OF HEPATOCELLULAR CARCINOMA

Although HCC is not a feature of the Li-Fraumeni syndrome, HCC characteristic hot-spot p53 mutations at codon 249 have been frequently observed in HCC high-incidence areas such as South Africa and China[46-48]. Epidemiological and *in-vitro* data revealed that the p53 mutation 249ser is specifically induced by aflatoxin B1[49,50]. In contrast to the HCC high-incidence areas p53 gene alterations in European HCC are rare (approximately 10–30%) and do not generally occur at the codon 249[51-53]. Therefore the frequency of the 'HCC-specific' p53 mutation p53-249ser appears to be a reliable indicator of aflatoxin B1 exposure of a population.

Molecular studies have indicated potential mechanisms which may account for a direct role of hepatitis B and C virus in hepatocarcinogenesis. The molecular events of HBV-mediated hepatocarcinogenesis have been extensively studied[54-56]. A variety of viral-cellular interactions which appear to have a role in malignant transformation of the hepatocytes have been observed:

1. *Cis*-acting growth-promoting mechanisms resulting from HBV integration (see above).

2. *Trans*-acting growth-promoting mechanisms involving HBV products (HBx, MHBs^t).

3. Integration-provoked genetic instability indirectly leading to changes endowing growth advantage.

4. Immune-mediated permanent cell death leading to continuous regeneration with a higher risk for mutations.

Much evidence for an X-gene-associated transformation has been reported. For instance transgenic mice containing a HBV-enhancer-X-gene construct develop HCC[57] and the transfected X-gene is capable of transforming immortalized hepatocytes[58]. X-gene products are promiscuous transactivators of genes which contain AP-1, AP-2 or NF-κB sites in their regulatory elements[59,60]. It has been shown that X-protein transactivates the proto-oncogenes c-myc and c-fos, which implies a link to hepatocarcinogenesis[60-62]. Besides the promiscuous gene transactivation other X-mediated mechanisms have been described which may also contribute to hepatocyte transformation (kinase activity, protease inhibition, p53-inhibition)[63-65]. Furthermore HBV codes for a set of transactivating proteins outside the X-gene sequences. Not wild-type, but C-terminal truncated preS2 polypeptides (MHBs^t) display an AP-1, AP-2 or NFκB site dependent transactivation function, similar to the X-protein[62,66-68].

HCV is a single-stranded RNA virus with no known DNA intermediate in its replication cycle. Therefore carcinogenesis through insertion of HCV-specific nucleic acid sequences into the genome of the hepatocytes can be excluded. However, the mechanisms of hepatocyte transformation by HCV remain obscure. With the present status of knowledge, the most plausible explanation of the link between HCV and hepatocarcinogenesis is that the virus causes chronic inflammation with the consequence of necrosis or apoptosis and subsequently the development of potentially neoplastic mutations associated with vigorous hepatic regeneration and nodule formation. A strong argument for this hypothesis is the fact that, at the time of presentation, nearly all of the patients with HCV-associated hepatocellular carcinomas are cirrhotic, in contrast to patients with HBV-associated hepatocellular carcinomas. However, a small number of patients with HCV-RNA positive hepatocellular carcinomas have also been reported, and there are data from liver-specific HCV-transgenic mouse models which suggest that some HCV proteins may have the capacity to induce cell transformation[69–72]. In addition to transgenic HCV-HCC mouse models, it has been shown by cell culture experiments that HCV may be directly involved in hepatocarcinogenesis. The hepatitis C core protein activates the human proto-oncogene c-myc[73] and the non-structural protein NS3 is capable of transforming NIH3T3 cells[74]. Although there is evidence that HCV can directly induce transformation of cells, the epidemiological data suggest that the transforming activity of HCV in humans is low; in particular much lower than the oncogenic potential of HBV.

OBESITY, DIABETES MELLITUS AND METABOLIC SYNDROME: INCREASINGLY IMPORTANT FACTORS FOR HEPATOCARCINOGENESIS IN DEVELOPED COUNTRIES

In general 15–50% of HCC cases remain idiopathic, suggesting also that other risk factors in addition to alcohol or viral hepatitis are responsible for some HCC. Obesity, insulin resistance and diabetes mellitus are strongly increasing diseases among populations in developed countries. Obesity is recognized as a significant risk factor for the development of many types of cancer. Primary liver cancer has been associated with obesity in two large population prevalence studies[75,76]. In the study from Denmark the relative risk of HCC was increased to 1.9 compared to with the general population[75] and, in a study from the US, liver cancer had the highest relative-risk increase of all of the cancers studied among the male group (4.52 times higher compared to reference group)[76].

A study examining the risk factors for HCC in 19 271 patients with cirrhosis who underwent transplantation showed that in multivariate analysis obesity remained an independent risk factor for HCC in patients with alcoholic and cryptogenic cirrhosis, in contrast to patients with viral hepatitis, autoimmune hepatitis or primary biliary cirrhosis[77].

Among 641 cirrhosis-associated HCC Bugianesi et al.[78] retrospectively identified 44 patients with cryptogenic cirrhosis and compared these patients in a case–control study with viral- and alcohol-associated HCC. The authors showed that patients with cryptogenic cirrhosis had significantly higher glucose, cholesterol, triglyceride plasma levels and increased parameters of insulin resistance compared to patients with viral- or alcohol-associated HCC. Since these alterations are features of non-alcoholic steatohepatitis, HCC may represent a late complication of NASH-related cirrhosis. Non-alcoholic fatty liver disease (NAFLD) has become one of the most common causes of chronic liver disease in developed countries. A recent population-based cohort study found that 34% of the adult population in the US has excessive fat accumulation in the liver[79]. However, a current study demonstrated that overall mortality and liver-related deaths among NAFLD patients were higher than in the general population, but HCC developed only in 0.5% of the 420 patients with NAFLD during a mean follow-up period of 7.6 years[80].

Diabetes has also been suggested as a primary risk factor for HCC, but the causal relationship is difficult to study, because liver disease itself can cause glucose intolerance and diabetes. Earlier studies reported no association between diabetes and HCC while recent studies have identified diabetes as a primary risk factor for hepatocarcinogenesis[36,81–85].

WHAT FACTORS ACCOUNT FOR THE STRIKINGLY INCREASING INCIDENCES OF HCC IN DEVELOPED COUNTRIES?

Recent reports from North America, Europe and Japan have shown that the incidence of HCC is strongly increasing[5,86–90]. In a population-based study Davila et al.[90] showed that the age-adjusted incidence of HCC among persons 65 years of age or older significantly increased from 14.2/100 000 in 1993 to 18.1/100 000 in 1999. In this study the proportion of HCV-associated HCC increased from 11% to 21%, whereas HBV-related HCC increased only from 6% to 11%. In multiple logistic regression analysis the risk for HCV-related HCC increased by 226% between the investigated time periods.

The prevalence of HCV-related HCC is considerably lower in the US and Western Europe than in Japan. By using molecular clocked long-term serial samples obtained from HCV carriers it has been estimated that HCV appeared in Japan around 1880, whereas emergence in the US was delayed until around 1910[91,92]. By statistical analysis is was suggested that the major spread time for HCV in Japan occurred in the 1930s, whereas widespread dissemination of HCV in the US occurred in the 1960s. These estimates of viral spreading are in agreement with epidemiological data and predict that the burden of HCC in Western developed countries will further increase in the next two to three decades, presumably to equal that currently observed in Japan.

Additional modifiable risk factors for HCV-associated HCC include alcohol consumption, obesity and diabetes mellitus[93]. With the rising incidence of the prevalence of HCV in developed western countries, the rising problems of supernutrition in these countries are emerging as increasingly important cofactors for the development of HCV-associated HCC. Since it has been shown that alcohol, tobacco and obesity are also synergistic primary risk factors for the development of HCC[94], it is tempting to speculate that in developed countries the currently rising problems of supernutrition will have a strong impact on the incidence of HCC in the future.

References

1.   Bosch FX, Ribes J, Diaz M, Cleries R. Primary liver cancer: worldwide incidence and trends. Gastroenterology. 2004;127(5 Suppl. 1):S5–16.
2.   Muir C, Waterhouse J, Mack T, Dowell J, Whelan S, editors. Cancer Incidence in Five Continents, vol V. World Health Organization, IARC Scientific Publications No 88, 1987.

3. Rustgi VK. Epidemiology of hepatocellular carcinoma. Gastroenterol Clin N Am. 1987;16:545–51.
4. Simonetti RG, Camma C, Fiorello F, Politi F, D'Amico G, Pagliaro L. Hepatocellular carcinoma. A worldwide problem and the major risk factors. Dig Dis Sci. 1991;36:962–72.
5. Deuffic S, Poynard T, Buffat L, Valleron AJ. Trends in primary liver cancer. Lancet. 1998;351:214–15.
6. El-Serag HB, Mason AC. Rising incidence of hepatocellular carcinoma in the United States. N Engl J Med. 1999;340:745–50.
7. La Vecchia C, Negri E, Parazzini F. Oral contraceptives and primary liver cancer. Br J Cancer. 1989;59:460–1.
8. Corrao G, Ferrari P, Zambon A, Torchio P, Arico S, Decarli A. Trends of liver cirrhosis mortality in Europe, 1970–1989: age-period-cohort analysis and changing alcohol consumption. Int J Epidemiol. 1997;26:100–9.
9. Roizen R, Kerr WC, Fillmore KM. Cirrhosis mortality and per capita consumption of distilled spirits, United States, 1949–94: trend analysis. Br Med J. 1999;319:666–70.
10. Sangiovanni A, Del Ninno E, Fasani P et al. Increased survival of cirrhotic patients with a hepatocellular carcinoma detected during surveillance. Gastroenterology. 2004;126:1005–14.
11. Benvegnu L, Gios M, Boccato S, Alberti A. Natural history of compensated viral cirrhosis: a prospective study on the incidence and hierarchy of major complications. Gut. 2004;53:744–9.
12. Niederau C, Fischer R, Sonnenberg A, Stremmel W, Trampisch HJ, Strohmeyer G. Survival and cause of death in cirrhotic and noncirrhotic patients with primary hemochromatosis. N Engl J Med. 1985;313:1256–62.
13. Eriksson S, Carlson J, Velez R. Risk of cirrhosis and primary liver cancer in alpha1-antitrypsin deficiency. N Engl J Med. 1986;314:736–9.
14. Polio J, Enriquez RE, Chow A, Atterbury CE. Hepatocellular carcinoma in Wilson's disease. Case report and review of the literature. J Clin Gastroenterol. 1989;11:220–4.
15. Adams PC, Speechley M, Kertesz AE. Long term survival analysis in hereditary hemochromatosis. Gastroenterology. 199;101:368–72.
16. Casporaso N, Romano M, Marmo R et al. Hepatitis C virus infection is an additive risk factor for development of hepatocellular carcinoma in patients with cirrhosis. J Hepatol. 1991;12:367–71.
17. Simonetti RG, Camma C, Fiorello F et al. Hepatitis C virus infection as a risk factor for hepatocellular carcinoma in patients with cirrhosis. Ann Int Med. 1992;116:97–102.
18. Tsukuma H, Hiyama T, Tanaka S et al. Risk factors for hepatocellular carcinoma among patients with chronic liver disease. N Engl J Med. 1993;328:1797–801.
19. De Bac C, Stroffolini T, Gaeta GB, Taliani G, Giusti G. Pathogenic factors in cirrhosis with and without hepatocellular carcinoma: a multicenter Italian study. Hepatology. 1995;20:1225–30.
20. Ryder SD, Koskinas J, Rizzi PM et al. Hepatocellular carcinoma complicating autoimmune hepatitis: role of hepatitis C virus. Hepatology. 1995;22:718–22.
21. Nashan B, Schltt HJ, Tusch G et al. Biliary malignancies in primary sclerosing cholangitis: timing for liver transplantation. Hepatology. 1996;23:1105–11.
22. Yu MC, Yuan JM. Environmental factors and risk for hepatocellular carcinoma. Gastroenterology. 2004;127(5 Suppl. 1):S72–8.
23. Neuberger J, Forman D, Doll R, Williams R. Oral contraceptives and hepatocellular carcinoma. Br Med J. 1986;292:1355–7.
24. Kew M, Song E, Mohammed A, Hodkinson J. Contraceptive steroids as a risk factor for hepatocellular carcinoma: a case control study in South Africa black women. Hepatology. 1990;11:298–302.
25. WHO Collaborative study of neoplasia and steroid contraceptives. Depot-medroxyprogesterone (DMPA) and risk of liver cancer. Int J Cancer. 1991;49:182–5.
26. Prentice RL. Epidemiologic data on exogenous hormones and hepatocellular carcinoma and selected other cancers. Prevent Med. 1991;20:38–46.
27. Tagger A, Donato F, Ribero ML et al. Case–control study on hepatitis C virus (HCV) as a risk factor for hepatocellular carcinoma: the role of HCV genotypes and the synergism with hepatitis B virus and alcohol. Brescia HCC Study. Int J Cancer. 1999;;81:695–9.

28. Grant B, Harford T, Dawson D, Chou P, DuFour M, Pickering R. Prevalence of DSM-IV alcohol abuse and dependence: United States 1992. Alcohol Health Res World. 1994;18:243–8.
29. Kaczynski J, Hansson G, Hermodsson S, Olsson R, Wallerstedt S. Minor role of hepatitis B and C virus infection in the etiology of hepatocellular carcinoma in a low-endemic area. Scand J Gastroenterol. 1996;31:809–13.
30. Kubicka S, Rudolph KL, Hanke M et al. Hepatocellular carcinoma in Germany: a retrospective epidemiological study from a low-endemic area. Liver. 2000;20:312–18.
31. Schoniger-Hekele M, Muller C, Kutilek M, Oesterreicher C, Ferenci P, Gangl A. Hepatocellular carcinoma in Austria: aetiological and clinical characteristics at presentation. Eur J Gastroenterol Hepatol. 2000;12:941–8.
32. Hellerbrand C, Hartmann A, Richter G et al. Hepatocellular carcinoma in southern Germany: epidemiological and clinicopathological characteristics and risk factors. Dig Dis. 2001;19:345–51.
33. Rabe C, Pilz T, Klostermann C et al. Clinical characteristics and outcome of a cohort of 101 patients with hepatocellular carcinoma. World J Gastroenterol. 2001;7:208–15.
34. Chen CJ, Liang KY, Chang AS et al. Effects of hepatitis B virus, alcohol drinking, cigarette smoking and familial tendency on hepatocellular carcinoma. Hepatology. 1991;13:398–406.
35. Mohamed AE, Kew MC, Groeneveld HT. Alcohol consumption as a risk factor for hepatocellular carcinoma in urban southern African blacks. Int J Cancer. 1992;51:537–41.
36. Hassan MM, Hwang LY, Hatten CJ et al. Risk factors for hepatocellular carcinoma: synergism of alcohol with viral hepatitis and diabetes mellitus. Hepatology. 2002;36:1206–13.
37. Chung WK, Sun HS, Park DH, Minuk GY, Hoofnagel JH. Primary hepatocellular carcinoma and hepatitis B virus infection in Korea. J Med Virol. 1983;11:99–104.
38. Tao QM. Epidemiology of persistent infection with hepatitis B virus in chronic liver disease. In: Hepatocellular Carcinoma in Asia. Kobe, Japan: Kobe University School of Medicine. 1985:3–6.
39. Bruix J, Barrera JM, Calvet X et al. Prevalence of antibodies to hepatitis C virus in Spanish patients with hepatocellular carcinoma and hepatic cirrhosis. Lancet. 1989;2:1004–6.
40. Colombo M, Kuo G, Choo QL et al. Prevalence of antibodies to hepatitis C virus in Italian patients with hepatocellular carcinoma. Lancet. 1989;2:1006–8.
41. Kiyosawa K, Sodeyama T, Tanaka E et al. Interrelationship of blood transfusion, non-A, non-B hepatitis and hepatocellular carcinoma: analysis by detection of anti-body to hepatitis C virus. Hepatology. 1990;12:671–5.
42. Beasley RP, Hwang LY, Lin CC, Chien CS. Hepatocellular carcinoma and hepatitis B virus: a prospective study of 22707 men in Taiwan. Lancet. 1981;2:1129–33.
43. Furuta T, Kanematsu T, Matsumata T et al. Clinicopathologic features of hepatocellular carcinoma in young patients. Cancer. 1990;66:2395–8.
44. El-Refaie A, Savage K, Bhattacharya S et al. HCV-associated hepatocellular carcinoma without cirrhosis. J Hepatol. 1996;24:277–85.
45. Shiratori Y, Shiina S, Imamura M et al. Characteristic difference of hepatocellular carcinoma between hepatitis B- and C-viral infection in Japan. Hepatology. 1995;22:1027–33.
46. Hsu IC, Metcalf RA, Sun T, Welsh JA, Wang NJ, Harris CC. Mutational hot spot in the p53 gene in human hepatocellular carcinomas. Nature. 1991;350:427–8.
47. Fujimoto Y, Hampton LL, Wirth PJ, Wang NJ, Xie JP, Thorgeirsson SS. Alterations of tumor suppressor genes and allelic losses in human hepatocellular carcinoma in China. Cancer Res. 1994;54:281–5.
48. Unsal H, Yakicier C, Marcais C et al. Genetic heterogeneity of hepatocellular carcinoma. Proc Natl Acad Sci USA. 1994;91:822–6.
49. Aguilar F, Harris CC, Sun T, Hollstein M, Cerutti P. Geographic variation of p53 mutational profile in nonmalignant human liver. Science. 1994;264:1317–19.
50. Aguilar F, Hussain SP, Cerutti P. Aflatoxin B1 induces the transversion of G-T in codon 249 of the p53 tumor suppressor gene in human hepatocytes. proc Natl Acad Sci USA. 1993;90:8586–90.
51. Debuire B, Paterlini P, Pontisso P, Basso G, May E. Analysis of the p53 gene in European hepatocellular carcinomas and hepatoblastomas. Oncogene. 1993;8:2303–6.

52. Volkman M, Hofman WJ, Müler M et al. p53 overexpression is frequent in European hepatocellular carcinoma and largely independent of the codon 249. Oncogene. 1994;9: 195–204.
53. Kubicka S, Trautwein C, Schrem H, Tillman H, Manns M. Low incidence of p53 mutations in European hepatocellular carcinomas with heterogeneous mutation as a rare event. J Hepatol. 1995;23:412–19.
54. Schröder CH, Zentgraf H. Hepatitis B virus related hepatocellular carcinoma: chronicity of infection – the opening to different pathways of malignant transformation? Biochim Biophys Acta. 1990;1032:137–56.
55. Robinson WS. Molecular events in the pathogenesis of hepdnavirus-associated hepatocellular carcinoma. Ann Rev Med. 1994;45:297–323.
56. Caselman WH. Transactivation of cellular gene expression by hepatitis B viral proteins: a possible molecular mechanism of hepatocarcinogenesis. J Hepatol. 1995;22(Suppl):34–7.
57. Kim CM, Koike K, Saito I, Myamura T, Jay G. HBx gene of hepatitis B virus induces liver cancer in transgenic mice. Nature. 1991;351:317–20.
58. Seifer M, Höhne M, Schaefer S, Gerlich WH. *In vitro* tumorigeniicity of hepatitis B virus DNA and HBx protein. J Hepatol. 1991;13:61–5.
59. Twu JS, Roden CA, Haseltine WA, Robinson WS. Identification of a region within the human immunodeficiency virus type I long terminal repeat that is essential for transactivation by the hepatitis B virus gene X. J Virol. 1989;63:2857–60.
60. Seto E, Mitchell PJ, Yen TSB. Transactivation by hepatitis B virus X protein depends on AP-2 and other transcription factors. Nature. 1990;344:72–4.
61. Colgrove R, Simon G, Ganem D. Transcriptional activation of homologous and heterologous genes by the hepatitis B virus gene product in cells permissive for viral replication. J Virol. 1989;63:4019–26.
62. Natoli G, Avantaggiati ML, Chirillo P: Induction of the DNA-binding activity of c-jun/c-fos heterodimers by the hepatitis B virus transactivator pX. Mol Cell Biol. 1994;14:989–98.
63. Wu JY, Zhou ZY, Judd A, Cartwright CA, Robinson WS. The hepatitis B virus-encoded transcriptional trans-activator hbx appears to be a novel protein serine/threonine kinase. Cell. 1990;63:687–95.
64. Takada S, Kido H, Fukutomi A, Mori T, Koike K. Interaction of hepatitis B virus X protein with a serine protease, tryptase TL2 as an inhibitor. Oncogene. 1994;9:341–8.
65. Wang XW, Forrester K, Yeh H, Feitelson MA, Gu JR, Harris CC. Hepatitis B virus X protein inhibits p53 sequence-specific DNA binding, transcriptional activity, and association with transcription factor ERCC3. Proc Natl Acad Sci USA. 1994;91:2230–4.
66. Caselman WH, Mayer M, Kekule AS, Lauer U, Hofschneider PH, Koshy R. A novel transactivator is encoded by hepatitis B virus preS/S sequences integrated in human hepatocellular DNA. Proc Natl Acad Sci USA. 1990;87:2970–4.
67. Lauer U, Weiß L, Hofschneider PH, Kelule AS. Transcription factors AP-1, AP-2 and NFkB are mediators of the HBV preS/S (MHBs) transactivator effect. Hepatology. 1991;14:120A.
68. Mayer M, Caselman WH, Schlüter V, Schreck R, Hofschneider PH, Baeuerle PA: Hepatitis B virus transactivator MHBst: activation of NFκB, selective inhibition by antioxidants and integral membrane localization. EMBO J. 1992;11:2991–3001.
69. Moriya K, Fujie H, Shintani Y et al. The core protein of hepatitis C virus induces hepatocellular carcinoma in transgenic mice. Nature Med. 1998;4:1065–7.
70. Moriya K, Nakagawa K, Santa T et al. Oxidative stress in the absence of inflammation in a mouse model for hepatitis C virus-associated hepatocarcinogenesis. Cancer Res. 2001;61:4365–70.
71. Lerat H, Honda M, Beard MR et al. Steatosis and liver cancer in transgenic mice expressing the structural and nonstructural proteins of hepatitis C virus. Gastroenterology. 2002;122:352–65.
72. Disson O, Haouzi D, Desagher S et al. Impaired clearance of virus-infected hepatocytes in transgenic mice expressing the hepatitis C virus polyprotein. Gastroenterology. 2004;126:859–72.
73. Ray BB, Lagging LM, Mayer K, Steele R, Ray R. Transcriptional regulation of cellular and viral promotors by the hepatitis C virus core protein. Virus Res. 1995;37:209–20.
74. Sakamuro D, Furukawa T, Takegami T. Hepatitis C virus nonstructural protein NS3 transforms NIH 3T3 cells. J Virology. 1995;69:3893–6.

75. Moller H, Mellemgaard A, Lindvig K, Olsen JH. Obesity and cancer risk: a Danish record-linkage study. Eur J Cancer. 1994;30A:344–50.
76. Calle EE, Rodriguez C, Walker-Thurmond K, Thun MJ. Overweight, obesity, and mortality from cancer in a prospectively studied cohort of US adults. N Engl J Med. 2003;348:1625–38.
77. Nair S, Mason A, Eason J, Loss G, Perrillo RP. Is obesity an independent risk factor for hepatocellular carcinoma in cirrhosis? Hepatology. 2002;36:150–5.
78. Bugianesi E, Leone N, Vanni E et al. Expanding the natural history of nonalcoholic steatohepatitis: from cryptogenic cirrhosis to hepatocellular carcinoma. Gastroenterology. 2002;123:134–40.
79. Browning JD, Szczepaniak LS, Dobbins R et al. Prevalence of hepatic steatosis in an urban population in the United States: impact of ethnicity. Hepatology. 2004;40:1387–95.
80. Adams LA, Lymp JF, St Sauver J et al. The natural history of nonalcoholic fatty liver disease: a population-based cohort study. Gastroenterology. 2005;129:113–21.
81. Yu MC, Tong MJ, Govindarajan S, Henderson BE. Nonviral risk factors for hepatocellular carcinoma in a low-risk population, the non-Asians of Los Angeles County, California. J Natl Cancer Inst. 1991;83:1820–6.
82. Adami HO, Chow WH, Nyren O et al. Excess risk of primary liver cancer in patients with diabetes mellitus. J Natl Cancer Inst. 1996;88:1472–7.
83. Wideroff L, Gridley G, Mellemkjaer L et al. Cancer incidence in a population-based cohort of patients hospitalized with diabetes mellitus in Denmark. J Natl Cancer Inst. 1997;89:1360–5.
84. El-Serag HB, Tran T, Everhart JE. Diabetes increases the risk of chronic liver disease and hepatocellular carcinoma. Gastroenterology. 2004;126:460–8.
85. Davila JA, Morgan RO, Shaib Y, McGlynn KA, El-Serag HB. Diabetes increases the risk of hepatocellular carcinoma in the United States: a population based case control study. Gut. 2005;54:533–9.
86. Okuda K, Fujimoto I, Hanai A, Urano Y. Changing incidence of hepatocellular carcinoma in Japan. Cancer Res. 1987;47:4967–72.
87. Taylor-Robinson SD, Foster GR, Arora S, Hargreaves S, Thomas HC. Increase in primary liver cancer in the UK, 1979–94. Lancet. 1997;350:1142–3.
88. La Vecchia C, Lucchini F, Franceschi S, Negri E, Levi F. Trends in mortality from primary liver cancer in Europe. Eur J Cancer. 2000;36:909–15.
89. El-Serag HB, Davila JA, Petersen NJ, McGlynn KA. The continuing increase in the incidence of hepatocellular carcinoma in the United States: an update. Ann Intern Med. 2003;139:817–23.
90. Davila JA, Morgan RO, Shaib Y, McGlynn KA, El-Serag HB. Hepatitis C infection and the increasing incidence of hepatocellular carcinoma: a population-based study. Gastroenterology. 2004;127:1372–80.
91. Tanaka Y, Hanada K, Mizokami M et al. Inaugural Article: A comparison of the molecular clock of hepatitis C virus in the United States and Japan predicts that hepatocellular carcinoma incidence in the United States will increase over the next two decades. Proc Natl Acad Sci USA. 2002;99:15584–9.
92. Mizokami M, Tanaka Y. Tracing the evolution of hepatitis C virus in the United States, Japan, and Egypt by using the molecular clock. Clin Gastroenterol Hepatol. 2005;3(10 Suppl. 2):S82–5.
93. Yuan JM, Govindarajan S, Arakawa K, Yu MC. Synergism of alcohol, diabetes, and viral hepatitis on the risk of hepatocellular carcinoma in blacks and whites in the US. Cancer. 2004;101:1009–17.
94. Marrero JA, Fontana RJ, Fu S, Conjeevaram HS, Su GL, Lok AS. Alcohol, tobacco and obesity are synergistic risk factors for hepatocellular carcinoma. J Hepatol. 2005;42:218–24.
95. US Department of Health and Human Services. Sixth annual report on carcinogens. Washington, DC: US Government Publication, 1991:92–12066.

24
New therapeutic approaches: anti-angiogenesis, immunotherapy

M. SCHUCHMANN

INTRODUCTION

Hepatocellular carcinoma (HCC) is a growing clinical problem making it up to the fifth most common cause of cancer. Usually arising from a cirrhotic liver – with an additional disease-specific risk of malignant transformation – cells of HCC are particularly resistant towards chemotherapy. Although the enigma of this particular resistance is only partially understood, a large body of data suggests that the process of oncofetal dedifferentiation enables hepatocytes to evade immune surveillance by refining their intracellular set of proteins, which orchestrate the subtle balance of apoptotic death and survival. Evading the immune surveillance by developing resistance to apoptosis is a classic principle, which is of particular importance in a number of malignancies including HCC, where increased levels of anti-apoptotic proteins such as c-FLIP and survivin, or decreased levels of pro-apoptotic proteins such as FADD, have been described. Another hallmark of HCC is its high degree of neovascularization.

Having the above in mind, three new therapeutic approaches to fight HCC are currently pursued: restoring an effective immune response towards tumour cells, restoring sensitivity of tumour cells towards apoptosis and the deadly attack of killer cells, and interfering with the tumour-driven neovascularization by anti-angiogenic means.

ANTI-ANGIOGENIC APPROACHES

Neovascularization is a prerequisite for tumour growth beyond a size of 2–3 mm in order to maintain the necessary supply of oxygen and nutrients. In addition it provides a route for tumour cells to be shed into the circulation.

Rapidly grown tumour vasculature differs from regular vessels with more fragile and fenestrated endothelial walls. It was Judah Folkman, in 1971, who first described the idea of blocking vessel formation as a therapeutic principle to fight tumour growth[1].

However, it took three decades until the monoclonal antibody bevacizumab, an anti-angiogenic biological, successfully entered the clinical stage as part of treatment of patients with colon carcinoma[2]. Bevacizumab targets soluble vascular endothelial growth factor (VEGF) and there is evidence from preclinical studies that, also in HCC animal models, direct interference with the VEGF system reduces tumour growth.

Poon et al. demonstrated that in patients with HCC high serum levels of VEGF – reflecting a heavily active neovascularization – are accompanied by a significantly reduced survival: median survival of patients with a VEGF level above 240 pg/ml was only 6.8 months compared to 19.2 months for those who had lower levels[3].

In line with this Musso et al. were able to demonstrate that the expression of negative regulators of angiogenesis in HCC such as endostatin inversely correlates with median tumour progression[4].

The VEGF ligand–receptor system, which is considered to be a dominant regulator of neoangiogenesis, can be modulated on several levels: antibodies which bind to the soluble ligand (e.g. the above-mentioned bevacizumab), as well as soluble receptors which prevent the ligand from binding to its receptors.

This concept was further investigated in small phase II trials in which patients with HCC were treated with bevacizumab either in combination with gemcitabine and oxaliplatin or as monotherapy. At the ASCO meeting 2005 data were presented which indicate decrease of tumour marker alpha-fetoprotein (AFP) in one-half of the patients with combination therapy[5] and stable disease for 4 months in 11 of 13 patients with monotherapy of bevacizumab[6] – results which underscore the need for larger and controlled randomized trials.

Another mode of antibody-mediated anti-angiogenetic action is the direct inhibition of receptor–ligand interaction by antibodies binding to the membrane-bound receptor – specifically the VEGF-receptor 2. This can also be accomplished by interfering with a soluble VEGF-receptor, as Raskopf et al. demonstrated nicely with an adenoviral transfer of an adenoviral-encoded dominant negative fragment of VEGFR-2[7].

However, one has to take into account that the limited efficacy in the tumour microenvironment is an intrinsic shortcoming of therapy with large molecules such as antibodies or soluble receptors. This observation further stimulated research on small molecules, which interact with the intracellular receptor kinase-domain receptors of the VEGF family and other angiogenic and oncogenic receptors. These receptor thyrosine kinase inhibitors (RTKI) are considered to penetrate into the cytoplasm of carcinoma cells where they compete with the ATP-binding site of the catalytic domain. They are orally active, small molecules that have a favourable safety profile and can be easily combined with other forms of chemotherapy or radiation therapy. Several RTKI have been found to have effective antitumour activity, and have been approved or are in clinical trials. There is now considerable hope that RTKI will also find their way into therapy of HCC and ongoing randomized phase III trials with substances such as sorafenib, a VEGF receptor 2 and raf inhibitor, might pave the way. In addition, substances such as vatalanib showed promising results in mouse models of HCC[8] (see Table 1).

Table 1

Inhibitor	Targeted tyrosine kinase	Tumour targeted	Study status
Sorafenib (BAY-43-9006)	B-Raf; VEGFR-2	HCC, renal, melanoma	Phase III
Semaxinib (SU 5416)	VEGFR-2; c-KIT; FLT3	AML	Phase I/II
Vatalanib (PTK787/ZK222584)	VEGFR-1, VEGFR-2	Colorectal, prostate, renal	Phase I/II
Sutent (SU11248)	VEGFR; PDGFR; KIT; FLT3	Renal, GIST	Phase I/II

Adapted from ref. 9.

Angiogenesis can be counteracted not only by interfering with VEGF binding but also by down-regulation of its production. Cyclo-oxygenase (COX)-2, a key enzyme required for the conversion of arachidonic acid to prostaglandins (PG), plays an important role in inflammation and cancer development[10]. Mounting evidence suggests that COX-2 regulates angiogenesis both *in vitro*[11] and *in vivo*[12].

COX-2 up-regulation has recently been demonstrated in cirrhosis and well-differentiated HCC, but less so in poorly differentiated HCC, suggesting that it is involved in the early steps of hepatocarcinogenesis[13]. Interesting data have also been obtained with COX-2 inhibitors, demonstrating in animal models that COX-2 inhibition suppresses the growth of HCC[14]. In line with these observations Tang et al. found a correlation of COX-2 expression with invasiveness of HCC and patient survival[15].

Thalidomide is another well-characterized substance which is currently being investigated regarding its effect on HCC: it down-regulates COX-2 expression and subsequently VEGF, and modulates the expression of adhesion molecules. However, in a phase II trial, treatment with thalidomide in combination with epirubicin resulted in stable disease in one-third of the patients only[5]. A study with increasing doses of thalidomide revealed a partial response in five out of 32 patients and stable disease in 31% of the study population, while the median survival time was only 6.8 months[16] (Table 2).

IMMUNOTHERAPY OF HCC

Although obviously attractive and promising, so far there are no firm clinical data demonstrating a benefit of immunotherapy for patients with HCC.

The first indication that a significant immune response is correlated with a favourable outcome came from a study of Wada et al., who demonstrated that patients with HCC highly infiltrated with lymphocytes showed a significantly better survival[18].

It is not clear why the immune response towards HCC tumour cells is primarily down-regulated. Analysis of tumour-infiltrating lymphocytes

Table 2

Substances	Indication	Phase	Web
Bevacizumab	Unresectable HCC, no metastasis	II	www.clinicaltrails.gov/ CT/show/NCT00055692
Bevacizumab	Unresectable HCC; additional chemoembolization	II	www.clinicaltrails.gov/ CT/show/NCT00049322
Celecoxib /epirubicin	HCC	I/II	www.clinicaltrails.gov/' CT/show/NCT00057980
Thalidomide/epirubicin	Unresectable or metastatic HCC	II	www.clinicaltrails.gov
Sorafenib	HCC	III	

Adapted from ref. 17.

indicated that a subgroup of suppressive $CD4^+CD25^+Foxp3^+$ T(reg) cells prevent a more vigorous immune response. Different approaches have been followed to overcome the immunological anergy. In a human trial with 21 patients Sangro et al., from the group of Prieto, could demonstrate that direct injection of adenoviral encoded interleukin 12 (IL-12) into tumour nodules induced a cellular anti-tumour response, and led to a decrease of AFP in five out of nine patients with HCC[19].

The first controlled randomized study on adjuvant immunotherapy for patients with HCC who underwent resection was published by Takayama et al.[20]. The authors revealed that the repeated reinfusion of autologous lymphocytes, which were activated *in vitro* by IL-2 and anti-CD3 stimulation, led to a significantly improved recurrence-free survival. Although overall survival did not differ significantly, the study clearly supported the view that boost the immunological tumour surveillance might have a role in future HCC treatment protocols. This was further underlined by recent results in a study by Kuang et al., who intradermally vaccinated a similar group of patients after HCC resection with autologous tumour lysate, IL-2 and GM-CSF. The 19 patients who were randomized for vaccination showed a significantly better recurrence-free and overall survival[21].

A dendritic cell-based vaccination approach was followed by Lee et al., who pulsed PBMC-derived dendritic cells and reinfused them weekly five times in patients with advanced HCC. Patients who in addition received monthly boosts showed a significantly better survival than those who were vaccinated only[22].

A more specific approach follows the idea of activating an HCC-specific response, which can be accomplished by strategies using tumour-associated self-antigens (for example, α-fetoprotein (AFP)).

In line with this, the group of Geissler investigated the option to elicit a specific anti-tumour response by a DNA-based vaccination strategy. They were able to demonstrate a significant anti-tumour response in a mouse model[23]. A major concern is the induction of an autoimmune response by vaccinating with antigens expressed not only in the tumour; indeed, in a subsequent study the authors observed a significant autoimmune reaction resembling an autoimmune hepatitis when they vaccinated mice against AFP upon partial hepatectomy[24].

However, a variety of specific and non-specific immunostimulatory strategies against HCC have been applied in preclinical experimental models with some promising results. The molecular characterization of HCC-associated tumour antigens such as AFP and the increased understanding of the immunological pathways involved in liver and tumour immunology paved the way to design promising gene-based cancer vaccines. The most promising of these techniques is based on the use of dendritic cells, which are able to process and present antigens to activate naive T cells and, when loaded with tumour antigens, can stimulate a specific and durable anti-tumour response. The first phase I and II immunotherapeutic clinical trials, based on dendritic cell immunotherapy and peptide vaccines, are ongoing in HCC patients.

SENSITIZING TOWARDS APOPTOSIS

Although the enigma of this particular resistance is only partially understood, a large body of data suggests that the process of oncofetal dedifferentiation enables hepatocytes to evade immune surveillance by refining their intracellular set of proteins, which orchestrate the subtle balance of apoptotic death and survival. Evading the immune surveillance by developing resistance to apoptosis is a classic principle, which is of particular importance in a number of malignancies including HCC, where increased levels of anti-apoptotic proteins such as c-FLIP[25] and surviving[26], or decreased levels of pro-apoptotic proteins such as FADD[27], have been described.

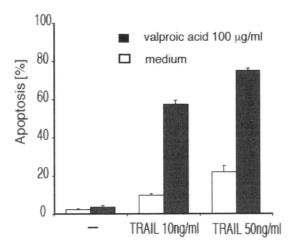

Figure 1 Valproic acid sensitizes human hepatoma cells towards TRAIL-induced apoptosis

In clinical practice only a subgroup of patients with early disease qualifies for curative treatment by resection or liver transplantation. In patients with progressive disease, restriction to the liver allows palliative treatment by transarterial chemoembolization. However, the chemoresistant nature of the tumour leads to a poor outcome for patients when the disease is advanced and extrahepatic dissemination of HCC has already occurred[28]. Improved efficacy of chemotherapy is desperately needed. In this context there is rising interest in the concept to integrate the group of histone deacetylase inhibitors (HDAC-I) in chemotherapy protocols for patients with malignancies[29]. Indeed, inhibition of histone deacetylase by sodium butyrate significantly enhanced the sensitivity of hepatoma cells to apoptosis[30]. Since sodium butyrate itself seems not to be the ideal candidate, due to its unfavourable pharmacokinetics, we tested the short-chain fatty acid valproic acid, an approved drug to treat patients with seizures, which turned out to have strong HDAC-I activity[31].

The combinatorial treatment of the hepatoma cell line HepG2 with VA and death receptor agonists led to a substantial increase of apoptosis induction. Our group observed 40–60% apoptotic cells with the combination of VA and death receptor agonist, even in concentrations which alone led to apoptosis in less than 10% of the cells. Although the underlying mechanism is not yet completely elucidated, down-regulation of the anti-apoptotic molecule c-FLIP might contribute[32].

CONCLUSION

Treatment of patients with HCC remains a clinical challenge. New approaches, which target the Achilles' heel of HCC (namely its resistance towards killer cells and apoptosis, as well as its hypervascularity), are about to enter the clinical stage. Due to the usually underlying liver disease, HCC patients will remain a difficult-to-treat and heterogeneous population, which will require a multimodal and interdisciplinary approach.

References

1. Folkman J. Tumor angiogenesis: therapeutic implications. N Engl J Med. 1971;285:1182–6.
2. Hurwitz H, Fehrenbacher L, Novotny W et al. Bevacizumab plus irinotecan, fluorouracil, and leucovorin for metastatic colorectal cancer. N Engl J Med. 2004;350:2335–42.
3. Poon RT, Ho JW, Tong CS, Lau C, Ng IO, Fan ST. Prognostic significance of serum vascular endothelial growth factor and endostatin in patients with hepatocellular carcinoma. Br J Surg. 2004;91:1354–60.
4. Musso O, Theret N, Heljasvaara R et al. Tumor hepatocytes and basement membrane-Producing cells specifically express two different forms of the endostatin precursor, collagen XVIII, in human liver cancers. Hepatology. 2001;33:868–76.
5. Zhu AX, Fuchs CS, Clark JW et al. A phase II study of epirubicin and thalidomide in unresectable or metastatic hepatocellular carcinoma. Oncologist. 2005;10:392–8.
6. Schwartz JD, Schwartz M, Lehrer D et al. Bevacizumab in hepatocellular carcinoma (HCC) in patients without metastasis and without invasion of the portal vein. ASCO Meeting 2005, Abstract 4122.
7. Raskopf E, Dzienisowicz C, Hilbert T et al. Effective angiostatic treatment in a murine metastatic and orthotopic hepatoma model. Hepatology. 2005;41:1233–40.
8. Liu Y, Poon RT, Li Q, Kok TW, Lau C, Fan ST. Both antiangiogenesis- and angiogenesis-independent effects are responsible for hepatocellular carcinoma growth arrest by tyrosine kinase inhibitor PTK787/ZK222584. Cancer Res. 2005;65:3691–9.

9. Arora A, Scholar EM. Role of tyrosine kinase inhibitors in cancer therapy. J Pharmacol Exp Ther. 2005;315:971–9.
10. Dubois RN, Abramson SB, Crofford L et al. Cyclooxygenase in biology and disease. FASEB J. 1998;12:1063–73.
11. Tsujii M, Kawano S, Tsuji S, Sawaoka H, Hori M, DuBois RN. Cyclooxygenase regulates angiogenesis induced by colon cancer cells. Cell. 1998;93:705–16.
12. Masferrer JL, Leahy KM, Koki AT et al. Antiangiogenic and antitumor activities of cyclooxygenase-2 inhibitors. Cancer Res. 2000;60:1306–11.
13. Cheng AS, Chan HL, To KF et al. Cyclooxygenase-2 pathway correlates with vascular endothelial growth factor expression and tumor angiogenesis in hepatitis B virus-associated hepatocellular carcinoma. Int J Oncol. 2004;24:853–60.
14. Kern MA, Schoneweiss MM, Sahi D et al. Cyclooxygenase-2 inhibitors suppress the growth of human hepatocellular carcinoma implants in nude mice. Carcinogenesis. 2004; 25:1193–9.
15. Tang TC, Poon RT, Lau CP, Xie D, Fan ST. Tumor cyclooxygenase-2 levels correlate with tumor invasiveness in human hepatocellular carcinoma. World J Gastroenterol. 2005;11: 1896–902.
16. Patt YZ, Hassan MM, Lozano RD et al. Thalidomide in the treatment of patients with hepatocellular carcinoma: a phase II trial. Cancer. 2005;103:749–55.
17. Graepler F, Gregor M, Lauer UM. [Anti-angiogenic therapy for gastrointestinal tumours]. Z Gastroenterol. 2005;43:317–29.
18. Wada Y, Nakashima O, Kutami R, Yamamoto O, Kojiro M. Clinicopathological study on hepatocellular carcinoma with lymphocytic infiltration. Hepatology. 1998;27:407–14.
19. Sangro B, Mazzolini G, Ruiz J et al. Phase I trial of intratumoral injection of an adenovirus encoding interleukin-12 for advanced digestive tumors. J Clin Oncol. 2004;22:1389–97.
20. Takayama T, Sekine T, Makuuchi M et al. Adoptive immunotherapy to lower postsurgical recurrence rates of hepatocellular carcinoma: a randomised trial. Lancet. 2000;356:802–7.
21. Kuang M, Peng BG, Lu MD et al. Phase II randomized trial of autologous formalin-fixed tumor vaccine for postsurgical recurrence of hepatocellular carcinoma. Clin Cancer Res. 2004;10:1574–9.
22. Lee WC, Wang HC, Hung CF, Huang PF, Lia CR, Chen MF. Vaccination of advanced hepatocellular carcinoma patients with tumor lysate-pulsed dendritic cells: a clinical trial. J Immunother. 2005;28:496–504.
23. Grimm CF, Ortmann D, Mohr L et al. Mouse alpha-fetoprotein-specific DNA-based immunotherapy of hepatocellular carcinoma leads to tumor regression in mice. Gastroenterology. 2000;119:1104–12.
24. Geissler M, Mohr L, Weth R et al. Immunotherapy directed against alpha-fetoprotein results in autoimmune liver disease during liver regeneration in mice. Gastroenterology. 2001;121:931–9.
25. Okano H, Shiraki K, Inoue H et al. Cellular FLICE/caspase-8-inhibitory protein as a principal regulator of cell death and survival in human hepatocellular carcinoma. Lab Invest. 2003;83:1033–43.
26. Morinaga S, Nakamura Y, Ishiwa N et al. Expression of survivin mRNA associates with apoptosis, proliferation and histologically aggressive features in hepatocellular carcinoma. Oncol Rep. 2004;12:1189–94.
27. Shin EC, Shin JS, Park JH, Kim JJ, Kim H, Kim SJ. Expression of Fas-related genes in human hepatocellular carcinomas. Cancer Lett. 1998;134:155–62.
28. Llovet JM, Burroughs A, Bruix J. Hepatocellular carcinoma. Lancet. 2003;362:1907–17.
29. Johnstone RW. Histone-deacetylase inhibitors: novel drugs for the treatment of cancer. Nat Rev Drug Discov. 2002;1:287–99.
30. Ogawa K, Yasumura S, Atarashi Y et al. Sodium butyrate enhances Fas-mediated apoptosis of human hepatoma cells. J Hepatol. 2004;40:278–84.
31. Gottlicher M, Minucci S, Zhu P et al. Valproic acid defines a novel class of HDAC inhibitors inducing differentiation of transformed cells. Histone deacetylase is a direct target of valproic acid, a potent anticonvulsant, mood stabilizer, and teratogen. EMBO J. 2001;20:6969–78.
32. Schuchmann M, Schulze-Bergkamen H, Fleischer B et al. Histone deacetylase inhibition by valproic acid down-regulates c-FLIP/CASH and sensitizes hepatoma cells towards CD95- and TRAIL receptor-mediated apoptosis and chemotherapy. Oncol Rep. 2006;15:227–30.

25

Special Lecture: Living donor liver transplantation: extended indications?

S. NADALIN, G. C. SOTIROPOULOS, M. MALAGÓ and
C. E. BROELSCH

INTRODUCTION

Liver transplantation (LT) nowadays represents the treatment of choice for
end-stage liver disease.

Due to improved immunosuppressive regimens, tissue preservation,
reduction of infectious disease, and better postoperative management,
orthotopic liver transplantation has achieved patient and allograft survival
rates that have expanded the indications for transplantation, as well as the
number of potential recipients awaiting liver transplantation[1].

Despite supportive legislation, media network systems, and the attempt to
raise public awareness, actual donor numbers have remained relatively
constant and do not meet the growing need for more organs.

In this regard living donor liver transplantation (LDLT) has emerged as the
only innovation to significantly expand the scarce donor pool in countries in
which the growing demands of organs are not met by the shortage of available
cadaveric grafts. Up to now almost 3500 adult-to-child and 2500 adult-to-adult
LDLT have been performed worldwide.

The application of LDLT is associated with several theoretical advantages:
(1) the transplantation can be performed on an elective basis before serious
decompensation of the recipient; (2) grafts are in excellent condition and
complications due to preservation injury are absent; (3) possibility of LT for
recipients who might otherwise not be eligible for standard deceased donor
liver transplantation (DDLT). The drawback of this procedure is represented
by the potential risk of death or serious complications to the donor and a series
of still-unsolved technical, physiological, and ethical questions.

The indications for LDLT are similar to standard DDLT in both adult and
paediatric patients. Nonetheless, clinical experience has shown that the
willingness to donate increases as the clinical conditions of the recipient
worsens. Consequently, there is a trend to extend the indications for LDLT,

especially in tumour patients, decompensated end-stage liver disease and post-hepatitis cirrhosis.

HEPATOCELLULAR CARCINOMA (HCC)

Until the start of the 1990s the results of DDLT because of HCC were very poor, since the main indication to LT was advanced HCC. As a result, HCC became a contraindication to DDLT until the introduction of the Milan Criteria (MC) by Mazzaferro et al. in 1996[2]: no extrahepatic metastases, no macroscopic vascular invasion, single tumour nodule ≤5 cm or three or more tumours ≤3 cm. Applying the MC, a 4-year survival of 83% and a disease-free survival at 4 years of 75% was reached[2]. Similar results were observed in LDLT in different centres. Unfortunately, the actual preoperative tumour screening and tumour staging is not always reliable; the consequence is that sometimes patients are overstaged before LT, with the exclusion of a high number of patients who could benefit from LT. Additionally the probability of dropping out because of tumour progression during the waiting time ranges between 40% and 50% at 2 years after diagnosis. To escape the dilemma of limited organ availability, LDLT is a good alternative, offering a short waiting time with consequently less dropout and reduced mortality in the waiting list.

The possibility of extending indications for LT beyond classic criteria is an extraordinary chance for these patients. The timely transplant, in contrast to deceased LT, reduces the effect of 'observation time' and the natural selection, and could result in a better selection of patients: (1) patients who initially meet the MC but experience dropout due to tumour progression while on the waiting list; (2)patients outside current listing criteria at the time of presentation as; well as (3) patients meeting the criteria but not able to wait because of end-stage liver cirrhosis may be considered in this debate.

Additionally, more than 50% of patients in the published series of LDLT for HCC were beyond MC.

For the above-mentioned reasons, Yao et al. proposed to expand the MC in the case of LDLT: single nodule ≤6.5 cm or three or more nodules ≤4.5 cm. The authors reported a 1- and 5-year survival of 90% and 75%, respectively[3].

It seems that the number of tumour nodules represents a less important factor than diameter, presence of vascular infiltration, and histological type associated with different grades of malignancy. Therefore, Lee et al. suggested extending the MC in selected cases with a higher number of tumour nodules, as long as the HCC were small without macrovascular invasion[4]. Recently, also, the size of the tumour has been under discussion. Gondolesi et al. recently reported good results also in the case of LDLT for large HCC[5,6]. Overall, in patients with HCC >5 cm ($n = 12$), there were no statistically significant differences in survival or in freedom from recurrence between recipients of living donor and deceased donor grafts. LDLT allows timely transplantation in patients with early or with large HCC. The current international trend to 'expand' the existing MC in the case of LDLT is based on several factors:

1. Current imaging techniques do not always allow appropriate staging of small HCC <2 cm, with high rates of false-negative results[7–10];

2. HCC is often multifocal and the difficulty of differentiating a multifocal HCC from regenerative nodules in an end-stage cirrhotic liver can make it impossible to allocate according to the MC 'two to three tumours all ⩽3 cm.'[7–10];

3. There is still no imaging method that can estimate micro vascular invasion, a factor correlated with bad prognosis and quick recurrences in most studies[9,11];

4. Many transplant centres based on pathological findings report acceptable overall and recurrence-free outcomes in patient groups exceeding the MC[11–18].

For all these reasons LDLT is becoming progressively utilized in several centres using 'extended indications'. Different criteria for patient selection are probably necessary in LDLT.

In conclusion, although complicated factors, such as donor voluntarism and selection criteria, limit the role of LDLT for HCC, LDLT allows more patients to undergo early transplantation, which results in a better outcome also in cases beyond MC.

DECOMPENSATE END-STAGE LIVER DISEASE

LDLT for patients with decompensate end-stage liver disease (UNOS 2A, MELD >30) is controversial. Nevertheless, these patients are most in need of a timely liver transplant. In our series, patient and graft survival rates were only 43%[19]. Notwithstanding the high mortality rate, no donors had regrets about the procedure, and all donors stated that they would donate again if presented with the same decision. LDLT represents a timely and effective alternative to DDLT in the case of decompensate end-stage liver disease. Nonetheless, the ethical concerns regarding risk of benefits for both donor and recipient should be discussed.

HCV CIRRHOSIS (HCV)

Approximately 170 million people worldwide have been infected with HCV. By the year 2020 current estimates suggest that nearly 14 million people will have cirrhosis due to chronic HCV. HCV-related disease accounts for more than half of the indications for LT in most transplant programmes. As waiting lists continue to expand, the time to transplantation is becoming increasingly prolonged. The current number of deaths on the waiting list is, at the moment, higher for patients with the diagnosis of chronic HCV infection than for other diagnoses. Liver cirrhosis, secondary to HCV, actually represents 30–50% of the indication to LT in European and American countries.

Relapse of HCV infection occurs virologically in 100% of LT recipients. Histological recurrence affects approximately 50% of recipients, with ensuing graft failure in 10% of patients by the fifth postoperative year. Additionally, 8–31% of patients with post-transplant HCV recurrence develop cirrhosis within 5–7 years, resulting in reduced long-term survival rates[20]. Based on these 'poor' results of DDLT it has been discussed whether HCV cirrhosis still represents a standard or an extended indication to LT.

In contrast to whole DDLT, survival outcomes and effects of recurrence following adult LDLT for HCV are not yet defined. Preliminary reports earlier showed a severe recurrence within the first year after transplantation, with a higher incidence of cholestatic hepatitis[21]. In this case the advantages of early transplantation may be offset by the risk of graft failure imposed by early recurrent disease. Nevertheless, an emerging strategy for preventing recurrent HCV infection is pre-transplant treatment to achieve viral eradication (especially in patients with HCC and compensated cirrhosis with a good viral profile: non-genotype-1 or genotype-1 with low viral load) followed by timed LDLT[22,23]. If such strategies become successful, LDLT may exhibit an advantage over DDLT.

ETHICAL CONSIDERATIONS

LDLT has always been accompanied by ethical concerns, mainly related to the risk imposed on the donor[24,25]. Over the past decade it has been proven that LDLT significantly increases the donor pool and that the outcome is equal to or even superior to DDLT. In this sense the risk benefit/ratio for the recipient is clearly in favour for LDLT[26]. Applying the principle of justice to LDLT is also complex, and nobody knows whether a procedure that violates the principle 'above all, do no harm' can be justified. Further, still-ongoing ethical discussions are concerned with questions such as who should receive a living donor transplant. While some argue that stable patients with chronic liver disease, before hepatic decompensation, benefit the most from LDLT, others maintain that very ill patients are precisely the ones who should be offered LDLT[27,28]. An extension of this argument is concerned with patients who cannot currently be placed on the waiting list due to advanced cancer, but in whom LDLT offers the only effective option.

However, who should donate then? LDLT is guided by two main principles: (1) donor morbidity and mortality must be kept to a minimum; and (2) graft and recipient survival should be as high as in full-size LDLT. The exact risk to the living donor, though, is not known. The evidence from several surveys and subjective assessments indicates that donor mortality is somewhere between 0.2% and 1%, and morbidity as high as 60%[29]. Trotter reported that a complete recovery required more than 3 months in 75% of all donors[30]. Despite all this, recent studies have shown a significant benefit for the donor. Liver donors reported satisfaction and an increased self-esteem. In a study by Karliova et al. 92% of all donors would decide to donate again[31]. A high degree of preoperative information enabled the donors to have a realistic view of the operation and its potential complications, and explained the overall positive retrospective rating.

Clearly, donor safety is paramount in LDLT, and the risks and benefits to the donors will undoubtedly be debated by ethicists.

CONCLUSIONS

In recent decades, LDLT has emerged as a clinically safe addition to DDLT. The widespread adoption of LDLT has the potential to decrease waiting list mortality. The advantages of LDLT are obvious: (1) transplantation can be performed on an elective basis before serious decompensation of the recipient; and (2) complications due to organ preservation are minimized or completely absent, and grafts are generally in excellent condition. Although the benefits are enormous, the physical and psychological sacrifice of the donors is immense, and the expectations for a good outcome for themselves, as well as for the recipients, are high. Donor safety has an absolute priority, and only the assurance of a low morbidity and zero mortality can justify this procedure.

The extension of the indication to LDLT should be drawn carefully, and individually based on both patient and donor safety. Nevertheless, LDLT opens new perspectives for patients with advanced HCC, decompensate end-stage liver disease and HCV cirrhosis.

References

1. Keeffe EB. Liver transplantation: current status and novel approaches to liver replacement. Gastroenterology. 2001;120:749–62.
2. Mazzaferro V, Regalia E, Doci R et al. Liver transplantation for the treatment of small hepatocellular carcinomas in patients with cirrhosis. N Engl J Med. 1996;334:693–9.
3. Yao FY, Ferrell L, Bass NM et al. Liver transplantation for hepatocellular carcinoma: expansion of the tumor size limits does not adversely impact survival. Hepatology. 2001;33:1394–403.
4. Lee KW, Park JW, Joh JW et al. Can we expand the Milan criteria for hepatocellular carcinoma in living donor liver transplantation? Transplant Proc. 2004;36:2289–90.
5. Gondolesi G, Munoz L, Matsumoto C et al. Hepatocellular carcinoma: a prime indication for living donor liver transplantation. J Gastrointest Surg. 2002;6:102–7.
6. Gondolesi GE, Roayaie S, Munoz L et al. Adult living donor liver transplantation for patients with hepatocellular carcinoma: extending UNOS priority criteria. Ann Surg. 2004;239:142–9.
7. Bigourdan JM, Jaeck D, Meyer N et al. Small hepatocellular carcinoma in Child A cirrhotic patients: hepatic resection versus transplantation. Liver Transplant. 2003;9:513–20.
8. Libbrecht L, Bielen D, Verslype C et al. Focal lesions in cirrhotic explant livers: pathological evaluation and accuracy of pretransplantation imaging examinations. Liver Transplant. 2002;8:749–61.
9. de Ledinghen V, Laharie D, Lecesne R et al. Detection of nodules in liver cirrhosis: spiral computed tomography or magnetic resonance imaging? A prospective study of 88 nodules in 34 patients. Eur J Gastroenterol Hepatol. 2002;14:159–65.
10. Jonas S, Bechstein WO, Steinmuller T et al. Vascular invasion and histopathologic grading determine outcome after liver transplantation for hepatocellular carcinoma in cirrhosis. Hepatology. 2001;33:1080–6.
11. Fernandez JA, Robles R, Marin C et al. Can we expand the indications for liver transplantation among hepatocellular carcinoma patients with increased tumor size? Transplant Proc. 2003;35:1818–20.
12. Kaihara S, Kiuchi T, Ueda M et al. Living-donor liver transplantation for hepatocellular carcinoma. Transplantation. 2003;75(Suppl. 3):S37–40.

13. Lo CM, Fan ST, Liu CL, Chan SC, Wong J. The role and limitation of living donor liver transplantation for hepatocellular carcinoma. Liver Transplant. 2004;10:440–7.

14. Todo S, Furukawa H. Living donor liver transplantation for adult patients with hepatocellular carcinoma: experience in Japan. Ann Surg. 2004;240:451–9; discussion 459–61.

15. Gonzalez-Uriarte J, Valdivieso A, Gastaca M et al. Liver transplantation for hepatocellular carcinoma in cirrhotic patients. Transplant Proc. 2003;35:1827–9.

16. Yao FY, Ferrell L, Bass NM, Bacchetti P, Ascher NL, Roberts JP. Liver transplantation for hepatocellular carcinoma: comparison of the proposed UCSF criteria with the Milan criteria and the Pittsburgh modified TNM criteria. Liver Transplant. 2002;8:765–74.

17. Roayaie S, Frischer JS, Emre SH et al. Long-term results with multimodal adjuvant therapy and liver transplantation for the treatment of hepatocellular carcinomas larger than 5 centimeters. Ann Surg. 2002;235:533–9.

18. Si MS, Amersi F, Golish SR et al. Prevalence of metastases in hepatocellular carcinoma: risk factors and impact on survival. Am Surg. 2003;69:879–85.

19. Testa G, Malago M, Nadalin S et al. Right-liver living donor transplantation for decompensated end-stage liver disease. Liver Transplant. 2002;8:340–6.

20. Moreno R, Berenguer M. Hepatitis C and liver transplantation. Ann Hepatol. 2002;1:129–35.

21. Thuluvath PJ, Yoo HY. Graft and patient survival after adult live donor liver transplantation compared to a matched cohort who received a deceased donor transplantation. Liver Transplant. 2004;10:1263–8.

22. Feliu A, Gay E, Garcia-Retortillo M, Saiz JC, Forns X. Evolution of hepatitis C virus quasispecies immediately following liver transplantation. Liver Transplant. 2004;10:1131–9.

23. Forns X, Garcia-Retortillo M, Serrano T t al. Antiviral therapy of patients with decompensated cirrhosis to prevent recurrence of hepatitis C after liver transplantation. J Hepatol. 2003;39:389–96.

24. Caplan AL. Proceed with caution: live living donation of lobes of liver for transplantation. Liver Transplant. 2001;7:494–5.

25. Shiffman ML, Brown RS Jr, Olthoff KM et al. Living donor liver transplantation: summary of a conference at The National Institutes of Health. Liver Transplant. 2002;8:174–88.

26. Malago M, Testa G, Marcos A et al. Ethical considerations and rationale of adult-to-adult living donor liver transplantation. Liver Transplant. 2001;7:921–7.

27. Miwa S, Hashikura Y, Mita A et al. Living-related liver transplantation for patients with fulminant and subfulminant hepatic failure. Hepatology. 1999;30:1521–6.

28. Seaberg EC, Belle SH, Beringer KC, Schivins JL, Detre KM. Liver transplantation in the United States from 1987–1998: updated results from the Pitt-UNOS Liver Transplant Registry. Clin Transplant. 1998;17–37.

29. Northup PG, Berg CL. Living donor liver transplantation: the historical and cultural basis of policy decisions and ongoing ethical questions. Health Policy. 2005;72):175–85.

30. Trotter JF. Living donor liver transplantation: is the hype over? J Hepatol. 2005;42:20–5.

31. Karliova M, Malago M, Valentin-Gamazo C et al. Living-related liver transplantation from the view of the donor: a 1-year follow-up survey. Transplantation. 2002;73:1799–804.

Index

Falk Symposium Series

Falk Symposium Series

Falk Symposium Series

Falk Symposium Series

Falk Symposium Series

148. Kruis W, Forbes A, Jauch K-W, Kreis ME, Wexner SD, eds. *Diverticular Disease: Emerging Evidence in a Common Condition.* Falk Symposium 148. 2006
ISBN 1-4020- 4317-1
149. van Cutsem E, Rustgi AK, Schmiegel W, Zeitz M, eds. *Highlights in Gastrointestinal Oncology.* Falk Symposium 149. 2006. ISBN 1-4020-5108-5
150. Galle PR, Gerken G, Schmidt WE, Wiedenmann B, eds. *Disease Progression and Disease Prevention in Hepatology and Gastroenterology.* Falk Symposium 150. 2006
ISBN 1-4020-5109-3